Models for Measuring Quality in Managed Care: *Analysis and Impact*

Medical

Outcomes

& Practice

Guidelines

Library II

Volume I

Models for Measuring Quality in Managed Care: *Analysis and Impact*

Edited by
Jonathan Seltzer, MD, MBA, and
David B. Nash, MD, MBA

F&G

Models for Measuring Quality in Managed Care: Analysis and Impact

Faulkner & Gray, Inc.
Eleven Penn Plaza
New York, NY 10001
http://www.FaulknerGray.com/healthcare

ISBN: 1–57987-001–5

Published by Faulkner & Gray's
Healthcare Information Center

Luci Koizumi, Sponsoring Editor
Margo Harris, Project Editor
Bob Cooper, Production Manager
Paul Hamann, BA, Production Editor
Beth Rosenthal, Managing Editor
David Beck, Publisher

PRINTED IN THE UNITED STATES OF AMERICA

TABLE OF CONTENTS

About the Editors and Authors vii
Acknowledgments xviii
Foreword xix

Introduction ***1***

The Evolution of Physician Quality Assessment
Robin L. Smith, MD, David B. Nash, MD, MBA, Craig P. Tanio, MD, MBA, and Jonathan Seltzer, MD, MBA

Section I: Formal Models for Measuring the Quality Of Managed Care

Chapter One: Establishing Accountability in Managed Health Care ***35***

National Committee for Quality Assurance
Cary Sennett, MD, PhD

Chapter Two: Framework for Accountability ***55***

Foundation for Accountability
Christina Bethell, PhD, MBA, and David Lansky, PhD

Chapter Three: Performance Measurement and Accreditation ***79***

Joint Commission on Accreditation of Healthcare Organizations
Jerod M. Loeb, PhD, and Deborah M. Nadzam, PhD, RN

Chapter Four: Advancing the Science and Practice of Health Outcomes Measurement ***101***

The Medical Outcomes Trust
Lyn Paget and Alvin Tarlov, MD

Chapter Five: In Search of a Few Good Performance Measures ***121***

CONQUEST
Ann G. Lawthers, ScD, and Heather Palmer, MB, BCh, SM

Chapter Six: Models for Assessing Physician and Health Plan Performance ***151***

American Medical Association
Gail H. Thomason and William F. Jessee, MD

Section II: Analysis and Response

Chapter Seven: The Physicians' Approach to Quality in Managed Care ***171***

The American Academy of Family Physicians
Susan Black, MD, and David Massanari, MD

Chapter Eight: Managed Care Quality Assessment for Organized Labor *183*
Service Employees International Union
Directed by Peggy Connerton

Chapter Nine: Employer Purchasers Push for the Ideal Organized Health Care Delivery System *203*
Washington Business Group on Health
Robert F. Cole, PhD

Chapter Ten: A Consumer Agenda *213*
The Consumer Coalition for Quality Health Care
Andrew Webber

Section III: Impact of Quality Measurement

Chapter Eleven: Measuring and Improving Organizational Performance *229*
Allina Health Systems
Bryan Bushick, MD, MBA

Chapter Twelve: Patient-Centered Models for Providing Quality *251*
Aetna U.S. Healthcare
Carol C. Diamond, MD, and Nicholas A. Hanchak, MD

Chapter Thirteen: Demonstrating and Communicating Quality *279*
Milliman and Robertson
Frederick W. Spong, MD, MBA

Chapter Fourteen: Transforming Quality Measures Into Value *297*
Ernst & Young, LLP
David Plocher, MD, and Linda Davis, RN

Chapter Fifteen: Public Release of Quality Data *321*
The Case of Pennsylvania
Ernest J. Sessa

Chapter Sixteen: Communicating Managed Care Quality *341*
The National Press
George Anders

About the Editors

Jonathan Seltzer, MD, MBA, MA

Director, Health Systems Research
Premier Research Worldwide

Jonathan Seltzer is responsible for conducting clinical trials in therapeutic economics, technology assessment, and clinical data auditing. Additionally, through Premier Research Worldwide's contractual agreement with Premier, Inc., a purchasing consortium of over 2,000 health care organizations, he has responsibility for Premier Research Worldwide's role in designing data collection health care process improvement tools. Seltzer has a strong interest in clinical quality improvement and participates as a consultant, peer reviewer, and editorial board member to several organizations actively involved with the examination of clinical quality in the era of managed care.

He maintains a faculty appointment at Thomas Jefferson University, where he previously served as the deputy director of the Office of Health Policy and managed the office's pharmacoeconomic and health care effectiveness projects. Seltzer is a board-certified cardiologist and received medical training at the Universities of Michigan, Maryland, and Chicago. He holds an undergraduate degree from Haverford College, an MBA and MA (applied economics) from the University of Michigan, and an MD from the University of Pennsylvania.

David B. Nash, MD, MBA, FACP

Associate Dean for Health Policy
Director, Office of Health Policy and Clinical Outcomes
Thomas Jefferson University

David Nash oversees research and policy work in the areas of outcomes management, medical staff development, and quality-of-care improvement and has published more than four dozen articles and edited eight books. Repeatedly named as one of the most influential policymakers in academic medicine, he serves on the Joint Commission on Accreditation of Healthcare Organizations National Performance Council and the American Medical Association Physician

Measurement Advisory Committee. He is the associate director of the National Pew Charitable Trust Managed Care Education Program, is one of the principal faculty members on quality-of-care issues of the American College of Physician Executives, directs the Physician Track of the National Managed Health Care Congress, and serves as a consultant to the Pennsylvania Health Care Cost Containment Council, the Hartford Foundation, the Agency for Health Care Policy and Research, and numerous other private and public interests. He is editor-in-chief of the *New Medicine*, and a member of the *Medical Economics* editorial board.

He has served as chair of the Center for Clinical Quality Evaluation and the Clinical Evaluative Sciences Council of the University HealthSystem Consortium. Nash received the Latiolais Prize by the American Managed Care Pharmacy Association for his leadership in disease management, formulary design, and pharmacoeconomics. He holds an undergraduate degree from Vassar College, a medical degree from the University of Rochester School of Medicine and Dentistry, and an MBA from the University of Pennsylvania, where he also was a Robert Wood Johnson Clinical Scholar.

About the Authors

George Anders

Senior Special Writer
The Wall Street Journal

George Anders is a Senior Special Writer in the health and technology group at *The Wall Street Journal*. He covers financial aspects of health care, with emphasis on page one features. He writes extensively about HMOs, doctors, hospitals, and the cost of medical technology. He is listed among the "highest rated journalists" in the United States by the annual *Forbes Media Guide 500*. Anders recently has written *Health Against Wealth* (Houghton Mifflin), a book covering the rise of the HMO industry and its impact on medical quality.

Christina Bethell, PhD, MBA, MPH

Director, Accountability Measurement
Foundation for Accountability

Christina Bethell is responsible for facilitating the development of accountability measures and is instrumental in ensuring the involvement of consumers, health care providers, and researchers in the identification and implementation of these measures. She has worked for over 12 years in the field of public health and health care policy, including her work with the Coro Foundation in its efforts with health care reform in the state of California. She has also worked at the federal level, assisting the American Association of Retired Persons in creation of a congressional consensus regarding the role of Medicaid in a reformed health system. Bethell has worked directly with inner-city communities and in conjunction with the Voluntary Hospitals of America to develop instruments for consumer evaluation of health care.

Susan Black, MD

Vice President and Director
American Academy of Family Physicians

Susan Black is the vice president of the American Academy of Family Physicians—the first woman to hold executive office in the 50-year history of that organization. She is also a director and the past chair of AAFP's Commission on Medical Education. Previously, Black served the AAFP as a congressional delegate and participated on its committees on health education and aging. She also was elected the president of the Massachusetts Academy of Family Physicians.

Black maintains a full-time practice in family medicine and participates in a number of professional and civic organizations; she has served as the chair of the Massachusetts Medical Societies Committee on Women in Organized Medicine as well as received the Lowell Woman of the Year Award in 1995.

Bryan Bushick, MD, MBA

System Vice President, Performance Measurement and Improvement
Allina Health System

Bryan Bushick is leading Allina's effort to better understand its overall clinical and operational performance and to apply the resulting knowledge toward improvement across all Allina business units. His responsibilities are complemented by his role as a senior examiner for the Malcolm Baldrige National Quality Award, with past service as a senior evaluator for the Baldrige Health Care Pilot. Prior to assuming his current systemwide responsibilities, Bushick maintained a series of senior management roles within Medica, an HMO with membership currently approaching one million that merged with HealthSpan Health Systems Corporation from Allina in 1994.

Robert F. Cole, PhD

Director, National Resource Network for Child and Family Mental Health Services
Washington Business Group on Health

Robert F. Cole is director of the National Resource Network for Children & Family Mental Health Services (NRN), a $2.3 million cooperative agreement with the federal Center for Mental Health Services to provide a nationwide training and technical assistance network for state and community recipients of federal dollars for mental health. Cole also serves as deputy director of the Mental Health Services Program for Youth, an eight-site demonstration program funded by the Robert Wood Johnson Foundation to improve services for children and adolescents with serious mental illness. Both programs are based at the Washington Business Group on Health (WBGH) in Washington DC. Cole has 20 years of experience in human services administration, including 10 years as area director for the Massachusetts Department of Mental Health.

Linda C. Davis, RN

Senior Manager
Ernst & Young, LLP

Linda Davis is senior manager in the East/Great Lakes Health Care Consulting Practice in Minneapolis. She has more than 18 years of managed care experience. Davis provides expertise across multiple functional areas including managed care product development, operations, medical management, demand management, as well as marketing and sales. Davis has developed PHOs and MSOs for a national physician practice management firm, designed and developed strategic approach to demand management for a major national managed care corporation, as well as planned and directed community health improvement initiatives for multiple regional and national health care organizations. Prior to working at Ernst & Young, Davis was senior director of population health at Health Partners in Minneapolis, where she initiated programs related to improving health status, consumer satisfaction, physician communication, and worksite health improvement.

Carol C. Diamond, MD, MPH

Medical Director
US Quality Algorithms

Carol Diamond is a medical director for US Quality Algorithms (USQA). She is responsible for developing research methodologies to measure and improve the quality of medical care in the Aetna/US Healthcare member population. Her research interests include preventive care and population-based health interventions. Prior to joining USQA, Diamond worked as a consultant for Johnson & Johnson and the Robert Wood Johnson Foundation, where she developed and evaluated private-sector and academic programs in chronic disease management.

Nicholas A. Hanchak, MD

President
US Quality Algorithms

Nicholas Hanchak is president of US Quality Algorithms, Inc., a subsidiary of Aetna/US Healthcare. He heads USQA's efforts to measure and improve the quality of care and service within Aetna/US Healthcare's medical delivery system. In addition, he coordinates efforts to assess the cost-effectiveness of Aetna/US Healthcare's managed care programs. He has led USQA's efforts in developing performance-based compensation models, performance report cards, and risk-adjustment methodologies for performance measurement. He also has been instrumental in creating tools to evaluate the effectiveness of patient management programs, as well as developing health data analysis systems to assess the quality of care provided by physicians and hospitals.

William F. Jessee, MD

Vice President, Quality and Managed Care
American Medical Association

William Jessee leads the AMA's efforts to support physicians in their managed care activities, as well as oversees the association's quality initiatives. He is also chair of the Board of Physician's Managed Care Services, Inc., which develops and manages physician-owned managed care organizations throughout the Midwest and Southeast. Jessee has long been associated with quality in health care; he has worked in executive positions for both nonprofit and for-profit health systems. He is a board member of the International Society for Quality in Health Care, the American Society for Health Care Quality, and the Commission on Professional and Hospital Activities. He has served as an adviser to the World Health Organization and the American Hospital Association and as a judge for the Secretary of Veterans' Affairs Robert W. Carey Quality Award. Jessee has authored more than 60 articles, books, and chapters and is especially well known for managed care strategies and quality of care.

David Lansky, PhD

President
Foundation for Accountability

David Lansky directs the Foundation for Accountability, a nonprofit organization dedicated to helping consumers, patients, and purchasers make more informed choices among the health care options they face. FACCT's primary task is to endorse a standardized set of quality measures that are based on the results of health care services and how individuals experience the health system. Previously, Lansky was the regional director of clinical information for Providence Health System, where he was responsible for outcomes research, measurement of consumer satisfaction, health-risk and health-status assessment, development of electronic member and patient records, and communicating with purchasers and the larger community about health care quality. Lansky also worked with the Jackson Hole Group, where he was responsible for national accountability measures under the "managed competition" model.

Ann Lawthers, ScD

Lecturer, Center for Quality of Care Research and Education
Department of Health Policy and Management
Harvard School of Public Health

For the past decade, Ann Lawthers has conducted research developing methods and measures to assess the quality of medical care. Her particular interests are the design and testing of performance measurement using both administrative databases and medical resources. At the Center for Quality of Care, Lawthers was a key member of the team responsible for development of the CONQUEST measures. Prior to this, she was the research director for the DEMPAQ project, where she oversaw the development and implementation of methods to evaluate the quality of care rendered to Medicare beneficiaries in primary care physicians' offices.

Jerod M. Loeb, PhD

Director Research and Evaluation
Chief Scientific Officer
Joint Commission on Accreditation of Healthcare Organizations

Jerod Loeb plays a leadership role in initiating the broad-scale collection and evaluation of performance measures from a variety of measurement systems across the United States. Prior to joining JCAHO he served as assistant vice president for science, technology and public health at the American Medical Association. He is the author or coauthor of more than 100 publications and serves as a peer reviewer and editor on numerous publications. He received an Established Investigator Award from the American Heart Association and was the 1995 recipient of the Orr E. Reynolds Award from the American Physiological Society. He holds a faculty appointment at Northwestern University Medical School.

David Massanari, MD

Director
American Academy of Family Physicians

As a director of the AAFP, a national membership organization representing 84,000 family physicians, residents, and students, David Massanari also chairs the AAFP Commission on Health Care Services, which oversees the AAFP's advocacy of social and economic issues that affect family physicians and their patients. Formerly, he chaired the AAFP's Commission on Legislation and Governmental Affairs. Massanari is also a clinical instructor in the department of family medicine at the University of Vermont College of Medicine. Massanari is a past president of the Maine Academy of Family Physicians and a past president of the Maine Academy of Family Physicians Foundation, a nonprofit educational foundation. He is board certified in family medicine.

Deborah M. Nadzam, PhD, RN

Director, Indicator Measurement
Joint Commission on Accreditation of Healthcare Organizations

Deborah M. Nadzam is responsible for overseeing IMSystem operations and is the project manager for integrating performance measures into the accreditation process. She also has responsibility for indicator development and testing. Additionally, she has experience as a quality assurance clinician, director of nursing information resources, and as a director of nursing research and quality assurance.

R. Heather Palmer, MB, BCh, SM

Director, Center for Quality of Care Research and Education
Department of Health Policy and Management
Harvard School of Public Health

Heather Palmer directs the research team funded by the Agency for Health Policy and Research that built CONQUEST 1.0, the prototype system for the collection, retrieval, and evaluation of clinical performance measurement sets. She collaborates on many research projects in the area of quality of care. Palmer serves as a board member for the Center for Clinical Quality Evaluation and the Massachusetts Peer Review Organization. Additionally, she serves on the National Performance Measurement Council of the Joint Commission on Accreditation of Healthcare Organizations, the American Medical Association

Expert Consultant Panel for Physician Performance Assessment, and the National Academy of Sciences/National Research Council on Study on Performance Measure and Data for Public Health Performance Partnership Grants.

Lyn Paget, MPH

Vice President
Medical Outcomes Trust

Lyn Paget is vice president of the Medical Outcomes Trust in Boston. This is a nonprofit, public service organization dedicated to improving health and health care by advancing the science and use of patient-based outcome measures. Prior to joining the Trust she worked as a consultant on contract to the Forum of Quality and Effectiveness in Health Care of the Agency for Health Care Policy and Research to support the development of clinical practice guidelines. She also has worked in professional training at the AIDS Project Los Angeles and as manager of the Tacoma-Pierce County Health Department AIDS Section.

David Plocher, MD

Partner, Health Care Consulting
Ernst & Young, LLP

David Plocher has 17 years of experience in the managed care field. Most recently, he has designed and implemented integrated delivery systems and advanced care management systems. He has worked on quality audits and accreditation with both the Joint Commission on Accreditation of Healthcare Organizations and the National Committee for Quality Assurance. He has performed on-site operations review in many health plans, studying nonclinical and clinical areas for improvement. Clinical areas included all features of care management and new designs were recommended in selected areas such as disease management, demand management, and member risk adjustment. Additionally, Plocher developed the first nationwide center of excellence network for solid organ and allogeneic bone marrow transplants as well as selection criteria and performance measures for Centers of Excellence for invasive cardiac procedures for a large insurance carriers.

Cary Sennett, MD, PhD

Vice President for Performance Measurement
National Committee for Quality Assurance

Cary Sennett has responsibility for overseeing NCQA's efforts to provide national leadership in initiatives to develop methods and tools to objectively assess the performance of managed care plans. Prior to joining NCQA, Sennett had quality leadership roles at Group Health Cooperative of Puget Sound, U.S. Healthcare's US Quality Algorithms subsidiary, and Aetna Health Plans. He is a frequent speaker and author on issues of quality measurement and quality improvement in health care and is a member of the editorial boards of The Joint Commission's

Journal on Quality Improvement and *Quality Management in Health Care*. Sennett is a board-certified internist with considerable training and experience both in the science and application of clinical measurement for quality improvement in managed care.

Ernest J. Sessa

Executive Director
Pennsylvania Health Care Cost Containment Council

Ernest Sessa has directed the Pennsylvania Health Care Cost Containment Council, an independent state agency, since 1987. Its mission is to stimulate competition in the health care market through the collection, analysis, and public dissemination of objective cost and quality health care data. Sessa oversees a staff of 50 employees and an annual budget of $3 million. The Pennsylvania Health Care Cost Containment Council is generally considered to be one of the more aggressive and innovative health data collection and public dissemination efforts in the United States. Sessa has supervised a series of comprehensive annual "Hospital Effectiveness Reports," the "Consumer Guide to Coronary Artery Bypass Graft Surgery," small market area analysis reports, a utilization study of major organ transplants performed in Pennsylvania hospitals, and statewide hospital financial and utilization reports.

Robin Smith, MD

Special Projects Consultant
Jefferson Medical College

Robin Smith, MD, is a special project consultant to the Department of Health Policy and Clinical Outcomes at Jefferson Medical College. She is the creator of the bimonthly "Managed Care Corner" editorial and recently was appointed to the editorial board of the *American Journal of Managed Care*. As a U.S. Quality Algorithms Managed Care Fellow, her interests lie in aspects of managed care including clinical practice guidelines, cost-effective practices, Medicare and Medicaid, and strategies to be successful in a managed care environment. Additionally, she participated in the design and evaluation of physician quality measures, informed decisionmaking, and physician-patient barriers.

Frederick W. Spong, MD, MBA

Senior Healthcare Management Consultant
Milliman & Robertson, Inc.

Frederick Spong has special expertise in physician education and communication, physician retraining, physician-patient communication, patient education and communication, and total quality management in health care. He has served managed care organizations, health care facilities, medical groups, and employers.

Additionally, he has been a medical director of a 150,000-member HMO as well as an associate medical director of an 800,000-member HMO. Spong is a board-certified internist and nephrologist.

Craig P. Tanio, MD, MBA

Associate Medical Director
Baltimore Medical System

Craig Tanio oversees the quality management, utilization management, credentialing, home health, social work, and patient education departments for an ambulatory health system comprised of a group of federally qualified community health centers serving 35,000 patients in east Baltimore. He currently is leading a team that is redesigning the primary care processes of the system. Tanio has worked as a management consultant for McKinsey and Company, as a health policy analyst for the Public Citizen Health Research Group, and as a research consultant for the Office of Technology Assessment and the American College of Physicians. He was a contributing author for a best-selling consumer guide on prescription drugs, *Best Pills Worst Pills*.

Alvin R. Tarlov, MD

President and CEO
Medical Outcomes Trust

Alvin Tarlov is executive director of the Division of Health Improvement at the Health Institute, New England Medical Center, Boston, where he applies his considerable research and work experience in health manpower and measuring medical outcomes. In 1994, he became chair of the board and president of the Massachusetts Health Data Consortium, a nonprofit organization. He also serves as president and CEO of the Medical Outcomes Trust, a public service organization that distributes standardized questionnaires that measure health-related quality of life. Since 1990, he has been both a professor of medicine at Tufts University and a professor of health promotion at Harvard School of Public Health. From 1984-1990 Tarlov was president of the Henry J. Kaiser Family Foundation. Before that, he served for 13 years as chair of the Department of Medicine at the University of Chicago.

Gail H. Thomason, JD

Division Counsel, Managed Care Quality
Office of Quality and Managed Care
American Medical Association

Gail Thomason supports the AMA's efforts to assist physicians in their managed care activities, particularly as they relate to the AMA's quality initiatives. She has assisted in the development and implementation of the AMA's American Medical Accreditation Program. Additionally, she runs the AMA's Center on Society Sponsored Managed Care Organizations, which provides information, expertise, and leadership to medical societies and physician leaders interested in developing medical society-sponsored managed care organizations. Thomason is also the author of *Managed Care and the Market: A Summary of National Trends Affecting Physicians*, which garnered the American Association of Medical Executives "Pinnacle of Success" Award in 1995.

Andrew Webber

Senior Associate for Quality Policy
Consumer Coalition for Quality Health Care

Andrew Webber is responsible for policy development and federal advocacy issues for the Consumer Coalition on Quality Health Care. Founded in 1993, the Consumer Coalition is a national organization of consumer groups advocating for programs and policies in the public and private sectors to evaluate, protect, and improve the quality of health and health care delivery for all Americans. Its present focus is to translate consumer views into policy positions that advance quality assurance and consumer protection initiatives under managed care. Prior to joining the Consumer Coalition, Webber served as executive VP of the American Medical Peer Review Association (AMPRA), now renamed the American Health Quality Association.

ACKNOWLEDGMENTS

Constructing a successful multiauthored, edited text is a complex undertaking. We are grateful to all of our contributors from across the country for their help in bringing this project to fruition. In addition, we would like to thank Joseph S. Gonnella, MD, the dean of Jefferson Medical College, and Thomas J. Lewis, the chief executive officer of Thomas Jefferson University Hospital, for their ongoing enthusiastic support over the last eight years. We would also like to thank Rita Salzmann for her administrative help. Clearly, without her there would be no book.

Finally, we owe our wives, Liza and Es, and all of our children, Cassie, Benjamin, Leah, Rachel, and Jacob, a collective overdue hug. We recognize our primary responsibilities are to all of them, and we never want to lose sight of that reality.

FOREWORD

Lost in the clamor for measurement of quality is the reality that less than a decade ago medicine was predominantly a cottage industry. Since quality of care was a vague agreement between physician and patient, there was no perceived need for valid and precise instruments to measure care. However, the past 10 years have witnessed a dramatic change in medicine: it has grown from cottage industry into industrial system, changed its name from medicine to health care, and moved from the privacy of doctor-patient to the theater of provider, consumer, business, and government.

Although the health care system has changed dramatically, it is unclear whether such change is positive or negative. It seems as if every positive story about managed care is followed by an equally negative one. The argument over the fate of American health care is, indeed, an emotional one, being argued anecdote by anecdote. Managed care companies reason that more people than ever are receiving better care. Yet, legislation regarding particulars of medical care now is seen in a majority of states; even the President of the United States has called for a federal effort directed at assuring quality of care.

Models for Measuring Quality in Managed Care: Analysis and Impact is the first single-source text that documents the opinions of the major participants in the above debate. After an introductory history of quality assessment, Section I introduces the philosophies and instruments of the major players in the measurement game—the National Committee for Quality Assurance, the Foundation for Accountability, the Joint Commission on the Accreditation of Healthcare Organizations, the Medical Outcomes Trust, CONQUEST, and the American Medical Association. Section II responds to the above measures through those most affected—patients and doctors—in opinions contributed by the American Academy of Family Physicians, the Service Employees International Union of the AFL-CIO, the Washington Business Group on Health, and the Consumer Coalition for Quality Health Care. Finally, the synthesis of the measures and responses is addressed in Section III wherein managed care organizations (Allina Health Systems and Aetna U.S. Healthcare); health care consultants (Milliman and Robertson and Ernst & Young LLP); the government, and the health care reporter for *The Wall Street Journal* discuss how measurement of quality in health care is conducted and communicated.

Ultimately, rigorous application of objective scientific tools to the measurement of quality will be a key ingredient in the mix that settles the question of how to optimally deliver health care to a population. The percentage of the mix and the specifics of the tools will be continuing food for thought.

Jonathan Seltzer, MD, MBA
David B. Nash, MD, MBA

Introduction

The Evolution of Physician Quality Assessment

Robin L. Smith, MD, David B. Nash, MD, MBA,
Craig P. Tanio, MD, MBA, and Jonathan Seltzer, MD, MBA

Measurement of clinical competency is not a new concept. However, as the health care delivery system increasingly becomes influenced by managed care, the methods used to assess physician performance are changing rapidly. Over 100 years ago the professional model dominated and physicians implicitly judged one another.

> "as one watches a man handle a patient, it is easy to tell whether or not he has had a proper training, and for this purpose fifteen minutes at the bedside are worth three hours at the desk."[1]

Today employers and patient groups are asking for objective information that will demonstrate the quality of a health plan and of individual physicians. The government, the single largest purchaser of health care, is seeking to track outcomes of clinical care to ensure quality. In response to purchasers' demands, managed care organizations (MCOs) are developing methods to identify and improve quality of care. Professional societies are endorsing quality through board certification—a process designed to discriminate between physicians who meet the standards and those who do not.

Although the different stakeholders in today's complex health care system have differing interests, they all share a need for measures of clinical competence that are accurate, valid, and reproducible. Such measures of a physician's clinical competence can be used not only to ensure clinical quality, but also to promote and improve the quality of care used in the correct manner. This chapter will examine how measurement of physician performance has changed over the last century. Subsequent chapters will demonstrate the performance assessment tools that are currently being used by the major players in today's health care market.

CREDENTIALING AND PRIVILEGING

The oldest tools used to assess clinical competence include credentialing and privileging. Credentialing is the process of assessing and validating the qualifications of a licensed independent practitioner to provide member health services in a health care network and/or its components, such as an individual hospital, managed care organization, or the like.[2] Membership on the medical staff of a network component or membership on the panel of another network does not guarantee appointment or subsequent reappointment to the practitioner panel. Large group practices, independent practice associations, and certain medical societies also perform some credentialing.

Credentialing generally is performed at initial appointment, initial delineation in granting of clinical privileges, and reappointment and renewal or revision of clinical privileges. The role of a credentialing committee becomes particularly important for specialties where practice guidelines are not explicit and in which practitioners have varied training backgrounds. In the case of percutaneous transluminal coronary angioplasty (PTCA), where requirements for use of new and changing technology are not stipulated, credentialing committees of individual hospitals may need to develop their own criteria in consultation with appropriate experts.

In contrast, privileging is the authorization granted by the hospital, health care network, or managed care organization, or a component of the network, to a practitioner to provide specific patient care services.[3] Granting of initial or continuing medical staff privileges should be based on assessments of applicants against professional criteria specified in the medical staff by-laws. The services authorized must fall within defined limits based upon the licensed individual practitioner's qualifications and current competence.

Every practitioner on the network panel, for example, must be granted clinical privileges by each component in which he or she will be providing patient care, whether or not that component is a fully accredited organization. For instance, a physician responsible for both exercise testing and echocardiographic imaging during exercise echocardiography would need to demonstrate competence in both areas. In the case of arthrocentesis and joint-soft tissue injection, because some joints are more commonly aspirated than others, certification and privileging of these sites may be given individually or in joint-size categories. Privileges awarded must be consistent with the organization's plan for service and its ability to support the care provided. Each of the attached guidelines emphasizes physician skill—that is, individual performance, taking into account individuals' unique learning curves—over such important but "softer" factors as type of training program and continuing education course in the privileging process.

Is there any precedent for truly assessing physician performance beyond a perfunctory review of academic and training "tickets" that have been "punched"? Seminal work by Gonnella and his colleagues,[4] through a longitudinal educational database, has shown the "connectivity" between performance during medical school and in the first year of residency. They tested the strength of association[5] for such "outcome" variables as board scores, board certification, and postgraduate clinical competence evaluations made by residency directors (in the areas of data gathering, processing skills, and socioeconomic aspects of patient care). While contending only that the "research glass" is half full, they have helped to lay the intellectual foundation for much of the assessment work done by specialty societies. In short, there is ample evidence at the trainee level that competence (of all types) can be measured, tested, and evaluated.

With all of the integration taking place, do we still need credentialing and privileging at every hospital and managed care organization? Is there any precedent for truly assessing physician performance, beyond a perfunctory review of academic and training "tickets" that have been "punched"?

Recent evidence would suggest that we still must be vigilant about the credentialing process to bar incompetents and frauds from obtaining practice privileges. In several highly publicized cases,[6] grossly negligent physicians went unreported by knowing colleagues willing to "wink" at grievous breaches of professional conduct. In one infamous case,[7] a physician was convicted of murder for botching an abortion and then letting the patient bleed to death. Astonishingly enough, he had a long history of patient complaints and malpractice cases and 38 counts of gross negligence against him from a lenient state hearing committee.

Surely these are some of the worst apples in the barrel, but sometimes the orchard produces a poor crop. Sekas and colleagues[8] retrospectively reviewed all 236 applications submitted for a gastroenterology fellowship program in 1995 for confirmation of research experience and cited publications. They found that misrepresentation on applications was common; more than one-third of the listed research activities could not be confirmed. An accompanying editorial[9] described this behavior and called for our continued vigilance in reviewing credentials and establishing disciplinary procedures that "leave no doubt about our personal and collective standard of integrity."

BOARD CERTIFICATION

Board certification remains the sine qua non of credentialing in the new marketplace. Indeed, as "burgeoning" health care costs have driven employers and public health programs to turn increasingly to managed care as a health care delivery method for their employees and beneficiaries, managed care's use of board certification to credential physicians has become an issue. How did we arrive at this current state of affairs? Let's look at the American Board of Internal Medicine as the prototype for certifying boards.

The American Board of Internal Medicine (ABIM) was established in 1936 with the sponsorship of the American College of Physicians (ACP) and the American Medical Association (AMA), and was given the responsibility of setting and maintaining the standards for certification in internal medicine and recognizing those who met them. The ABIM is the largest of 24 boards that comprise the Confederation of the American Board of Medical Specialties (ABMS).[10] According to Harry Kimball, MD, the president and chief executive officer of the ABIM in Philadelphia PA, the Board has only one real product—namely, its certificate.[11] The process of certification, including the principles, goals, and procedures, involves a variety of component products. The purpose of certification is to improve the quality of health care to patients by assuring that certified internists possess the knowledge, skills, and attitudes required for the provision of excellent care.

The Board exists as an independent self-governing group that has set standards for internists who voluntarily desire to be certified. The Board does not have a responsibility to advocate for one or another group or issue, nor does it develop a detailed curriculum about specific content, nor does it conduct continuing education courses or publish educational materials. Finally, the Board does not regard certification or its standard as a way of influencing or manipulating the composition or supply of physicians. The Board sets standards and will certify all physicians who meet them. The Board's examinations derive their importance and influence from the fact that they can objectively and reliably measure a candidate's knowledge base and, to a reasonable extent, are able to test the ability of candidates to apply this knowledge to clinical problemsolving.[12] However, there are very few studies that clearly link board certification with the delivery of higher quality care. One study in particular found a "clinically modest trend suggesting that board certified physicians provide more comprehensive preventive care compared to non-certified internists."[13] But, this same study found more similarities than differences between ABIM-certified and noncertified internists on questions of practice patterns, patient satisfaction, and patient outcomes.

According to the American Society of Internal Medicine,[14] board certification in internal medicine does not guarantee physician characteristics that may be extremely important to patients, such as listening ability, time spent with a patient, availability when a patient is sick or facing an emergency, and the length of the physician-patient relationship. Neither does it measure the ethical nature of a physician's practice, the value of life experience, the ability of the physician to participate as part of a health care team, practice performance through a peer review process, or the devotion and satisfaction of patients. Finally, board certification only reveals, "what a doctor knew at a particular point in time and cannot measure what has been learned or forgotten in the interim."[15]

The ASIM contends that board certification should be considered one measure of competence, but other measures may provide an additional, and often more accurate, assessment. These other attributes, in addition to the ones already mentioned, include:[16]

1. Evidence of extensive continuing medical education,
2. Appointments to peer review or quality assurance committees,
3. Evidence of a large, busy practice of satisfied patients,
4. Documentation of good standing in the medical community,
5. Clinical privileges granted by a hospital medical staff, and
6. Outcome measures of a physician's competence.

The American Society of Internal Medicine believes there may be alternatives to board certification.[17] In its survey of 62 managed care plans, the ASIM found that some plans might consider accepting alternatives to board certification as a condition for a physician's participation. Over 70 percent of the plans surveyed said they would "consider accepting other standards that would demonstrate competence in Internal Medicine as a minimum qualification for participation." Over 65 percent of the plans said they would accept the completion of the training requirements necessary to qualify for the board exam; 62 percent said they would accept successful completion of a residency program in internal medicine. Few other alternatives received approval by a margin close to 50 percent.

As employers begin to examine health care plans to demonstrate their quality of care, one tangible mechanism to meet this demand, in the absence of better outcome measures, is the credentialing criterion of board certification. Board certification is perceived by both employers and patients as a beginning attempt to answer the questions of quality of care. According to the American Medical Association,[18] in 1993 almost 40 percent of all physicians were not board certified. Again, as employers begin to look at health care plans to demonstrate their quality of care, one tangible mechanism to meet this demand, in the absence of better outcome measures, is the credentialing criteria that includes board certification. This criterion was perceived by both employers and patients to begin to answer the question of quality of care.

Greene and Miller have observed that employers are beginning to ask plans to indicate the percentage of board-certified physicians in their particular panel of physicians. Plans, in turn, are beginning to aggressively market the fact that their participating physicians are board certified.[19] As a result, we now are faced with the dilemma of the noncertified physician. The AMA policy supports the view that all board certification "is a voluntary undertaking and that physicians who practice competently should be able to practice without specialty board certifications."[20]

Although managed care organizations still are using board certification as their gold standard for assuring appropriate credentials, they agree to include only those providers who will render good medical care additional criteria and to institute surveillance systems.[21] The credentialing process will help the managed care organization determine which providers are suitable to become participating members in the plan. Contracting with providers who meet all of the credentialing standards is indeed one method of reducing potential liability for the conduct of a participating provider. "A solid credentialing program, integrated effectively with an ongoing quality improvement system, assists the managed care organization to identify and screen out incompetent physicians and shield the managed care organization from liability."[22] In addition, a strong, consistently applied credentialing program also will provide a record of fairness and objectivity to counter provider challenges that they have been denied participation unfairly. In short, the credentialing process is one of the pivotal elements in demonstrating and maintaining good quality participating providers.

FORCES DRIVING CHANGES IN CREDENTIALING AND PRIVILEGING

Writing in *The Wall Street Journal* editorial page, Kleinke[23] said, ". . . with a trillion dollars in annual health care spending on the table, the most startling aspect of the drive toward provider accountability is its belatedness. The current industrialization of medicine, ushered in by the appearance of tools for measuring and managing its practitioners, echoes what every major U.S. industry experienced several decades ago." Credentialing and privileging does not give us information about physicians' performance once in practice. Nearly five decades of experience with the hospital-based clinical privileging and credentialing model has produced some very disheartening evidence about physicians' collective performance. Brennan and colleagues, in a broad review of tens of thousands of inpatient charts across more than 50 hospitals,[24] found that there is a substantial amount of injury to patients from medical mismanagement, and many injuries are the result of substandard care. Subsequent studies by the same team[25] suggest that many adverse patient events are potentially preventable. A heavy emphasis on systems analysis and education, coupled with practice guidelines, are among the mechanisms suggested by Brennan et al[26] that hold promise for remediation of patient injury. Although most physicians would acknowledge mistakes by trainees as an inevitability, one study found that only 54 percent of house officers ever discuss their mistakes with the attending physicians and only 24 percent told the patients or families.[27]At the trainee level, there is little formal exposure to the concepts of risk management, professional liability, and quality assurance in residency despite self-reports of high levels of interest.[28]

Coupled with the aforementioned focus on assessment of physician performance are many marketplace drivers for changes in credentialing, privileging, and hospital-medical staff relations. These forces include, but are not limited to:[29]

1. The requirement for hospitals to develop cross-disciplinary service products and market them at a competitive rate (raising questions about the relevancy of traditional medical staff departmental structures).

2. Quality for the evaluation of physician performance, as narrowly defined by the medical staff, ignores the impact of inefficient practice patterns and a destructive personal style.
3. The shift to problem resolution by interdisciplinary task forces trained in total quality management (TQM) tends to reduce traditional medical staff meetings to redundancy or to occasions for defending old prerogatives.
4. Peer review and confidentiality of medical staff transactions will be challenged as greater emphasis is placed on interdisciplinary data collection, problem resolution, and public accountability.
5. Medical staff structures mandated by accrediting bodies, Medicare conditions of participation, and state-licensure regulations are likely to adapt slowly to innovations that individual hospitals might find attractive. The resulting tension may be a drag on the adaptation needed for efficiency and quality enhancement.
6. To keep primary care physicians in the outpatient setting where they practice most efficiently, medical staffs may cede more responsibility to mid-level practitioners such as nurse midwives, certified nurse surgical assistants, and nurse practitioners hired either by the hospital or by individual physician groups to be supervised by hospital-based specialists.
7. The need of the hospital and the medical staff to create a cost-efficient continuum of care—from prevention to prehospital, inhospital, and posthospital—will mandate relationships that facilitate information flow, quality assessment, and performance evaluation. The traditional medical staff is focused on the inpatient setting. Review of care outside the hospital is regarded as an intrusion on a sacred preserve.
8. Physicians and hospitals already have begun to recognize their least efficient members. Specifically, competitive demands will lead to the identification of a "first team" that will get the contract, thereby blocking out less efficient or suboptimal practitioners. The traditional egalitarian approach will be replaced by the need to meet a standard of cost and outcome predictability as the price of playing the game. *The reliability of credentialing in predicting optimal performance will emerge as a key factor in marketing and in the negotiation of reimbursement rates.*
9. The coalescence of practice into physician networks related by contract will shift the locus of credentialing and peer review away from the medical staff. Medical staff self-governance guided by by-laws will compete with economic relations defined by contract.
10. As managed care organizations are being evaluated and accredited by the National Committee for Quality Assurance in Washington DC, there is an increased pressure for mechanisms to ensure that their

providers are meeting the standards that have been set to evaluate their plan. NCQA has criteria beyond the traditional hospital credentialing and privileging process and beyond a query from the state Board of Medical Examiners or Department of Professional Regulations.

11. The tools and process of peer assessment, a cornerstone of assuring and evaluating the quality of the medical care across all practice settings as well as a key component of the clinical credentialing and privileging process, have fallen under attack.

ADDITIONAL QUALITY ASSESSMENT TOOLS

Recognizing that credentialing, privileging, and board certification are inadequate alone to assess physician performance and contribute to quality improvement, additional measurement tools have been designed. These include continuing medical education, board recertification, peer rating, peer review, patient satisfaction surveys, and physician profiling to name a few. In subsequent chapters it will be shown in greater detail how these measures have been adapted to effectively assess physician performance in today's health care market and what additional tools are being developed.

Continuing Medical Education

A major structural measure used to assure that physicians maintain their cognitive skills has been the presence of continuing medical education. State licensing boards require a minimum amount of CME I credits. However, research calls into question the effectiveness of much of current continuing medical education efforts practiced today. The vast majority of CME practiced today consists of journal reading and conferences. The effectiveness of journal reading on changes in knowledge and performance has not been studied at all by peer-reviewed research. Formal CME conferences or activities in and of themselves have been found by many studies to have little or no effect on changing physician performance. Strategies found to be effective in changing physician knowledge and physician performance include physician reminders, patient-mediated interventions, outreach visits, opinion leaders, and multifaceted activities.[30, 31] However, most of these strategies are institutional or system-initiated activities rather than individually motivated activities. As such, they do not fit the traditional professional model of continuing medical education and have not been widely implemented.

Board Recertification

After post-graduate training, what happens to an internist's cognitive skills? The literature shows that the knowledge and skills of practicing specialists can decay with time. One study that looked at practicing internists' scores on questions from a 1988 ABIM certifying examination showed a significant inverse correlation between examination scores and the number of years elapsed since certification. Knowledge declined sharply within 15 years of certification. If a passing cutoff used for the certifying examination had been applied to these practitioners who had been certified 15 years previously, approximately 68 percent of these individuals would have failed the examination.[32]

As a result, there has been a recent evolution in the board certification process to offer time-limited board certificates offered by most specialties. Time-limited certification has become a means for specialty boards to set and assure standards of clinical competence throughout a physician's career. The ABIM has attempted to implement a continuing improvement model in its execution of the recertification process by developing a process that promotes learning rather than attempts to screen out the "bad apples."

The ABIM has organized its recertification program in three steps:

- A self-evaluation process consisting of five modules of 60 clinically relevant questions from recent certifying exams—using an absolute standard method;
- A peer assessment of clinical competence, comprising eight components of clinical competence including clinical judgment, medical knowledge, clinical skills, humanistic qualities, professional attitudes and behavior, medical care, continuing scholarship, and moral and ethical behavior in the clinical setting; and
- Full certification is granted after a candidate is deemed eligible from the first two steps and has passed a final recertification examination given over one day.[33]

Data on the recertification process show an interesting trend toward specialization in the career of a primary care physician. The American Board of Family Practice was the first specialty certification to mandate recertification in 1969, and as such has had the longest experience with this process. A review of the performances of six cohorts of family physicians in the last 20 years showed significant declines in the cohorts' performance on each recertification examination. The authors of this review suggest that "it is possible that as the practice life of a family physician evolves the focus of the practice becomes narrower, and this narrowed focus results in a decline in performance on an examination, half of which covers the breadth of the specialty."[34] A retrospective cohort study of 335,438 physicians in active practice confirmed that more self-defined generalists became specialists (6.2 percent) than self-defined specialists became generalists (2.2 percent).[35] This trend needs to be recognized by managed care organizations when privileging primary care physicians over a career, especially when market trends may push them to grant as broad a privileging package to a primary care physician as possible. Indeed, the ABIM is allowing subspecialists to recertify in their internal medicine subspecialty without needing to recertify in internal medicine, with the understanding that they will no longer be regarded by the ABIM as a certified internist. How specialists will respond to this option given current market pressures will be interesting to observe.

Peer Ratings

Peer ratings have been another major method for assessing cognitive as well as humanistic and global skills. Global performance ratings have been used frequently to evaluate performance of medical students and residents. These ratings have been found to be reliable in the training setting[36] and in clinical practice[37] where a sufficient number of observers are used. One study piloted a brief professional associates rating questionnaire that judged clinical skills on two dimensions: cognitive/clinical management skills and humanistic qualities/psychosocial skills. It found that ratings from at least 11 professional associates, including physicians and nurses, are needed to provide a reliable assessment. The ratings were not found to be biased substantially by the method of selection of the peers or the relationship between the rater and the subject. Because of their reliability, these ratings scales are being considered as an evaluative mechanism for recertification of practicing physicians by several specialty boards, including the ABIM.

Peer Review

Peer review has been a cornerstone in current medical quality assurance efforts. The peer review process is mandated by federal law and conducted through peer review organizations (PROs). Considerable money and energy has been spent in federal, state, and private peer review of the quality of care of individual patients.[38] Despite this effort, there are serious limitations with the current use of peer review, including poor interrater reliability and failure to detect and refer substandard cases for review. Other barriers identified with peer review include inaccurate descriptors for the variety of patient and physician management plans and wide differences in judgments about patient care. These problems are not limited to federal PROs but come up with almost any current use of peer review.

Most peer review involves examination of the medical record using one of two types of methods. Explicit review relies on predetermined criteria; however, its use has been limited because of the complexity and heterogeneity of medical care. Implicit review relies on a physician's global judgment of quality without predetermined criteria and has become the community standard.[39]

However, implicit review has several limitations. Peer review using implicit criteria has been shown to be useful only when judging groups of patients. Using peer review to review the care of a single patient is useful only when care is egregiously bad and the relevant standard is obvious.[40] A study of implicit review on inpatients found particular unreliability in its use to evaluate appropriateness of hospital resource use and patient's readiness for discharge,[41] two of its more common uses. Another study found fault on the part of a PRO in its initial screening process—to detect and refer for PRO physician review two of three records that this one study judged substandard when compared with an independent panel of credible judges on the quality of care.[42] These shortcomings also were found in the outpatient setting.

Proposed methods to improve the process include more objective assessment procedures, use of multiple reviewers, higher standards for reviewers, elimination of systematic reviewer bias, use of outcome judgments, and adoption of practice guidelines.

Patient Satisfaction Surveys

Humanistic competence—defined as measuring a physician's ability to perform the human element of the profession including communication with patients, empathy, and rapport-building—is a critical component of clinical care. While explicit measures of humanistic competence have been underdeveloped compared to measures of technical and cognitive competence, there has been tremendous advances in such measures in recent years.

The development of patient satisfaction surveys is an attempt to measure quality of care from the patient's point of view, one component of which is patient satisfaction. The patient's experience, including interactions with institutions, health care professionals, and prescribed regimens, can be accurately assessed only by patients themselves. The patient experience is affected by multiple interactions with members of the entire health care team and system, not just with an individual physician. As a result, such surveys are most reliable when comparing individual physicians in a single system.

Since 1987, the Picker/Commonwealth Program for Patient-Centered Care, located at Beth Israel Hospital in Boston MA, has been a leader in research that explores patients' needs and concerns. These researchers found that patients, rather than being focused on the amenities of care (as previously presumed), are most concerned about issues of clinical relevance. Most patient concerns fall into the following dimensions of care:[43]

- access to care—including the ability to make a timely appointment, office waiting time, and telephone access;
- physical care, comfort, and alleviation of pain;
- emotional support;
- coordination of care and integration of services;
- involvement of family and friends;
- respect for patients' values, preferences, and expressed needs;
- transition and continuity;
- communication and interpersonal interaction between patient and physicians and the patient and other providers of care;[44] and
- the perceived technical quality of care seems to play a lesser role in affecting satisfaction.[45]

Almost all managed care organizations now are using patient satisfaction surveys. These surveys fulfill several internal needs including responding to employer requests for such information, marketing, strategic planning, and provider profiling and payment. The use of such data has a factor in determining bonus reimbursement and has been used to determine whether a physician remains in an HMO network.[46] Indeed, the National Committee for Quality Assurance, the principal body accrediting HMOs, requires that a managed care plan use satisfaction surveys to evaluate quality of care and service delivery.

There is a move by several organizations to try to design a satisfaction survey instrument that can be utilized nationwide to obtain consistent results. NCQA issued a standardized Annual Member Health Care Survey for members of managed care organizations in 1995, which will be incorporated into its next version of its Health Plan Employer Data and Information Set (HEDIS) 3.0. The Agency for Health Care Policy and Research is bringing federal government input into the process by an ambitious work that is attempting to develop a national validated tool for consumer satisfaction that will be appropriate for managed care and non-managed care settings. Different components of the effort are being field tested.[47]

Physician Profiling

A rapidly evolving addition to physician performance assessment is physician profiling. A profile is a measure of outcomes at the physician level. Traditionally, outcomes had been examined on a case-by-case basis due to limitations in the availability of data and the capacity for data collection, storage, and analysis. However, advances in information technology now allow rapid collection and analysis of data on hundreds and thousands of patients. The majority of current efforts aimed at variations in clinical outcomes have examined outcomes on a aggregate level, whether it is by states, cities, HMOs, multispecialty group practices, or hospitals. Physician profiling is an attempt to look at outcomes at the individual physician practice level.

The measurement of physician-specific outcomes is an attempt to assess whether the goals of health care are achieved and to assess the quality of care rendered by that physician. Such an analysis requires several components:

- a standard outcome, representing outcomes that are ordinarily achieved;
- an expected outcome, calculated from the rate at which the standard outcome occurs and then adjusted for differences unique to the physician's group of patients being assessed;
- a measurement of the actual outcome of the physician's practice;
- a comparison of the actual outcomes to the expected outcome; and
- an analysis to determine whether the difference is too small to be important or solely could be due to chance.

Ideally, a profile would contain the following components:

- it would be nonjudgmental;
- outcomes would be based on the patient panel that a physician sees;
- there would be disease-specific outcomes;
- outcomes would be adjusted by severity of disease;
- outcomes would be based on data that are accurate;
- outcomes would be initially fed back to physicians in the form of user-friendly reports with explanations of methodology;
- the use of profiles would allow physicians to improve quality;
- profiles would not be released to the public without adequate education about the limitations of such methodologies; and
- profiles would not pick out individual physicians for problems that may be more indicative of system problems.

The most important aspect of a profile is the actual outcomes that are selected for inclusion. Choosing the outcomes as well as the standards set for these outcomes are the foundation of the entire profile. Outcomes selected should summarize important aspects of care and should not just be selected based on ease of measurement. Physician-specific outcomes should measure events that physicians have control over. They should summarize the care being evaluated and be valid reflections of the aspects of care they measure. They also should reflect occurrences that can be observed reliably and can be reproduced.

Another important aspect to understand in a profile is exactly what a specific outcome is measuring. Variation in a clinical outcome may be the result of variation of multiple variables in a health care system, only one of which is the physician's competence. Studies that have looked at outcomes of procedures such as CABG and artificial joint replacement have determined that there are other important aspects of the health care "system" that affect patient care—including the competence of other individuals on the health care team performing the surgery and process factors including the degree of coordination that exists between these various members.

One method of adjusting for variation caused by patient characteristics is the use of casemix adjusting. The use of casemix adjustments is critical to obtaining meaningful outcome measurements and cannot be limited to simply age and sex adjusters alone. For example, in one study adjustment for patient characteristics decreased the observed variation in referral profiles by 50 percent. Three-quarters of the physicians identified as statistical outliers with the use of an age/sex-adjusted measure were no longer identified as such with use of a casemix adjusted measure.[48] Techniques and technologies used to casemix adjust is a rapidly evolving field that has been well reviewed.

The number of outcomes that actually are measured is key to determining whether the differences are statistically significant or solely due to chance. Because physician profiling examines individual physician practices, there can be serious problems with small sample sizes. There are only a limited number of diseases and outcomes in a specific practice that will give enough numbers to provide the statistical power to look at significant differences by physicians. As a result, common events and diseases need to be selected when looking at individual physicians.

Another limitation in profiling methods is the source of data used to develop the profile. Most profiling methods have used insurance claims data because of their easy accessibility. However, there are serious quality errors in such claims data. There is a lack of medical detail necessary for good casemix adjustment as well as a high rate of coding error with claims data. For example, one study showed that the coding for a relatively straightforward diagnosis—diabetes mellitus—had a 10 percent error rate on claims data.[49] Diagnoses that are more complex to code, such as angina, unstable angina, congestive heart failure, and peripheral vascular disease, were shown to be identified by claims data less than 50 percent of the time than they were present in the medical record.[50] Primary data collection efforts that delve into the medical record are characterized by higher accuracy; however, they are much more costly. The computerized medical record obviously holds a great deal of promise in overcoming this limitation.

How a physician profile is used naturally depends on the objectives of the organization developing the profile. However, any program should have at least two objectives: measurement of the quality of care and facilitation and translation of the measurement into specific actions that will result in the improvement of the quality of care.

Older methods of quality assurance focused on the outlier approach—where "bad apples" were identified and either eliminated and punished. An example of this is the federal government's program of PROs, which primarily focused before 1993 on identifying and punishing individual cases of clinical error. The Institute of Medicine found that the PRO program spent over $300 million a year in this effort without demonstrable improvement in the overall quality of care.

Newer methods of quality improvement have focused on using such data and feeding back information to physicians, along with positive incentives, in a program that encourages continuous quality improvement. Organizations that have incorporated this philosophy into their oversight programs include the National Committee for Quality Assurance and the Joint Commission on Accreditation of Healthcare Organizations.

Profiles ideally should be fed back to physicians in the form of user-friendly reports with explanations of methodology and should allow physicians to understand them and develop methods that will allow them to improve quality. Organizations using physician profiles should not pick out individual physicians for problems that may be more indicative of entire system problems. Instead, they should use profiling to discover systemic problems and work on processes in the entire health care system that will improve the quality of care. Physician profiling may reveal deficiencies in skill sets that will need to be addressed through continuing education means.

Attempts at profiling physicians already are occurring. In a 1993 survey, the American Medical Association found that 39 percent of physicians surveyed were subject to clinical profiling. In 1993 it was reported that 45.5 percent of all U.S. physicians were subject to either clinical or economic profiling.[51] In general, most clinical profiling has focused on cost control looking at the patterns of care instead of specific clinical decisions. Such patterns have shown widespread variation in resource use by physicians. For example, in one study, Florida physicians used almost 50 percent more resources than Oregon physicians per hospital admission.[52]

In addition, governments are beginning to release physician-specific data. The Health Care Financing Administration first began to release hospital-specific mortality data in 1987 but has not released physician-specific information as of yet. However, both Pennsylvania (voluntarily) and New York state (as a result of a court order) have published physician-specific profiles. There naturally has been a great deal of concern about making physician-specific information public. Many professional societies such as the American Society of Internal Medicine have recommended that only aggregate performance data be released primarily because of the limitations that statistical power and proper casemix adjustments give to physician-specific data. Certainly, the public nature of such data can be threatening to an individual physician and not foster a state of continuous quality improvement. However, the state has a responsibility to the consumers to provide them with such information. In fact, much of the impetus toward developing physician profiling was brought on by HCFA's initial efforts to release mortality data followed by other government efforts. This tension between public accountability and quality improvement has not been adequately resolved yet.

Managed care organizations have taken a lead in developing physician profiles. The AMA found that physicians employed by health maintenance organizations were the most likely to be subject to clinical profiling (48 percent), followed closely by physicians holding independent practice association contracts (47 percent).[53] Ninety-six percent of preferred provider organizations maintained profiles of their providers in 1990.[54] For example, U.S. Healthcare, a managed care organization, uses measures of access to care, capability to provide care, aspects of technical performance, aspects of cognitive performance, appropriateness of care, patient satisfaction of care, processes of care, outcomes of care, and costs of care.

As physician profiling can be a powerful tool to assess physician performance, there are several research efforts to improve the process and expand the topics. One of the initial efforts to develop a profile on ambulatory physicians was the Developing and Evaluating Methods to Promote Ambulatory Care Quality (DEMPAQ) project. DEMPAQ was a three-year demonstration project funded by HCFA and administered by Harvard University and PROs of the State of Maryland and the District of Columbia to develop an evaluative system for physician office care. There were two review methods used—Medicare claims profiling and medical record review. Quality indicators were developed for both types of data and a computer algorithm was used to generalize physician profiles. Three types of patient-level profiles were developed:

- office practice, including physician caseload, distribution of patient visits, and primary patient characteristics;
- condition-specific, including selected samples of patients with certain conditions and the use of services that contributes to good management of patients; and
- preventive care, including influenza immunizations, sigmoidoscopy, colonoscopy, pap smears, and mammograms.

Researchers have continued this work in such areas as diabetes. For example, the Ambulatory Care Quality Improvement Project (ACQIP) is a collaborative effort to collect data on the processes and outcomes of care for patients with diabetes mellitus. Parties involved in the pilot project include HCFA, the American Diabetes Association, Delmarva Foundation for Medical Care, Alabama Quality Assurance Foundation, Iowa Foundation for Medical Care, and physicians in Alabama, Iowa, and Maryland.

One institution compared the practices of family practitioners and internal medicine physicians on the treatment of congestive heart failure using the AHCPR heart failure guidelines to measure quality of care in an ambulatory setting. Chart reviews were conducted and surprisingly unexplained clinical variation in the outpatient diagnosis and therapy of heart failure between the two practices studied were noted. The objective documentation of left ventricular hypertrophy (LVH) was underutilized in the diagnosis of heart failure as well as treatment with ACE inhibitors. Additionally, inappropriate use of calcium channel blockers were noted.[55] This information is critical for practitioners to know how they are performing compared to their colleagues so that continuous quality improvement may ensue.

Another example is the Center for Research in Ambulatory Health Care Administration (CRAHCA) Physician Profiling Project funded by the Robert Wood Johnson Foundation. Physicians learn which services other physicians in their specialties perform. Physicians then are able to compare their profiles with state- and national-level medians. One of the first demonstration projects was to profile ambulatory care practice patterns and collect patient demographics. The project is testing the Ambulatory Care Group (ACG) classification system on data selected from 130 nonacademic practices representing over 5,000 physicians in four demonstration states: Florida, Minnesota, New York, and Washington. Data are being collected through the practice's billing system.

MCOs: DIFFERENT PLANS, DIFFERENT CRITERIA

As managed care organizations grow in number, there is a parallel need for mechanisms that encourage quality in systems that offer financial incentives to use health care resources in a cost-effective manner. In short, across the country, managed care plans are experimenting with new kinds of internal performance assessment systems that identify problems and inefficiencies and purport to encourage quality improvement. As health plans use the physician performance information garnered from these systems to set compensation and recredential physicians, it is easy to see what pitfalls may develop.

For example, this grab bag of criteria used to set compensation and to recredential—including plans' use of physician performance information—complicated by the complexity in MCO/physician arrangements has resulted in chaotic, if not confusing, credentialing parameters.[56] As Gold and her colleagues[57] observed:

> These arrangements with physicians are expected to vary with the plan's management philosophy and strategic objectives and various characteristics of the plan's market area, including the degree of competitiveness, the maturity of the managed care market, physician receptivity to managed care and the accepting of financial risk, and the regulatory environment. . . . Each plan presumably chooses a set of approaches to its arrangements with physicians that, in combination, maximizes its probability of achieving its strategic objectives subject to any constraints imposed by market characteristics or other factors. For example, plans that capitate primary care physicians and place them at risk for specialty referrals and inpatient care through a withhold account, may be expected to place particular emphasis on monitoring physicians to ensure that the financial incentives do not result in under-service. On the other hand, plans operating in areas where physicians are resistant to accepting much financial risk may rely particularly heavily on nonfinancial mechanisms such as utilization management to influence practice patterns.[58]

Indeed, in follow-up studies[59] under the auspices of the Physician Payment Review Commission (PPRC) and the Medical College of Virginia and Mathematica Policy Research, 138 managed care plans were selected from 20 metropolitan areas nationwide to receive a detailed survey about their arrangements with plan physicians. Respondents from all three types of plans (HMOs, IPAs, and PPOs) said they emphasized careful selection of physicians, although the group or staff HMOs tended to have more demanding requirements such as board certification or eligibility. Sixty-one percent of the plans responded that physicians' previous patterns of cost or utilization of resources had little influence on their selection, 26 percent said these factors had a moderate influence, and 13 percent said they had a large influence.

Table 1 summarizes the procedures used in recruiting physicians in the aforementioned survey done by the PPRC.

When selecting physicians, the group or staff HMOs tended to have more demanding requirements than the other types of plans. Ninety percent of group or staff HMOs, but only 48 percent of the network or IPA HMOs and 41 percent of

Table 1. Procedures Used by Managed Care Plans To Recruit Physicians

Procedure	All Plans (N = 108)	Group or Staff HMOs (N = 29)	Network or IPA HMOs (N = 50)	PPOs (N = 29)
			percent	
Selecting physicians				
Require board certification or board eligibilityυ	57	90	48 †	41 †
Require privileges at network hospital or ability to obtain them	82	86	88	69 ‡
Require agreement to take predetermined number of patients or not to practice outside plan §	37	48	48	7 ¶
State that the effect of previous costs or utilization patterns on the decision was large	13	4	18 ‖	14
Contracting with physicians				
Verify license and credentialsυυ	100	100	100	100
Consult National Practitioner Data Bank, sources on substance abuse, or both	92	86	94	93
Visit physician's office, review facility, and screen care through medical records‡‡				
Do all three	43	38	66 ‖	7 ¶
Do none of these	27	34	8 †	52 ¶
Review quantitative data from indemnity claims, hospital discharge data, or both	37	24	38	48 ‖
Meeting four criteria for orienting new physicians‡‡	30	69	22 †	3†‡

υ Other plans may allow exceptions.
† P<0.01 for the comparison with group or staff HMOs.
‡ P<0.10 for the comparison with network or IPA HMOs.
§ Only 100 plans responded (27 group or staff HMOs, 45 network or IPA HMOs, and 28 PPOs).
¶ P<0.01 for the comparison with network or IPA HMOs.
‖ P<0.10 for the comparison with group or staff HMOs.
υυ Only 102 plans responded (25 group or staff HMOs, 48 network or IPA HMOs, and 29 PPOs).
†† Because they are much more likely to hire than to contract with physicians who practice in their facilities, group, or staff HMOs may find these steps unnecessary or address the underlying concerns in different ways (e.g. by contacting references).
‡‡ The four criteria are as follows: plan has orientation meetings specifically for medical staff, 75 percent or more of physicians participate, top management is involved, and less than 75 percent of time it devoted to administrative issues. Of all plans, 5 percent met none of the criteria, 17 percent one, 23 percent two, 26 percent three, and 30 percent four.

Reprinted with permission from The New England Journal of Medicine, *1995; 333:1680.*

the PPOs, required board certification or eligibility. Both types of HMO were more likely than the PPOs to require that new physicians either have privileges at network hospitals or be able to obtain them. Both types of HMOs also were more likely than the PPOs to require physicians to provide care for a predetermined number of patients or to practice only within the plan. A minority of the plans used quantitative information about physicians' performance and practice style in selecting new physicians. However, 63 percent of all the plans and 73 percent of the network or IPA HMOs took into account qualitative information such as professional reputation and patterns of care.

Before signing a contract with a new physician, virtually all plans verified the physician's license and credentials and almost all screened for reportable disciplinary actions, substance abuse, or similar problems. Sixty-six percent of the network or IPA HMOs visited the physician's office, reviewed whether the facility met set standards, and screened care by reviewing medical records. Only 7 percent of the PPOs took all these steps and 52 percent took none of them. Ninety-three percent of the plans had a formal process for recredentialing physicians, although 62 percent began to do this only in 1991 or later in response to accreditation requirements. Clearly, then, the scope and content of the credentialing and recredentialing process is changing dramatically under the market leverage of managed care.

Woolhandler and Himmelstein[60] observed that the current system may pressure doctors to exploit patients' trust for financial gain. For example, the practice profiles garnered from the unprecedented amounts of specific physician performance information being collected may encourage quality improvement but just as easily may be used to punish physicians or exclude them from specific managed care programs. The authors state:[61]

> As fee-for-service medicine withers, risk selection by HMOs will become a zero-sum game presaging fierce competition among doctors to avoid sick patients. Doctors who attract patients, for example, experienced surgeons, minority group physicians, medical school faculty members and those who care for the poor risk being ostracized from plans and even physician groups. The gulf between clinical excellence and professional success will widen.

Their contention led to front-page articles in places like *USA Today* where physicians and patients agonized about the implications of so-called physician "gag rules" and the like. State licensing boards also are joining the fray as they consider these perverse incentives.[62]

Is this what we wanted from the managed care credentialing and privileging process? As the ASIM has noted,[63] if plans reward physicians for doing more procedures in the office rather than demonstrating excellence in performing them, is this quality or is it a method of minimizing referrals? Is patient satisfaction, which some physicians argue is seldom critical to clinical outcome, an appropriate performance measure? Do other measures, often used by managed care plans to address issues such as cost control, utilization reduction, access, market expansion, and cooperation with the health plan (those issues outlined in the work of Gold et al), have anything to do with quality? Some observers contend that these measures appear to focus primarily on getting physicians to practice in ways that are congruent with the goals of the managed care plan, not necessarily for quality of care.

As a result of all of the aforementioned concerns, many national groups (ASIM among them) are calling for a balance between clinical quality, cost control, access, patient satisfaction, and the business concerns of the managed care entities. They believe that no single measure should be given more weight than direct assessments of clinical skills in disease-specific patient outcomes when evaluating physician performance.

Other observers argue that managed care plans should consult with their enrolled physicians on the appropriate weights to be assigned to measures of clinical skills, patient outcomes, patient satisfaction, and other elements that may be included in a program for assessing physician performance. This is a partially veiled call for increased physician vigilance and leadership with regard to these issues. Arguably, most rank and file physicians are not expert in these areas, and this new challenge may call for advanced training for a new cadre of physician quality leaders.

Most researchers would support the notion that physician performance assessment programs should provide physicians with nonjudgmental, comparative clinical performance information derived not from individual patients but from population-based data analysis and adjusted quality measurements to promote internal and quality improvement.[64] This requires, however, that plans provide educational feedback on a timely and routine basis in the form of user-friendly reports with explanations of methodology to facilitate review by physicians. Plans should allow opportunity for practice adaptation before initiating any adverse action toward a medical practice. Of course, this carries a price that many plans may not be willing to pay.[65] Also, many of these tools are still in the experimental stage.

In recognition of the concerns outlined above, other groups within organized medicine have rallied to this important public policy challenge. For example, the American Medical Association has convened an expert consultant panel concerned with physician performance assessment.[66] The first meeting of this expert panel convened in late 1995 with the bulk of the work scheduled for calendar year 1997 and beyond.

In late 1995, the AMA designed the Physician Profiling Project to examine existing profiling programs and to explore the appropriate role for the AMA in this arena. Several profiling entities in the private sector have asked the AMA to obtain physician input in the development of profiling methodologies to transform claims-based profiling into clinically focused databases, to propose pilot projects on specific patient populations or diseases, and to construct continuing medical education programs based on these profiles. Officially, the AMA appears encouraged by these possible partnerships to enhance the quality of medical care and promote standards setting and professionalism as part of the physician performance assessment program. Potential opportunities beyond profiling to the broader area of physician performance assessment also are being considered.

Internally, the AMA has created the Commission on Clinical Preventive Practice (CCPP). This internal working group is charged with creating a pilot program to assess the delivery of preventive services within an outpatient physician practice as one measure of physician performance. The CCPP has been dedicated to developing a pilot instrument based on the *Guide to Clinical Preventive Services* of the United States Preventive Services Task Force. Pilot testing of this CCPP instrument is scheduled to begin in 1996.

Finally, as the physician performance assessment initiative progresses, one major thrust will involve the evaluation and dissemination of practice parameters and their conversion into clinical algorithms. In short, it appears as though organized medicine supports the translation of complex clinical guidelines into easy-to-follow checklists or clinical algorithms, also sometimes called review criteria. One then can apply these review criteria to office-based practice to establish standards for actual performance evaluation. In December 1995, the AMA board of trustees authorized an experimental phase of a program to include the development of a physician performance assessment instrument and process to be pilot tested in 1996. This program is now called the American Medical Accreditation Program (AMAP).

The Joint Commission on Accreditation of Healthcare Organizations also has rallied to the challenge. The JCAHO has impaneled the Council on Performance

Measurement,[67] whose task, in part, will be to evaluate current performance measurement systems and make recommendations as to their enhancement. The Council will consider such variables as risk-adjustment methodologies, validity, and literature support.

There are, at minimum, four major future issues concerning the ability to truly promote clinical competence in patient care. These issues include (1) the process of credentialing within integrated systems of care; (2) the growth of private-sector efforts to verify credentials and improve the process; (3) the role of the organizational structure of physician's work on the privileging and credentialing process; and finally, (4) new evidence concerning communication between patients and physicians and its unique role in the credentialing process.

PHYSICIAN PERFORMANCE ASSESSMENT WITHIN INTEGRATED SYSTEMS

Certainly as we learn more about the impact of organizational and managerial factors on the quality of care in health care organizations we may be able to construct new models and new structures that will streamline and improve the credentialing and privileging process. In a major recent review, Flood[68] found that over a 25-year period we have barely begun to understand the relationship underlying the quality-of-care model that relies on structure, process, and outcome. Flood contends that, "Without clear insights at this level, setting up incentives or imperatives may reproduce the structural characteristic but not its intended effect: better care without undue cost. The legal system and health policy need to recognize the choices and trade-offs made in clinical decisions associated with providing adequate quality of care and services and in using reasonable resources to achieve that quality."[69] Current research that purports to examine relationships between organizational design and quality of outcomes is, in Flood's words, scant and crude. What we do know, however, is that when physicians respond to capitation by using utilization management techniques, they adopt the tools previously used only by insurers. This physician-initiated management approach represents a fundamental transformation in the practice of medicine, and its impact on the privileging and credentialing process has yet to be explored.[70]

Zablocki has found that hospitals in particular "are finding that their inclusive medical staff-credentialing models originally designed to attract qualified physicians and boost patient admissions now can result in networks that are too costly and administratively cumbersome to compete in a managed care market."[71] Networks, which are striving to obtain managed care contracts and increasing numbers of covered lives, need to be more selective by necessarily limiting membership to qualified and cost-conscious practitioners willing to play by the new managed care rules. When the networks start to become more exclusive, they head in treacherous and uncharted waters. These networks may undertake several different strategies for constructing credentialing and privileging procedures, including being highly selective at the outset; relatively open at the outset and pruning the physician ranks gradually; or relatively open on a permanent basis. Surely, each of these aforementioned strategies has its pluses and minuses. Yet many contend that regardless of the strategy used, networks may end up with 10 to 15 percent more capacity than needed.[72] Clearly, network size and subspecialty composition are difficult issues.

While there simply is not sufficient current information to predict how networks will grapple with these important challenges, one of the potential solutions, at least in part, is the development and use of specialty referral guidelines. Little is known about how care is coordinated between two or more physicians, patient perceptions of specialist versus generalist care, or the impact of reimbursement changes on the referral relationship. In response, specialist physicians at academic medical centers and professional societies are beginning to create their own referral guidelines. However, this trend has not been widely embraced by primary care specialties, who are concerned that strict referral procedures will impinge on their clinical autonomy.

Credential Verification Organizations (CVOs)

Many private- and public-sector efforts are under way to better organize the approach to physician credentialing and privileging. For example, the need for rapid and correct credentialing has set off a mini boom in the market for an entire new industry—labeled Credential Verification Organizations (CVOs). "Indeed, CVOs have become so popular that NCQA has decided to certify these verification organizations so HMOs will be able to contract out selected functions without jeopardizing their own accreditation status. NCQA mailed its new standard to interested CVOs in October of 1995, and expects to release the first group of CVO certification determinations in the fall of 1996."[73]

JCAHO has recognized that appropriate use of the AMA Physician Masterfile by an organization would meet verification requirements in the medical staff standards of the "Accreditation Manual for Hospitals" and in the credentialing standards in other JCAHO accreditation manuals. Typically, managed care organizations dedicate a great deal of internal resources to the process of credentialing and privileging. Each initial credentialing file may include an average of 30 pieces of paper, taking roughly five work hours to gather and assemble, and could cost anywhere from $300 to $400 per provider. The CVOs range in size from mom-and-pop-style paper chasers to giant national firms like Equifax, whose new Credentials Verification Division aims at assembling a complete file on every one of the nation's 600,000 practicing physicians.[74]

Table 2 outlines the private- and public-sector organizations currently involved in assessing physician performance and participating in the privileging and credentialing process.

Table 2. Organizations Assessing Physicians and/or Physician Practices

Organization	Focus of Physician Review
NCQA National Committee for Quality Assurance	Standards fall into six categories: • Quality Improvement • Physician Credentials** • Member's Rights and Responsibilities • Preventive Health Services • Utilization Management** • Medical Records** ***Categories most likely to lead to direct interaction and/or assessment of physicians.*
AAAHC Joint Accreditation Association for Ambulatory Health Care	Accredits ambulatory health care organizations and has a project with the CMA for Ambulatory Review in California. Ambulatory Health Care Standard categories include: • Credentialing • Peer Review • Clinical Records • Facility Safety • Patient Care and Monitoring • Hospital Transfer Protocols
JCAHO Joint Commission on Accreditation of Health Care Organizations	• Standards for Ambulatory Health Care • Standards for Health Care Networks
URAC Utilization Review Accreditation Commission	• Accredits companies performing external utilization review. • Standards forthcoming on accreditation standards for PPOs. • PPO standards do not include direct assessment of physicians.
HCFA Health Care Financing Administration	Interviews physicians participating under Medicare risk contracts to make sure that they understand their HMO contracts and reimbursement arrangements. HCFA relies on health plans to credential physicians and assess their performance.
MGMA Medical Group Management Association	Provides assessment manual for medical groups.
Medical Liability Carriers	Review multiple aspects of physician practices.
Managed Care Organizations	Assess multiple aspects of physician performance. Most MCOs use NCQA standards as a baseline, but some have developed their own regional standards that go beyond NCQA.
Board of Family Practice	Process for board re-certification includes medical record review that is performed by the physician.
American College of Radiology (ACR)	ACR has deemed status from the Food and Drug Administration to accredit mammography facilities. Additional standards available for ultrasound and diagnostic radiology.

Table 2 (cont).

Organization	Focus of Physician Review
College of American Pathologists (CAP)	Accredits hospital and reference labs as well as outpatient labs that are part of hospital systems. Smaller labs are referred to COLA. CAP provides proficiency testing, self-assessments, and checklists for educational purposes but does not assess individual physician performance.
IPA Association of California	Has developed the IPA Clinical Operations Manual to guide health plans in meeting NCQA standards
State Medicaid Programs	• Most states have minimal requirements for physician participation in Medicaid • Med-Cal, however, requires primary care sites to be reviewed unless they are accredited by CMA-AAHC or JCAHO. • The Oregon Health Plan also has specific standards for physicians.
Credentialing Verification Organizations (CVOs)	• Verify physician credentials for MCOs and hospitals. • Many of these organizations also perform on-site medical record reviews for HMOs

Reprinted with permission of the AMA, 1996.

The National Practitioner Data Bank

Probably the most important public-sector effort to improve the credentialing process was the formation of the National Practitioner Data Bank (NPDB), which was mandated by the Health Care Quality Improvement Act (HCQIA) passed by Congress in 1986 for the purpose of preventing incompetent practitioners from moving from state to state without detection. The NPDB is a database that contains adverse information regarding certain health care practitioners. The provisions regarding the NPDB contain both reporting and inquiry requirements, most of which is beyond the scope of this text. However, at a minimum, health care entities including hospitals and networks must report certain information to the NPDB through their state licensing boards. Health care entities must report any professional review action that adversely affects the clinical privileges of a physician or dentist for a period of longer than 30 days. Currently, information reported to the NPDB is confidential and may not be disclosed except in connection with peer review and as necessary to carry out the requirements of the HCQIA legislation. It is highly likely that the scope of control and level of detail currently contained within the NPDB will expand and take on added future significance.

In spite of the CVOs, JCAHO, NCQA, and the National Data Bank, there still remain future issues concerning our ability to truly promote clinical competence in patient care including the process of credentialing within integrated systems of care. The growth of private-sector efforts to verify credentials and improve the process, the role of organizational structure of physician's work on the privileging and credentialing process, and the role patient-physician communication should play in the credentialing and assessment process for physicians are yet to be determined.

SPECIALIST PERFORMANCE ASSESSMENT

There is no question that the scope of medical knowledge has exceeded the capabilities of any single physician at that specialty where care is needed. Specialty care is perhaps more important now than at any previous time in our history. However, specialization, which is organ-system specific, may conflict with other indicators of high-quality care, such as patient accessibility, continuity of care, and open physician-patient communication.[75] Population-based data can be used to evaluate primary care physicians; however, specialist performance must be based on the population of patients referred to the specialist by primary care physicians. Evaluation of the surgical specialists usually focuses on their performance on procedures and at times their diagnostic workups. It is therefore crucial that severity-of-illness adjustments must be made to balance differences in referral patterns between specialists. For example, the effectiveness of obstetrical care is being evaluated by c-section rates for each specialist as compared to their regional peers. Length-of-stay measures for appendectomies and laparoscopic cholecystectomies converted to open cholecystectomies can be indicators of quality for general surgeons. These data may be used as feedback in order for specialists to measure their practices against their peers and as national benchmark standards for continued quality improvement. Another specialty performance appraisal system designed to measure quality of care without using administrative data is the primary care satisfaction survey of the specialist. Referring physicians who interact with specialists are well positioned to pass judgment on the quality of care that specialists offer their patients. Primary care physicians are evaluating the specialists' communication and appointment availability as well as questions about quality care and integration of care. Questions may include:

- Does this specialist provide you with complete written information about the specialty visit in a timely manner?
- Is this specialist available to discuss cases?
- Is there an effort on behalf of the specialist to coordinate care with you?
- How is the specialist's technical, diagnostic, and management skills?

Under this evolving measurement system, specialty appraisal and compensation are becoming more dependent on primary care physician opinions. Specialists resent this shift in power as well as the emerging interface and overlap between primary and specialty care. Without the appropriate outcomes data, we can not address the question: "Who should do what?" To this end, the Agency for Health Policy and Research, in its recent conference,[76] brought together experts to review this interface and focus on conceptual models and methodological issues of concern to both clinicians and consumers. To clarify future directions for research, several areas of practice and policy relevance were focused on, including:

- clarification of provider roles and responsibilities;
- the effect changing health systems has on communication between providers and patients;

- the effects of economic incentives on referral patterns and utilization of specialists; and
- how patient perceptions regarding the need for specialty care influence patient satisfaction and ultimately health outcomes.

Some data have been collected to help define the roles and competencies of specialists and generalists and determine who does what best. One interesting finding is the difference between generalists' and specialists' perceptions of what constitutes quality. For example, some of the survey methodologies used to derive most of the minimum volume standards for procedure performance in the attached guidelines reveal differences in definition of competence as assessed by a generalist and a specialist. In its surveys, the Amercian College of Physicians solicited the opinions of program directors, general internists, and cardiologists to determine how many electrocardiograms a physician needs to have read to achieve competency. The median number recommended by program directors and general internists was 100 EKGs, while the median number recommended by cardiologists was 750.[77] On the other end of the scale is a recommendation by the 17th Bethesda Conference of Cardiology that cardiology fellows should read 3,500 EKGs in order to obtain competence.

Although the specialist is apt to be much more knowledgeable about the specific organ-system pathology, the generalist is apt to be more knowledgeable about the patient, the family, and social or economic factors that may affect the medical problem, suggesting that the generalist/specialist overlap, although seemingly duplicative, may not necessarily be as negative as purported. Proponents of specialty care feel that elimination of direct access to the specialist is, at best, unnecessary, and at worst, invokes a harmful delay in the care of the patient. Proponents of the generalist system of care feel that self-referral undermines the general practitioners' unique insight into the patient's illness, fragments continuity of care, and ultimately results in poor-quality medical management. Furthermore, on a systemwide basis, care by a generalist promotes high-quality care "by limiting over-medicalization by permitting an efficient division of tasks between generalists and specialists and by freeing specialists to develop their special knowledge and by containing the cost of medical care."[78]

For instance, with respect to the question of diabetes management, examination of Medicare claims data from 2,980 practices shows that using four well-accepted measures of quality of care (hemoglobin A1C measurement, ophthalmologic evaluation, cholesterol measurement, and blood glucose measurement), there did seem to be a difference in care among self-described general practitioners, family practitioners, and internists.[79] This finding has been contraindicated in the recently published Medical Outcomes Study (MOS), which also assessed functional outcome as well as seven-year mortality. The MOS, an observational study, found "no consistent advantages associated with any specialty" in the case of diabetes. The principal caregivers in this study were family practitioners, general internists, cardiologists, and endocrinologists. (It should be noted that in the subset of patients with diabetic foot ulcers, care by an endocrinologist did demonstrate a significantly better outcome than those cared for by general internists or family practitioners).[80]

Other specialty/generalist areas also have been examined. Ayanian et al report that in the treatment of myocardial infarction for a patient under 75 years old, cardiologists are more likely than internists or family practice practitioners to provide proper care defined by use of thrombolytic agents within six hours, aspirin within 24 hours, beta blockers as long-term therapy, avoidance of prophylactic lidocaine, and avoidance of deltiazem for Q-wave myocardial infarction with pulmonary congestion.[81] However, some objections have been raised as to the methodology by which these authors reached their conclusions.[82, 83] Likewise, Horner et al demonstrate an unadjusted increased survival estimate of patients with ischemic stroke who are managed on a neurology service as opposed to other services.[84] Those investigators, as well as an editorial, point out that this difference is not purely because of physician specialty; in large part it is dependent upon casemix and severity of illness.[85, 86] (The difference in adjusted estimated survival was not significant.)

Recent work by Federman et al concerning skin care demonstrated that the minority of internal medicine residents and attending internal medicine physicians can accurately diagnose common dermatologic disorders.[87] They also cite unnecessary procedures performed by nondermatologists. Other studies have even suggested that skin care by primary care physicians is not cost-effective. However, others argue that primary caregivers are quite capable of handling "about 80 percent of skin disorders," although additional training would be required for most of the primary care physicians.[88]

Markson et al found that there was a three-year delay in the institution of zidovudine therapy for AIDS patients who received their care from a non-AIDS specialist compared with those AIDS patients who received their care from AIDS specialists.[89] Likewise, Paauw finds that when using standardized patients, primary care physicians (both internists and family practice) had very poor recognition of Kaposi's sarcoma, oral hairy leukoplakia, and diffuse lymphadenopathy.[90]

Specialty versus generalist care also has been examined in two very common conditions—lower back pain and low-risk birth. In the former, outcomes such as time to return to work and complete recovery from back pain were similar whether care was received from primary care practitioners, chiropractors, or orthopedic surgeons.[91] With respect to 4,865 low-risk pregnancies, there seemed to be no significant difference in neonatal outcome between family physicians and obstetricians. However, there were differences in the rate of the use of interventions during delivery.[92]

CONCLUSION

What are some of the pressing issues facing us regarding the development of measures of clinical competence and their use in the credentialing and privileging process? There are four major developments in this area:

- Continuing to improve the accuracy, reliability, and validity of all measures of clinical competence and developing methods that rely on multiple interrelated markers to assess clinical competence.
- Understanding the relationship between volume and outcomes with technical procedures and determining the appropriate minimal volume standards where a threshold effect is thought to occur.
- Incorporating measures of physicians' interpersonal skills and humanistic competence through the development of patient satisfaction surveys.
- Continuing to improve efforts to assess clinical outcomes and performance and link them to the credentialing and privileging process through provider profiling.

Clinical competence has multiple dimensions and therefore cannot be captured through just one measure. However, current measures have the validity and accuracy to appropriately assess clinical competence in technical, cognitive, and humanistic areas when multiple measures are combined. Continued advances in the technology of such measures will allow better refinement and discrimination of clinical competence in the future. We soon may see the increased use of new technologies such as virtual reality or simulator technology that will allow more precise training and assessment of procedural skills. Simulator technology has been used in anesthesiology to test and improve the management of critical situations.[93] One of its values is that it can hone physician's ability to deal with critical, unexpected, and unusual situations.[94] Another value is that simulations can be standardized and provide another valid means of assessing technical skills. As the information revolution continues to develop, one can expect more widespread use of such simulator technology. Likewise, one may expect the development of more explicit volume standards as research into this area continues.

Measuring clinical competence means not only the assessment of clinical skills in multiple areas but an assessment of the outcome of care being produced by an individual physician and health care system. Advances in information technology has decreased the barriers to the measurement of such clinical outcomes. While clinical profiles were first developed to meet the needs of consumers and government, they hold their greatest promise for internal use within health care systems. When individual physicians receive real-time, valid data on their performance they can begin to see the effects of changes in their practice quickly. The advent of computerized medical records will only accelerate the reliability of such profiles and the potential to improve care. As such, the accurate measurement of clinical competence through profiling represents an opportunity for clinicians to retain the responsibility for the quality of health care—which, as most physicians would agree, is where this responsibility should squarely rest.

REFERENCES

1. Gonnella JS, Hojat M, Erdman JB, Veloski JJ. *Assessment Measures in Medical School, Residency, and Practice*. Springer Publishing, NY, 1993.
2. JCAHO. "Joint Commission Perspectives," *The JCAHO Newsletter*. Vol 15 #1, Jan/Feb 1995.
3. *Ibid.*
4. Gonnella JS, Hojat M, Erdman JB, Veloski JJ. "What have we learned, and where do we go from here?" *Acad Med* 1993; 68: 579-587.
5. Hojat M, Gonnella JS, Veloski JJ, Erdman JB. "Is the glass half full or half empty? A reexamination of the associations between assessment measures during medical school and clinical competence after graduation." *Acad Med* 1993; 68: 569-576.
6. The Quality Letter. "Credentialing and peer review foul-ups remind hospitals of need for vigilance and accountability." *The Quality Letter*, Bader and Assoc., November 1995.
7. *NY Times* (ed). "The Doctor Left Free to Murder," August 21, 1995.
8. Sekas G, Huston WR. "Misrepresentation of academic accomplishments by applicants for gastroenterology fellowships." *Ann Int Med* 1995; 123: 38-41.
9. Kimball HR. "Credentials misrepresentation: Another challenge to professionalism" (ed). *Ann Int Med* 1995; 123: 58-59.
10. Kimball HR. "Current ABIM programs: Certification, recertification and clinical competence. Physician Assessment in the 21st Century: ABIM's Role." ABIM Report of the 1995 Summer Conference, Philadelphia PA, October 1995.
11. *Ibid.*
12. *Ibid.*
13. ASIM. "The use of board certification to credential internists." American Society of Internal Medicine, Washington DC, August 1995.
14. *Ibid.*
15. *Ibid.*
16. *Ibid.*
17. *Ibid.*
18. Rubin HR, Rogers WH, Kahn KL, Rubinstein LV, Brook RH. "Watching the doctor watchers: How well do peer review organization methods detect hospital quality problems?" *JAMA* 1992; 267: 2349-2354.
19. Greene HL, Miller YR, "The dilemma of the non-certified physician. Physician Assessment in the 21st Century: ABIM's Role." ABIM Report of the 1995 Summer Conference. Philadelphia PA, October 1995.

20. "Physicians Without Specialty Board Certification," p. 1. Council on Medical Education Report 6, I-95, AMA, Chicago IL 1995.
21. Younger P, Conner C, Cartwright KK. *Physician Credentialing and Peer Review Answer Book.* Aspen Publishers Inc., Gaithersburg MD, 1995.
22. *Ibid.*
23. Kleinke JD. "Medicine's industrial revolution" (ed). *The Wall Street Journal,* August 21, 1995, p A8.
24. Brennan T, Leape L, Laird N, Herbert L, et al. "Incidence of adverse events and negligence in hospitalized patients." *NEJM* 1991; 324:370-376.
25. Leape L, Brennan T, Laird N, Lawthers A, et. al. "The nature of adverse events in hospitalized patients." *NEJM* 1991; 324:377-384.
26. *Ibid.*
27. Wu A, Folkman S, McPhee S, Lo B. "Do house officers learn from their mistakes?" *JAMA* 1991; 265:2089-2094.
28. Tuteur P. "Internal medicine chief residents want changes in medical education." (Resident forum) *JAMA* 1990; 264:175.
29. Lang DA, Kadzielski MA, Liset JR. "Managing Medical Staff Change Through Bylaws and Other Strategies." American Hospital Assoc. Chicago IL, 1995.
30. Davis DA, Thomson MA, Oxman AD, Haynes RB. "Evidence for the Effectiveness of CME. A Review of 50 Randomized Controlled Trials." *JAMA* 1992; 268:1111-1117.
31. Davis DA, Thomsom MA, Oxman AD, Haynes RB. "Changing Physician Performance. A Systematic Review of the Effect of Continuing Medical Education Strategies." *JAMA* 1995; 274: 700-705.
32. Ramsey PG, Carline JD, Inui TS et al. "Changes Over Time in the Knowledge Base of Practicing Internists." *JAMA* 1991;266:1103-1107.
33. Glassock RJ, Benson JA, Copeland RB et al. "Time-Limited Certification and Recertification: The Program of the American Board of Internal Medicine." *Annals Int Med* 1991; 114: 59-62.
34. Leigh TM, Young PR. Haley JV. "Performances of Family Practice Diplomates on Successive Mandatory Recertification Examinations." *Acad Med* 1993;68:912-919.
35. Christakis NA, Jacobs JA, Messikomer CM. "Change in Self-Definition from Specialist to Generalist in a National Sample of Physicians." *Ann Intern Med* 1994: 121:669-675.
36. Carline JD, Pauw DS, Thiede KW, Ramsey PG. "Factors affecting the reliability of ratings of students' clinical skills in a medicine clerkship." *J Gen Intern Med* 1992; 7: 506-510.

37. Ramsey PG, Wenrich MD, Carline JD, Inui TS, Larson EB, Logerfo JP. "Use of Peer Ratings to Evaluate Physician Performance." *JAMA* 1993; 269:1655-1660.

38. Dans PE, Weiner JP, Otter SE. "Peer Review Organizations: Promises and Potential Pitfalls." *New Engl J Med* 1985; 313:1131-7.

39. *Ibid.*

40. Rubenstein LV, Kahn KL, Reinisch EJ, Sherwood MJ, Rogers WH, Kamberg C, et al. "Changes in Quality of Care for Five Diseases Measured by Implicit Review," 1981 to 1986. *JAMA* 1990; 264:1974-9.

41. Hayward RA, McMahon LF, Bernard AM. "Evaluating the Care of General Medicine Inpatients: How Good is Implicit Review?" *Annals Int Med* 1993; 188:550-556.

42. Rubin HR, Rogers WH, Kahn KL, Rubinstein LV, Brook RH. "Watching the doctor watchers: How well do peer review organization methods detect hospital quality problems?" *JAMA* 1992; 267: 2349-2354.

43. Gerteis M, Edgman-Levitan S, Daley J, Delbanco TL. *Through the Patient's Eyes: Understanding and Promoting Patient-Centered Care*. Jossey-Bass, San Francisco CA 317 pp.

44. Weaver MJ, Ow CL, Walker DJ, Degenhardt EF. "A Questionnaire for Patients' Evaluations of their Physicians' Humanistic Behaviors." *J Gen Intern Med* 1993; 8:135-9.

45. Barr DA. "The Effects of Organizational Structure on Primary Care Outcomes under Managed Care." *Ann Int Med* 1995; 122:353-359.

46. Gold M, Hurley R, Lake T, et al. "Arrangements Between Managed Care Plans and Physicians: Results from a 1994 Survey of Managed Care Plans." Washington DC: Mathematica Policy Research, Inc. Feb 1995.

47. Packer-Tursman. "Refining Measurement Tools" in: *1996 Medical Quality Management Sourcebook*. Faulkner and Gray, 1995, pg 664.

48. Salem-Schatz S, Moore G, Rucker M, Pearson SD. "The Case for Casemix Adjustment in Practice Profiling: When Good Apples Look Bad." *JAMA* 1994; 272:871-4.

49. Weiner JP, Parente ST, Garnick DW. et al. "Variation in Office-Based Quality. A Claims-Based Profile of Care Provided to Medicare Patients With Diabetes." *JAMA* 1995; 273: 1503-1508.

50. Jollis JG, Ancukiewicz M, DeLong ER, Pryor DB, Muhlbaier LH, Mark DB. "Discordance of Databases Designed for Claims Payment versus Clinical Information Systems. Implications for Outcomes Research." *Ann Int Med* 1993; 119: 844-850.

51. Emmons DW, Wozniak G, Otten R, Baker N. "Data on Employee Physician Profiling." *Journal of Health and Hospital Law* 1993, 26(3); 73-82.

52. Welch HG, Miller ME, Welch WP. "Physician Profiling. An Analysis of Inpatient Practice Patterns in Florida and Oregon." *N Engl J Med* 1994; 330:607-12.
53. Emmons DW, Wozniak GD. "Socioeconomic Characteristics of Medical Practice," 1993. American Medical Association, Chicago IL 1994.
54. Hoy E, Curtis R, Rice T. "Change and Growth in Managed Care." *Health Affairs* 1991, 10(4) 18-36.
55. Chodoff, P, Bischof RO, Nash DB, Lane C. "The AHCPR Guidelines on Heart Failure: Comparison of a Family Medicine and an Internal medicine Practice With the Guideline and an Educational Intervention to Modify Behavior."
56. Gold M, Nelson L, Lake T, Hurley R, Berenson R. "Behind the curve: A critical assessment of how little is known about arrangements between managed careplans and physicians." *Med Care Res* Rev 1995; 52: 307-341.
57. *Ibid.*
58. *Ibid.*
59. Gold MR, Hurley R, Lake T, Ensor T, Berfenson R. "A national survey of the arrangments managed-care plans make with physicians." *N Engl J Med* 1995; 333: 1678-83.
60. Woolhandler S, Himmelstein DU. "Extreme risk—the new corporate proposition for physicians." *N Engl J Med* 1995; 333: 1706-1707.
61. Levy D. "Docs urged to ignore 'gag rules.'"*USA Today*, Dec. 27, 1995, p 1.
62. Prager LO. "State licensing boards consider curbing financial incentives." *AM News*, Oct. 16, 1995, p 1.
63. ASIM. "Assuring appropriate patient care under capitation arrangement." American Society of Internal Medicine, Washington DC, August 1995.
64. ASIM. "Assessing physician performance in managed care. American Society of Internal Medicine," Washington DC, August 1995.
65. ASIM. "Assuring appropriate patient care under capitation arrangement." American Society of Internal Medicine, Washington DC, August 1995.
66. American Medical Association. Physician Profiling Project.
67. Joint Commission on Accreditation of Healthcare Organizations. Council on Performance Measurement Minutes from the Sept. 18, 1995 meeting. Oakbrook Terrace IL.
68. Flood AB. "The impact of organizational and managerial factors on the quality of care in health care organizations." *Med Care Review* 1994; 51: 381-428.
69. *Ibid.*
70. Kerr EA, Mittman BS, Hays RD, Siu AL, Leake B, Brook RH. "Managed care and capitation in California: How do physicians at financial risk control their own utilization?" *Ann Int Med* 1995; 123: 500-504.

71. Zablocki E. "Building a high-quality, cost effective physician network." *The Quality Letter* 1995; 7: 2-10.
72. *Ibid.*
73. Rovner J. Credentialing HMO Physicians. "HMO's stand on the quality of their networks." *HMO Magazine*, Nov/Dec 1995, p61-68.
74. *Ibid.*
75. Barr DA. "The effects of organizational structure on primary care outcomes under managed care." *Ann Int Med.* 1995;122(5):353-59.
76. Gaus CR, Clancy CM. "Research at the Interface of Primary Care." *JAMA.*1995;274(18)1419.
77. ASGE Training and Practice Committee. "Methods of granting hospital privileges to perform gastointestinal endoscopy." *Gastro Endoscopy.* 1992;38:765-767.
78. Sweeney B. "The referral system prevents overmedicalisation and keeps costs down." *BMJ.* 1994;309:1180-81.
79. Weiner JP, Parente ST, Garnick DW, Fowles J, et al. "Variation in office-based quality." *JAMA.* 1995;273(19):1503-1508.
80. Greenfield S, Rogers W, Mangotich M, Carney MF, Tarlov AR. "Outcomes of patients with hypertension and non-insulin-dependent diabetes mellitus treated by different systems and specialties." *JAMA.* 1995;274(18):1436-1444.
81. Ayanian JZ, Hauptman PJ, Guadagnoli E, Antman E, et al. "Knowledge and practices of generalist and specialist physicians regarding drug therapy for acute myocardial infarction." *NEJM.* 1994;331(17):1136-1142.
82. Barry HC. "Knowledge of drugs for myocardial infarction: generalists versus specialists" (editorial). *NEJM*;1995;332(7):472.
83. Justice AC. "Knowledge of drugs for myocardial infarction: generalists versus specialists" (editorial). *NEJM*;1995;332(7):472-473.
84. Horner RD, Matchar DB, Divine GW, Feussner JR. "Relationship between physician specialty and the selection and outcomes of ischemic stroke patients." *Health Services Research.* 1995;30(2):275-287.
85. Menken M. "Commentary: Generalist and specialist care of stroke: Is there a better way?" *Health Services Research.* 1995;30(2):289-290.
86. Eisenberg JM. "Commentary: Are differences in outcomes due to differences in doctors or their patients?" *Health Services Research.* 1995;30(2):291-294.
87. Federman D, Hogan D, Taylor R, Caralis P, et al. "A comparison of diagnosis, evaluation, and treatment of patients with dermatologic disorders." *J Am Acad of Dermatology.* 1995;32(5), Part 1:726-729.
88. Wynn P. "Who's the most cost-effective provider of skin care?" *Managed Care.* September 1995;47-50.

89. Markson LE, Cosler LE, Turner BJ. "Implications of generalists' slow adoption of zidovudine in clinical practice." *Arch Int Med.* 1994;154:1497-504.

90. Paauw DS, Wenrich MD, Curtis JR, Carline JD, Ramsey PG. "Ability of primary care physicians to recognize physical findings associated with HIV infection." *JAMA*. 1995;274(17):1380-1382.

91. *Ibid.*

92. Carey TS, Garrett J, Jackman A, McLaughlin C, et al. "The outcomes and costs of care for acute low back pain among patients seen by primary care practitioners, chiropractors, and orthopedic surgeons." *NEJM*. 333(14):913-917.

93. Hueston JA, Mansfield CJ. *J Fam Pract*. 1995;40(4):345-351.

94. Schwid HA, O'Donnel D. "Anesthesiologists' management of simulated critical incidents." *Anesthesiology*. 1992; 76:495-501.

Chapter 1

National Committee for Quality Assurance

Establishing Accountability in Managed Health Care

Cary Sennett, MD, PhD

The National Committee for Quality Assurance (NCQA) is a not-for-profit, nongovernmental agency whose mission is to evaluate and report on the quality of managed care organizations. Founded originally as part of the Group Health Association of America and the American Managed Care and Review Association, NCQA leadership recognized that it could establish real accountability in the managed care industry only if it was separate from it. With funding from the Robert Wood Johnson Foundation, NCQA began operating as an independent entity in 1990, governed by a self-perpetuating board representing the various stakeholders to its work: purchasers (both public and private), consumers, experts in health care law and quality assessment, and heath plans.

NCQA's overriding objective is to assure that there is valid, reliable, and comprehensible information available in the marketplace to assist purchasers and consumers in making choices based on value. NCQA believes that competition can be a powerful tool to stimulate improvements in the quality and performance of health plans, but meaningful competition—based on value rather than on price alone—depends upon the availability of relevant, understandable, and timely information for those who make choices. NCQA believes that pressure in a market in which such information exists will drive health plans to higher levels of performance and that the public will benefit as health plan success in the marketplace depends upon a firm's ability to demonstrate it is best able to meet the care and service needs of the population it serves.

This chapter briefly reviews what has been learned about the issues that matter to those who purchase and consume managed care services and outlines NCQA's complementary strategies to respond to them. It then describes some of the policy issues the author thinks are most challenging to resolve and closes with some recommendations that might help move forward collective efforts to establish accountability.

WHAT INFORMATION IS NEEDED TO ESTABLISH ACCOUNTABILITY IN MANAGED CARE?

Any discussion of organizational efforts to provide information to help discipline the marketplace has to begin with some discussion of the information needs of those whose behavior drives that market. This is a subject for a paper itself, but the author will do no more here than briefly summarize what NCQA has learned—from its working relationships with purchasers (both private and public); from focus groups with consumers (again, both privately insured and publicly insured); and from the experts with whom NCQA has worked (and whose work it has read) whose findings both complement and reinforce NCQA's.

How do consumers define quality? Consumers appear to agree that the quality of, or value provided by, a managed care organization depends upon a reasonable balance of cost, coverage, choice of physician, accessibility of care, and technical (clinical) and service excellence. Consumers' value judgments begin with economic concerns—cost and coverage. Concerns about physician choice clearly emphasize the critical role the consumer believes the physician plays as a determinant of overall quality. Concerns about accessibility and technical and service excellence reflect anxiety about the restrictions to access (and rules that may be designed to serve health plan economic, rather than patient, interests), which are for many consumers the defining characteristic of managed care organizations. NCQA's experience working with large corporations like Xerox, Ford, Digital Equipment Corporation, and many others, as well as with public purchasers including the Health Care Financing Administration, the federal Office of Personnel Management (OPM), the California Public Employees' Retirement System (CalPERS), and many state Medicaid programs, is that the issues that matter to these "bulk purchasers" of managed care are much the same.

As a result, there is a demand for information about the cost and coverage offered by different health plans and about the composition of their physician or provider networks. To a significant extent, these data are routinely available.

While efforts to standardize these data (and to organize them in a way that might facilitate comparison) are worthwhile, NCQA's efforts have focused on gaining a better understanding of these other concerns and trying to create information where there has been almost none.

Not surprisingly, concerns about the restricted set of providers have created demand for information about the quality of the providers in the physician and hospital networks, as well as a demand for assurance that contracting decisions reflect consideration of provider clinical performance at least as much as provider financial performance. Concern about restricted access to specific services (for example, through utilization management protocols or through financial incentives to providers to limit the availability of high-cost services) has created a demand for information about the availability of care and for assurance that utilization management and provider compensation systems are well designed and adequately controlled so that access to necessary care is not unduly restricted.

These overriding concerns eventually find expression in questions about the effectiveness of clinical care. Although consumers, in general, do not feel comfortable assessing clinical effectiveness (the technical quality of care), they want assurance—from experts they can trust—that the care that's needed will be provided and that that care will be delivered with skill. Challenged by information, however—for example, in mock report cards NCQA and others have provided to consumers in focus groups—consumers show considerable sophistication. There is evidence that consumers are not only able to, but that many are willing or even eager to, process detailed information about the technical quality of clinical care. There is every reason to believe that ability will grow as more information stimulates consumers to learn about the issues and as that information is provided in a context that enables that learning.

Purchasers and consumers are interested in how well a health plan maintains health and prevents illness. Although there are very real concerns about what might happen to the sick member, there is considerable enthusiasm for the role of managed care firms as health maintenance organizations. Purchasers and consumers affirm an interest in knowing how committed various firms are to health maintenance and how successful they are in translating that commitment into results.

There is clear and significant interest in how other people experience contact with the health plan and its delivery system—how satisfied members are with the quality of care and service encounters. The challenge is to meet the information needs of different types of consumers; most people are interested in the satisfaction of others "like them." There is, however, considerable skepticism about health plan reports of member satisfaction. Consumers see the potential to manipulate survey processes and are cynical about plan reports of high levels of member satisfaction.

RESPONDING TO PURCHASER AND CONSUMER NEEDS: DEVELOPING INFORMATION ABOUT THE QUALITY AND PERFORMANCE OF MCOs

The information needs of consumers and purchasers are many and diverse. This implies some need to consider where and how to focus efforts to design systems to respond to them.

As Avedis Donabedian pointed out long ago, efforts to evaluate the quality of care delivered by an organization can focus on elements of organizational structure (which define the theoretical limits of an organization's capacity to deliver high-quality care), on aspects of organizational process (evaluation of which creates considerable potential knowledge about the extent to which organizational capacity is being employed effectively), and/or on the outcomes an organization actually achieves. It appears there is not yet a better framework for thinking about the evaluation of health plan quality.

Conceptually, it is clearly most satisfying to evaluate the outcomes organizations achieve. This is, after all, the "bottom line"—organizational structure may exist, but if it is not well utilized it will not achieve quality, and processes may be in place but may not operate as they are designed to. For these reasons, outcomes assessment seems the natural place to focus efforts to evaluate the quality of health plans.

There are many reasons, however, why outcomes measurement cannot be expected to achieve its promise—at least in the short run.

First, there are what one might call "biological constraints." Many outcomes—especially clinical outcomes like disease-related morbidity and mortality—proceed over very long timelines. As David Eddy—one of the nation's leading thinkers in this field—has pointed out, "it takes five years to calculate a five-year mortality rate." More than that, it may take 20 or 30 years before the consequences of untreated hypertension or hypercholesterolemia are manifest as the vascular complications (or as reductions in patient functional status) that are the real outcomes of these conditions.

The long timelines over which the biology of disease proceeds create three problems. First, there is a real practical issue: to estimate such outcomes implies a need to track individuals over time, but the ability is limited profoundly by the nature of current health care datasets. But there are theoretical concerns as well that will not be overcome by better information systems. Business users typically want information that is current. There are unanswered questions about the utility of information that summarizes success over long timelines. And there are real issues about accountability—who is accountable for an outcome—in an environment in which individuals typically change health care systems frequently.

There are other "biological" issues that limit the potential usefulness of pure outcomes measures. Most clinical outcomes depend not only on quality of care but quite substantially upon the characteristics of the individual at risk for some outcome. Thus, a five-year mortality rate for breast cancer depends not only on the care delivered to a woman with breast cancer, but also on the stage at which the cancer was detected and upon certain characteristics of the cancer itself. Until better techniques to adjust for differences in biological/patient risk have been developed—and until the data required to support the use of those techniques are routinely available—we need to be very concerned that differences in observed outcomes may be telling us more about the nature of the population being served than about the quality of care delivered in that system. In the worst case, there is the risk of complete misinformation: the risk that the system that serves the sickest patients (who are drawn to it because they know it to be the highest quality system available to them through firsthand observation) will appear to have the worst outcomes. In this case, information will lead consumers to draw exactly the wrong conclusion, and choices will be worse than were no information available at all.

In addition to the biological issues that might limit enthusiasm for outcome measures, there are also statistical issues that need to be kept in mind. Chief among these is a problem of small numbers: many outcomes, especially adverse outcomes like death, occur infrequently in most populations, and many of the conditions for which we would like information are relatively rare (even a relatively common clinical condition like diabetes mellitus affects only about one in every 30 Americans). And given that most health plans in the United States are small—the median health plan has only about 40,000 enrollees—many outcome measures will assess the rates at which rare events occur in very small populations. Such measures will have very limited power to detect meaningful differences among health plans. Thus, although we may have valid measures of very important outcomes, these measures may not be very useful for the purpose of comparing the quality of health plans.

Finally, and probably most importantly, the ability to develop useful outcome measures to discriminate among health plans is limited by a set of information system constraints. These constraints are several and quite problematic in the short term: much of the data needed to support measurement—especially data about the patient's experience—are not routinely collected; much of the data that are collected are in paper records, and the cost of data retrieval is quite high; much of the data collected electronically is of very low quality, lacking the clinical detail necessary for refined performance measurement; there is limited ability to link datasets within most health plans; and there is profoundly limited ability to link health plan datasets with other sources of data (other health plan, or public, datasets) that might permit longitudinal assessment to proceed. There is no reason to believe that these issues cannot be resolved—and NCQA is working affirmatively to try to encourage their resolution—but it must be recognized that these issues limit what is possible in 1997 and the very-near term beyond that.

Given this, NCQA thinks that a quality evaluation system that depends exclusively on outcome measures is not realistic at the moment. NCQA's response has not been to forego outcome measurement. Rather, it has been an effort directed at accomplishing three things:

1. **Combining standards based-review—to assess organizational capability and organizational control—with performance measures and using the sort of performance measure ("process" or "outcome") that makes most sense, given what it is we want to know.** NCQA's deeply held belief is that movement here needs to be driven by pragmatism and not ideology; it is taking the first steps in a field in which much of the infrastructure required for perfection is missing. NCQA greatly fears the potential to be hamstrung by what cannot be and has committed to taking best advantage of what can be.
2. **Moving rapidly—but incrementally—toward the ideal.** While one should never take their eyes "off the prize," the perfect system for evaluating health plans requires environmental change (for example, the development and diffusion of better information systems), which will take place only slowly. NCQA's strategy has been to put into place evaluation systems that represent those that are "best achievable," to work in parallel to stimulate environmental change that will enable better systems to operate, and then to modify and enhance the evaluation systems that are in place. NCQA believes pragmatic incrementalism needs to be the rule that governs this process, but that it never should be willing to accept the status quo.
3. **Working to influence the environment, to make rapid progress possible.** NCQA believes that organizations committed to developing better systems of evaluation should not only take best advantage of what is, but also should use their influence to create new possibilities for what can be. NCQA is working aggressively to identify the barriers to better evaluation systems—and proposing solutions as to how they can be overcome. NCQA also is developing and implementing strategies that will address the major deficiencies in current measurement systems (including HEDIS). One of the obligations that attends a commitment to incremental improvement is a commitment to do what can be done to accelerate improvement. While much of its work has focused on evaluation itself, increasingly NCQA's view has broadened to the systems environment that defines the limits of the possible and to what needs to be done to make that environment more hospitable to evaluation.

EVALUATING THE SYSTEMS UPON WHICH THE DELIVERY OF HIGH-QUALITY CARE DEPENDS: NCQA ACCREDITATION

NCQA believes that the best strategy for responding to the diverse needs of purchasers and consumers for information that will help them evaluate the quality of managed care organizations is to use both the processes of standards-based review (accreditation) and performance measurement in a way that is efficient and parsimonious. As a result, standards-based review is, and will continue to be, a cornerstone to NCQA's efforts to evaluate managed care organizations. NCQA's accreditation program is a strategy for evaluating whether a health plan can document that it operates in a manner expected to result in care and service that meets the needs of its membership. NCQA accreditation is organized around standards that represent statements of excellent managed care business practice—developed and maintained by industry experts in managed care and quality improvement—in six functional domains:

1. **Quality Management and Improvement:** Can the health plan demonstrate that it is working to improve quality? Can it document that is has necessary structures and processes in place, that they are adequately resourced, and that they are operating as they were designed to operate? Can the health plan document that is has achieved improvements and that these improvements are sustained?
2. **Utilization Management:** Can the health plan document that it has the structures and processes in place to assure that utilization of care will be appropriate? Is there adequate protection against underservice in a health plan that creates financial incentives to providers to limit the delivery of care? Are decisions about medical appropriateness informed by clinical science? Are decisions made by individuals with sufficient expertise to make them? Are decisionmaking processes systematic and consistent? Are they timely? Does the health plan have well-defined and fair processes for resolving disputes about the appropriateness of care?
3. **Credentialing:** Does the health plan have a rigorous process for establishing that providers have the credentials they represent they have or that are necessary to the delivery of the care they provide? Can the health plan document that its credentialing activities conform to that process; that is, is there evidence that credentials have been verified, and verification noted by accountable health plan management? Does the health plan incorporate information from ongoing performance reviews of providers into recredentialing decisions?
4. **Preventive Health:** Can the health plan document that it is effectively using preventive care to maintain the health of its enrolled population? Is there evidence that guidelines for preventive care are devel-

oped and communicated to providers and to patients as appropriate? Is there evidence of monitoring of the success of preventive care? Is there evidence of improvement where monitoring suggests an opportunity?

5. **Members' Rights and Responsibilities:** How does the health plan document that it recognizes and respects the rights of its membership? Is there a statement of rights and responsibilities that has been communicated to the member? Is there evidence that the plan diligently has tried to educate its member about important policies and procedures? Are there effective complaint and grievance processes? Do they motivate action? Is there closure?
6. **Medical Records:** Is the medical record documentation adequate? Is essential information in the chart? Is it organized? Is it legible? Is there evidence that patient information (laboratory results, consultant notes) is reviewed by the primary care physician? Is there evidence of continuity of care and follow-up? Is there evidence that care is appropriate: both that necessary care is given and that unnecessary care is not?

The accreditation process itself is a rigorous and intensive review. It involves both offsite and onsite review of materials a health plan has prepared to provide evidence that it meets NCQA standards, extensive review of other source materials (committee meeting minutes, memoranda, and so on), review of grievance and credentialing files, and interviews with senior managers of the plan and with participating physicians. The review team summarizes its findings in a report handed to the Review Oversight Committee (ROC), a group that includes senior-level physician executives from the managed care industry.

The ROC determines the plan's accreditation status based on the findings of the report and then communicates its decision to the plan. If there is additional information the plan feels has not been considered, the plan can bring that to NCQA's attention. The committee then reviews the decision and makes a final determination. Plans receive one of four accreditation decisions. The best is a three-year accreditation—"full accreditation." Plans may receive certification for one year—either "one-year accreditation" or a somewhat lower "provisional accreditation." Typically, between 10 and 15 percent of the plans reviewed are denied accreditation outright. It's important to note that accreditation is voluntary; no plan has to undergo accreditation before it feels ready, yet many plans fail. Even so, it is important to recognize that the plans that failed have at least stepped up to the plate.

Cost of preparation

Typically health plans will apply for accreditation and then spend 12 to 18 months preparing for the site review component. Part of that time is spent preparing the materials the review team will evaluate. Often, considerable time is spent strengthening the systems the survey team will assess. The immediate outcome of an NCQA survey is a certificate that will help a high-quality health plan compete in the marketplace. But an important outcome for most plans that undergo review is an organization that is stronger and better able to meet the care and service needs of the population it serves. To the extent this is so, NCQA accreditation is not only an instrument for quality evaluation, it is also a critical element of national efforts to improve the quality of managed care. It is likely that this is the reason an increasing number of large corporations are requiring that contracted health plans undergo NCQA review. One—Digital Equipment Corporation—recently has set the bar even higher. In the future, health plans will have to reach "full accreditation" status in order to serve Digital Equipment employees.

EVALUATING HEALTH PLAN RESULTS: THE HEALTH PLAN EMPLOYER DATA AND INFORMATION SET (HEDIS)

Accreditation produces summary information about health plan capability and control: an explicit evaluation of whether a health plan is capable of doing the things it must in order to deliver high-quality care and service and whether it can document that it is, in fact, doing those things successfully. Performance measurement provides information complementary to that: it is NCQA's work to assess the actual results that health plans achieve. NCQA's long-term vision for performance measurement is one in which the full range of information about health plan performance is available to let purchasers and consumers make comparisons and to support health plan efforts to improve. To achieve that vision, NCQA has focused its efforts in five areas:

1. developing, and progressively enhancing, a precisely specified set of measures (HEDIS, the Health Plan Employer Data and Information Set) that can serve as an industry standard, responsive to the needs of purchasers and consumers;
2. developing an audit process to assure that production of HEDIS data conforms with the precise specifications laid out by NCQA and that HEDIS data are credible to purchasers and consumers. As HEDIS data become more and more available, it will be critical to assure that results do not misrepresent performance and lead users to incorrect conclusions;
3. bringing quality data together to make it more accessible, and more comprehensible, to users and to permit benchmarking and analysis;
4. investigating the information needs of consumers to assure that future generations of HEDIS will be even more responsive to those; and
5. identifying and addressing environmental constraints to enable better measurement in the future.

HEDIS has grown out of a widespread desire for standardization and capacity expansion in the area of health plan performance assessment. A decade or so ago, health plans were bombarded by requests for results information; typically, many employer customers wanted to know the same things. At the same time, employer purchasers were receiving information from many health plan suppliers, with no assurance that statistics with the same names (e.g., mammography rate) were being calculated in a way that permitted comparison across plans. The system wasn't working very well for customer or supplier. The need for measurement standards seemed clear to all.

A group of purchasers, health plans, and a benefits consulting firm collaborated to lay out a set of measurement standards that would bring to this world of confusion some orderliness. The product of this collaborative work was HEDIS 1.0, completed in 1989. HEDIS 1.0 did not gain widespread acceptance. In 1992, the developers of HEDIS brought it to NCQA and asked it to assume ownership and responsibility for enhancement and maintenance.

NCQA organized a collaborative effort that brought a broad range of purchaser and health plan representatives together to expand the scope and utility of the measurement set. NCQA's first product—HEDIS 2.0—was released in November 1993. HEDIS 2.0 included some 60 statistics (actually, there are many more, as some "statistics" are tables with many statistics included) that focused on a broad array of issues ranging from clinical process to financial performance. HEDIS 2.0 seemed well suited to the needs of a broad range of purchasers and—although challenging—seemed appropriate for implementation across a broad range of managed care organizations.

HEDIS 2.0 diffused very rapidly into the marketplace. Clearly responding to a void, HEDIS has become a virtual marketplace necessity—an increasing number of purchasers are requiring plans to report HEDIS data, and survey estimates suggest that almost 90 percent of HMOs now are producing at least some HEDIS statistics. HEDIS is the basis for most health plan report cards, and HEDIS data have figured prominently in national press efforts to rank health plans.

As important as this first-generation product has been, NCQA clearly understood that HEDIS 2.0 did not address all of the issues that matter to purchasers and consumers. HEDIS did not assess the quality of care for publicly insured populations. The clinical measures in HEDIS 2.0 are narrowly focused on prevention. And there are issues of scientific method—particularly related to risk adjustment—that are not considered in the 2.0 specifications, but clearly need attention.

As a consequence, NCQA began to lay out a strategy for making HEDIS a dynamic document—a set of ever-improving, ever more responsive measures that would move incrementally but assuredly to address the broad range of information needs for all covered populations in a rigorous and cost-effective way. A first step was to adapt the specifications for application to the Medicaid population. With financial assistance from the David and Lucile Packard Foundation and the efforts of a broadly constituted "Medicaid workgroup," NCQA addressed many of the technical and conceptual issues that were needed to make HEDIS relevant to this population. Medicaid HEDIS was released early in 1996; survey data suggest that the vast majority of state Medicaid program directors intend to incorporate Medicaid HEDIS specifications into regulatory and oversight processes in the near future.

TABLE 1. Committee on Performance Measurement (CPM)

Wade M. Aubry, MD Blue Cross Blue Shield Association	**Patricia MacTaggart** State of Minnesota
Bruce Bradley General Motors Corporation	**Arnold Milstein, MD** William M. Mercer and Co. Pacific Business Group on Health
Kathryn Coltin Harvard Pilgrim Health Care	**Michael Rallston, MD** Kaiser Permanente
Peggy Connerton, PhD Service Employees International Union	**Louise Novotny** Communications Workers of America
Carol Cronin *Health Pages* Magazine	**Alan Peres** Ameritech
Helen Darling (Cochair) Xerox	**William L. Roper, MD** Prudential HealthCare
Joyce Dubow American Association of Retired Persons	**Sara Rosenbaum** George Washington Center for Health Policy Research
David Eddy, MD, PhD Independent Consultant/Researcher	**Cary Sennett, MD, PhD** National Committee for Quality Assurance
Jeffrey R. Harris, MD U.S. Centers for Disease Control and Prevention	**Dean Smart** California Public Employees' Retirement System
George J. Isham, MD (Cochair) HealthPartners	**Mark Smith, MD** Henry J. Kaiser Family Foundation
Jeffrey Kang, MD Health Care Financing Administration	**Mike Tarre** IBM Corporation
Robert Krughoff *Washington Consumers' CHECKBOOK* Magazine	**Richard E. Ward, MD** Henry Ford Health System

Carolyn Cocotas
Assistant Vice President of New Measurement
NCQA Staff Director for the CPM and Development

But the real challenge was not adapting HEDIS for new populations. It was creating a process for its ongoing expansion and designing that process to assure higher levels of customer responsiveness, a solid base in scientific method, and parsimony (cost-effectiveness). The response to that was HEDIS 3.0—not only a broader information set, but a process to assure the ongoing evolution of HEDIS to meet those broader objectives.

HEDIS 3.0 was developed under the direction of the broad-based Committee on Performance Measurement (CPM) and financed by contributions from both public (a contract with HCFA) and private sources (grants from the Henry J. Kaiser Family Foundation and from the pharmaceutical firms Merck, Pfizer, and SmithKline Beecham). The CPM (see Table 1), which includes public and private purchasers, consumers, labor unions, health plans, and measurement experts, was constituted to create a vehicle for the various constituencies most interested in moving performance measurement systems forward to debate the issues and to work together toward their common objective.

The CPM spent several months reaching agreement on its priorities for measurement and developing a process that would assure that its first product—HEDIS 3.0—reached the state of the art. It agreed to approach the development of HEDIS in a way unlike its predecessors; rather than developing HEDIS measures, the CPM saw that it could best achieve its objectives by drawing on the knowledge and experience of the many others who understood the sciences of measurement and medicine. To engage those others in its work—and to assure that those others understood the need for information to which their performance measures had to respond—the CPM drafted and distributed a public call for measures, which included a statement of its priorities for measurement and a description of the attributes it wanted performance measures to have. This call for measures was distributed to more than 1,700 organizations throughout the health care industry to try to reach into every nook and cranny and bring into the HEDIS 3.0 development process the best of what was available.

The public call brought forth over 820 measures from almost 200 organizations—a response that had the potential to overwhelm the CPM's resources. Fortunately, the committee was able to draw upon substantial expertise from some of the leading scientific organizations in the country. With assistance from the RAND corporation, Harvard University, the U.S. Centers for Disease Control and Prevention, the federal Agency for Health Care Policy and Research, and the Health Care Financing Administration, the committee was able to systematically and progressively evaluate submitted measures against three criteria sets that defined the essential requirements for HEDIS measures:

1. **Relevance.** The CPM was interested in measures only to the extent that those measures addressed some need for information relevant to purchasers and/or consumers. Direct measures of relevance were not available, so measures were inferred to be relevant by determining the extent to which they addressed health care problems known to be common; associated with significant morbidity, mortality, and/or cost; and for which there was known or suspected to be considerable variation (both from optimality—identify important opportunities for improvement—and across organizations—identify meaningful differences across health plans and thereby permit discrimination). In addition, measures were relevant to the CPM to the extent that they addressed issues that were "controllable" by a health plan. An issue could be very important—and current levels of performance nationally could be far from optimal—but if the issue was not something that a health plan could reasonably be expected to influence, then a measure that addressed that issue was not appropriate for inclusion in HEDIS.

2. **Scientific soundness.** The CPM was interested in measures that addressed important issues, but recognized that measures needed to have certain technical properties in order to be useful for the purposes for which HEDIS was designed. Clearly, measures needed to be reliable, valid, and risk-adjustable; they needed to measure what they were designed to measure in ways that were reproducible; and they needed to be designed in ways that could eliminate confounders. Many potential measures were eliminated from consideration for HEDIS 3.0, however, even though they were felt to be valid and reliable. To be useful for HEDIS—to be able to inform choice—measures needed to be able to distinguish between health plans. That meant measures had to be designed in ways that assured they had sufficient statistical power to detect the sort of differences between plans that are known or suspected to exist. Many measures that were clearly relevant proved

not to have necessary statistical power; important as these measures were, they were not appropriate for HEDIS.

3. **Feasibility.** The CPM was committed to producing a set of measurement specifications that was workable in 1997. Although refusing to be bound tightly by current constraints, the committee was unwilling to put forth specifications that placed a stake at an impossible distance. The CPM was aware of the burden that performance measurement places on health plans—and was aware that comparable levels of accountability are not required of many of the organizations that compete with managed care plans. The CPM also knew that every dollar spent on measurement is a dollar potentially diverted from patient care. The committee's overriding objective, of course, was to drive measurement to a new level. The feasibility criteria set was intended to assure that the committee's efforts resulted in a set that was as cost-effective as could be, given its primary objective.

The first product of the CPM's work was HEDIS 3.0. HEDIS 3.0 considerably broadens the scope of HEDIS and brings public- and private-sector health care measurement together. It accomplishes standardization of member satisfaction assessment and for the first time makes patient-reported health status measurement a component of a national measurement activity.

HEDIS 3.0 measures are organized in the eight "domains" in which purchasers and consumers have noted that measures needed to focus:

1. Effectiveness of care: is care achieving the gains in health expected?
2. Accessibility and availability of care: is care available to those who need it, without inappropriate barriers and delay?
3. Satisfaction with the experience of care: is the experience of care satisfying as well as clinically effective?
4. Cost of care: is care of high value?
5. Stability of the health plan: is the health plan stable—or will one experience the sort of change that could disrupt care?
6. Informed health care choices: is the health plan successful at helping members to be active and informed partners in health care decisions?
7. Use of services: how are resources used? Is there evidence of too much—or too little—care?
8. Plan descriptive information: how is the plan organized? What type of doctors participate and how many?

In total, there are approximately 75 measures in the HEDIS 3.0 Reporting Set (see Table 2).

(*text continued on page 51*)

Table 2. HEDIS 3.0 Reporting and Testing Set Measures

Effectiveness of Care

●Advising smokers to quit ●Beta blocker treatment after a heart attack	●Follow-up after hospitalization for mental illness	●Continuity of care for substance abuse patients ●Substance counseling for adolescents
●The health of seniors	●Number of people in the plan who smoke	●Availability of medication management and psychotherapy for patients with schizophrenia ●Patient satisfaction with mental health care
●Eye exams for people with diabetes ●Flu shots for older adults ●Flu shots for high-risk adults ●Flu shots for older adults	●Smokers who quit ●Flu shots for high-risk adults	
●Cervical cancer screening ●Breast cancer screening ●Childhood immunization status ●Adolescent immunization status ●Treating children's ear infections ●Prenatal care in the first trimester ●Low birthweight babies ●Check-ups after delivery	●Use of appropriate medications for people with asthma ●Cholesterol management of patients hospitalized for coronary artery disease ●Aspirin treatment after a heart attack ●Outpatient care of patients hospitalized for heart failure ●Controlling high blood pressure ●Prevention of stroke in people with atrial fibrillation	●Family visit for children 12 years of age or younger ●Failure of substance abuse treatment ●Screening for chemical dependency ●Appropriate use of psychotherapeutic medications ●Continuation of depression treatment
	●Colorectal cancer screening ●Follow-up after an abnormal pap smear ●Follow-up after an abnormal mammogram	●Monitoring diabetes patients ●Chlamydia screening ●Prescription of antibiotics for the prevention of HIV-related pneumonia
	●Stage at which breast cancer was detected ●Assessment of how breast cancer therapy affects the patient's ability to function	

Access /Availability of Care

●Availability of primary care providers ●Children's access to primary care providers	●Availability of dentists ●Adults' access to preventive/ambulatory health services ●Initiation of prenatal care ●Availability of obstetrical/prenatal care providers	●Problems with obtaining care
●Availability of mental health/chemical dependency providers ●Annual dental visit	●Low birthweight deliveries at facilities for high-risk deliveries and neonates ●Availability of language interpretation services	

Note: Measures in the shaded region are from the Testing Set.

Table 2. HEDIS 3.0 Reporting and Testing Set Measures (cont.)

Satisfaction with the Experience of Care

●Member Satisfaction Survey (numerous measures) ●Survey descriptive information	●Disenrollment survey ●Consumer Assessments of Health Plans (CAHPS) ●Satisfaction with breast cancer treatment	
Health Plan Stability ●Disenrollment ●Provider turnover ●Narrative information on rate trends, financial stability, and insolvency protection	●Indicators of financial stability ●Years in business/total membership	
Use of Services ●Well-child visits in the first 15 months of life ●Well-child visits in the third, fourth, fifth, and sixth year of life ●Adolescent well-care visit	●Birth and average length of stay, newborns ●Frequency of ongoing prenatal care ●Mental health utilization—percentage of members receiving inpatient, day/night, and ambulatory services ●Readmission for specified mental health disorders	●Use of behavioral health services
●Frequency of selected procedures ●Inpatient utilization—nonacute care ●Inpatient utilization—general hospital/acute care ●Ambulatory care	●Chemical dependency utilization—inpatient discharges and average length of stay ●Chemical dependency utilization—percentage of members receiving inpatient, day/night care and ambulatory services	
●Cesarean section and vaginal birth after cesarean rate (VBAC-rate) ●Discharge and average length of stay—maternity care	●Mental health utilization—inpatient discharges and average length of stay ●Readmission for chemical dependency ●Outpatient drug utilization	

Note: Measures in the shaded region are from the Testing Set.

Table 2. HEDIS 3.0 Reporting and Testing Set Measures, (cont.)

Cost of Care	
	●Health plan costs per member per month
●High-occurrence/high-cost DRGs ●Rate trends	
Informed Health Care Choices	
●Language translation services	●Counseling women about hormone replacement therapy
●New member orientation/education	
Health Plan Descriptive Information	
●Board certification/residency completion ●Provider compensation ●Physicians under captitation ●Recredentialing ●Pediatric mental health network ●Chemical dependency services ●Arrangements with public health, educational, and social service organizations ●Weeks of pregnancy at time of enrollment ●Family planning services	●Preventive care and health promotion ●Quality assessment and improvement ●Case management ●Utilization management ●Risk management ●Cultural diversity of Medicaid membership ●Unduplicated count of Medicaid members ●Enrollment by payer (member years/months) ●Total enrollment

Note: Measures in the shaded region are from the Testing Set.

These measures represent a pragmatic mix of process and outcome measures and depend upon data collected from patient surveys; drawn from medical records; and extracted from claim, encounter, pharmacy, and enrollment datasets.

HEDIS 3.0 is the first step into the future. With it, the CPM created a new construct—the HEDIS testing set—as a means by which to bring promising measures to maturity. The testing set includes approximately 30 measures that address issues of considerable relevance, but for which there was a perceived need for empirical evaluation of scientific strength or feasibility. NCQA will be working with researchers and health plans to study and refine these measures. It is NCQA's hope that they will be available for inclusion in future generations of HEDIS; they are a first step toward enriching the environment from which future versions of HEDIS will be drawn.

HEDIS 3.0 also includes a chapter unique to the history of HEDIS. Volume IV of HEDIS 3.0 is an analysis of the constraints limiting the development of performance measures and a set of recommendations for actions to move us forward. It is a systematic and deliberate attempt to influence the information systems environment and to create a world in which efforts to develop performance measures will not be limited by the availability and utility of data. It is also an attempt to provide guidance to health plans to permit more strategic and more rational investment in information management capability. The CPM was concerned about the apparently hectic nature of HEDIS releases and hoped by laying out a roadmap for the future to make the transition to new HEDIS measures feel more predictable and less discontinuous.

MOVING QUALITY INFORMATION TO USERS: "QUALITY COMPASS"

HEDIS is rapidly expanding the nation's ability to measure "the things that matter." That is clearly a necessary, but perhaps not so clearly, an insufficient condition for market discipline. While we cannot hope to make value-based choices without better information about the quality and performance of managed care plans, the existence of an increasing amount of data alone will not enable that either. What is needed is timely and low-cost access to that data and reporting in a manner that permits a potential mountain of data to become useful information.

It is in this spirit that in mid 1996 NCQA launched "Quality Compass," a national database of comparative information about the quality of the nation's managed care plans. The launch marks a quantum leap in efforts to make information about health plan quality more accessible to employers, consultants, consumers, and health plans. Reports from NCQA's "Quality Compass" include NCQA accreditation status information and data from HEDIS Version 2.5.

"Quality Compass" reports allow informed comparison among hundreds of health plans. This likely will make quality become a key competitive factor. Bringing together data from hundreds of plans—that collectively cover nearly 28 million Americans—allows NCQA for the first time to generate national averages, regional averages, and benchmarks for various aspects of plan performance. These statistics are included in the reports and will help employers and plans set performance goals, monitor improvement, and establish overall accountability. NCQA will report these national figures regularly to track improvement in the managed care industry.

Reports from NCQA's "Quality Compass" allow users to compare plans with one another, against national and regional averages, and against the top performing plans—identified as benchmarks. "Quality Compass" reports will help put HEDIS and accreditation information into the hands of those charged with selecting health plans for their organization by integration and will present information to them in ways that help guide interpretation and choice. For small and mid-size companies who did not have access to comparative data about health plan quality in the past, "Quality Compass" makes available previously costly information. Now a larger audience will be able make purchasing decisions with the aid of performance data.

"Quality Compass" also represents a dramatic new efficiency for purchasers, consultants, and health plans. With "Quality Compass," employers and consultants have a comprehensive, economical source for HEDIS and accreditation information. In years past, employers and consultants seeking performance information from dozens or even hundreds of individual plans typically were faced with an exhausting, expensive, and frustrating process. At the same time, health plans have faced the dim prospect of responding to numerous and varied requests for performance information from each of their employer clients.

To assure its timeliness, information in "Quality Compass" will be updated at least twice a year, including the national and regional benchmark information, which now is available over the Internet through NCQA's World Wide Web site (http://www.ncqa. org). To minimize the likelihood of errors in submitted data, all of which were submitted voluntarily, "Quality Compass" data were collected from health plans using an electronic data submission tool, and only HEDIS 2.5 data from 1995 were accepted. A few plans submitted data that had been audited by an independent third party. External audit is critical for the future and eventually will become an NCQA requirement.

Consumers will have access to NCQA's "Quality Compass" reports through a variety of channels, including employers and unions that make the information available to their employees and members, as well as libraries that purchase the reports. In addition, the media is expected to play a key role in presenting the data to consumers and helping them understand it.

Health plans likely will use "Quality Compass" both to help guide internal quality improvement efforts and to highlight plan strengths in their marketing materials. NCQA is issuing "Quality Compass" advertising guidelines to ensure appropriate use of the data in marketing activities.

In 1997, HEDIS 3.0 measures will be added to the "Quality Compass" database. NCQA Accreditation Summary Reports also will be integrated this year. In the future, reporting capabilities will be enhanced by providing users with direct, electronic access to the database and with the software tools to query it.

THE FUTURE OF HEALTH PLAN EVALUATION

NCQA accreditation clearly represents the gold standard in health plan evaluation and HEDIS is unquestionably the reference set for health plan performance assessment in 1997. Yet there is still much to be done and much happening as a result. NCQA is confident there will be progress. Whether that progress will be rapid and efficient, however, is less certain.

The past few years have been marked by new interest in accountability in managed care. That interest has spawned a number of new organizations whose mission is to create systems that assure accountability. In addition, other firms already in the business of health care evaluation have expanded the scope of their efforts to include managed care firms.

This has the potential to be of great value to the public, for there is no question that current systems are inadequate to meet the current need. But we should recognize that there may be a downside to this and work to assure that the common agenda is not threatened by efforts to accelerate progress.

The risk, of course, is that the effort will sink under its own weight—that multiple firms with overlapping initiatives will operate nonsynergistically and drive the cost of evaluation to a prohibitive level with little additional return. This risk exists both with regard to standards-based evaluation (accreditation) and with regard to the development of performance measures. The latter, though, is especially of concern as the tendency is for such measures to appear to be complementary (while accreditation programs are more clearly redundant). Thus, in the face of inadequate information and multiple sets of performance measures, the purchaser customer of a health plan is especially likely to require the reporting of measures from each of multiple sets.

In general, this could mean that each purchaser customer will have more and better information to guide choice. On the other hand, it may mean that every health plan has to produce virtually every measure extant—as one purchaser/customer asks for one combination, another asks for another, until every measure in every set is required by at least one health plan customer. This will expand the reporting burden on health plans exponentially; at some point that burden will pass the point of diminishing returns.

If we are not to encourage competition in the "market for measures," then how can customer responsiveness be assured in the pluralistic world in which we live? First, this author would argue that this is not a "market" in which competition is the best strategy to serve the public. Competition works well and, in fact, is possible only when customers are able to evaluate the extent to which the goods and services produced by competing firms meet their needs. In the market for measures, there is very limited ability to assess—and very little interest in assessing—the operating characteristics of performance measures. More than that, such marketplace assessment will take a long time. NCQA does not think that the public's interest will be best served by releasing into the marketplace a profusion of new measures and letting competitive processes eliminate useless measures over time.

Rather, the best policy at least for the foreseeable future is to work toward national standardization—to create a single set of measures that will meet 80 percent of the need. Such a standard will, by definition, fail at some margin. However, experience suggests that such a strategy will be very efficient. The objective, of course, is not to reduce the burden on health plans, but to invest the public's limited resources wisely.

This policy may need to be transitional only. Extensive customization may be possible when information systems are in place that make the marginal cost of producing additional performance information quite a bit smaller than it is today. At the moment, however, it seems wise to recommend that those who are driving the accountability agenda drive it toward uniformity and efficiency.

Of course, from NCQA's perspective it seems natural to suggest that HEDIS serve as the core for any national set of managed care performance indicators. HEDIS is deeply anchored in the industry. Experience has established that HEDIS statistics do meaningfully discriminate among health plans, and HEDIS 3.0 will extend the gains secured in the first three years of its predecessor's lifetime. To suggest a central role for HEDIS in the future of national measurement standards is not, of course, to suggest that there is no room for the work of others. NCQA believes quite the opposite to be true; the best way to assure that HEDIS matures rapidly and responsively is to bring into the set the most capable measures others have developed. That was the hallmark of the HEDIS 3.0 development process and it is the right path for the future, according to NCQA.

Therefore, NCQA hopes to see broadly distributed innovation. There is not only room for, but NCQA believes the success of the effort depends upon, the development of additional measures by those who are close to the purchasers and consumers who seek better information than they have now.

Ideally, however, those measures' development processes will be connected in some way to assure that duplication of effort is minimized and to maximize the likelihood that completed measures will be of comparable quality and interact synergistically. Carefully—even if informally—managed, there is unprecedented opportunity to move forward. But, absent coordination and collaboration, we see motion, not progress.

Chapter 2

Foundation for Accountability

Framework for Accountability

Christina Bethell, PhD, MBA, and David Lansky, PhD

The Foundation for Accountability (FACCT) is dedicated to helping Americans make better health care decisions. Americans make decisions at many levels of interaction with the health care system—selecting a health plan, selecting a medical group or hospital, selecting a treatment option, and even selecting a lifestyle or self-care regimen. FACCT seeks to provide tools to improve the ability of the individuals and organizations who rely on and pay for the health care system to base the multitude of health care decisions they make on relevant information about quality. FACCT does this by identifying and endorsing consumer-relevant measures of quality, encouraging the adoption of these measures in the field, and striving to ensure that their information is effectively communicated and used by consumers.

FACCT's position is that direct accountability to patients, consumers, and purchasers for attributes of quality they care about is a critical component of any well-functioning health care system and individual caregiving relationship. Without information, accountability is not possible. With information, the most important goals of accountability may be achieved:

- patients, consumers, and purchasers of health care will have a vehicle for becoming more active partners in evaluating, influencing, and improving America's health care system;

- health systems and communities will have information to identify and pursue opportunities to improve; and
- innovation to prevent and manage illness will be encouraged in all areas of the health care system and by providers and patients alike.

Several core assumptions underlie FACCT's work:

1. **Basic reform of the health care system is needed.** The system must continue to undergo basic reform toward a patient-centered and comprehensive view of health. To perform well on measures such as those endorsed by FACCT, health care systems will need to (a) work in close partnership with patients and communities to prevent and manage illness, (b) successfully coordinate the full continuum of care, and (c) have the capacity to manage the health of populations and individuals—whether they are well, at-risk, or living with complex, chronic health problems. The economic and organizational incentives of these systems should encourage direct accountability to those who use and pay for care and should actively seek innovative ways to continuously improve the well-being of the people served. Merely pushing the insurance premium through different hands will not improve the health of Americans. Ultimately, the examination of the results of care should play a central role in determining the success of system reforms currently under way.
2. **A focus on human health should exist at all levels of the system.** An accountability system focused on measuring changes and improvements in the functioning of people encourages the health care system to explicitly and visibly focus on the most essential goal of health care—to improve the ability of individuals to live long, full, and productive lives. Decisions ranging from what health benefits to include in a health plan, to what treatments to recommend and provide, to what performance measures to use for purposes of accountability best serve people when they are anchored by the primary goal of improving the daily and long-term health and functioning of individuals, families, and communities.
3. **Accountability measures should reflect the needs and values of patients.** FACCT's overarching philosophy is that informed consumers should drive health system accountability and, ultimately, the design and reform of the health care system. The accountability measures used to inform consumers should reflect their needs and values. Americans are paying for, using, and depending upon the health system for the most intimate and vital services. They are its customers and have a critical need to know how well it is meeting their personal and collective objectives; therefore, they should be defining its goals.

4. **Quality improvement and innovation are supported by an accountability system.** Accountability measures provide a device for focusing people's thinking on what the health system should achieve as well as reward those organizations that best achieve these objectives. They have the potential to compel those within the health care system as well as patients, consumers, and purchasers toward innovation in improving performance.

What FACCT Does

FACCT does four things:

1. Proposes an accountability framework.
2. Identifies and endorses measures based on a process that includes:
   - a targeted consumer-input process,
   - a targeted scientific-input process,
   - an open consumer and scientific public review process,
   - a health systems input process, and
   - a technical review and endorsement process.
3. Encourages and supports the adoption of FACCT measures by:
   - standard setting and accrediting bodies,
   - purchasers of health care,
   - public interest and community organizations, and
   - health systems, health plans, medical groups, and other providers.
4. Supports the effective presentation and use of FACCT measures to consumers and purchasers by conducting and supporting work that can assist sponsors of quality information to develop effective educational materials and decision aids for those who use and pay for health care.

Table 1.

WHAT FACCT DOES	*WHAT FACCT DOES NOT DO*
Proposes an accountability framework	Accredit health care plans or systems
Identifies and specifies sets of accountability measures using both consumer and scientific input	Collect data and publish comparative profiles on health plans or systems
Encourages adoption of measures in a variety of settings	Conduct large scale new measurement development activities
Works to ensure appropriate use and communication of information to consumers	

Status of FACCT Activities

Status of Measure Identification and Endorsement

As of winter 1996, FACCT has identified and endorsed five sets of measures in the following topical areas:

Condition-specific measurement sets:

- Major Depressive Disorder
- Diabetes
- Breast Cancer

Population-wide measurement sets:

- Health-risk behaviors
- Satisfaction with health plans

These measurement sets represent approximately 35 measures and three major domains of quality:

- **Results** (e.g. quality of life; functional status; clinical severity; progression of illness; ability to engage in work, school, or other daily activities);
- **Steps to Good Care** (e.g. application of essential processes of care, appropriateness of treatments); and
- **Satisfaction** (patient satisfaction with access, technical quality, interpersonal communication, involvement in treatment decisions, etc.).

While each condition-specific measurement set is meant to be taken as a comprehensive view of quality for that topical area, the sets do not attempt to identify measures for all aspects of the care process (as might be done in practice guidelines). Table 2 provides a summary of FACCT's diabetes measurement set. The measures for all sets endorsed so far draw on data from many sources, including:

- Patient self-reported survey data;
- Clinical encounter data (e.g. laboratory records, medical records);
- Administrative data;
- Condition-specific registries (e.g. cancer registry, diabetes registry); and
- Data obtained directly from physicians.

The FACCT process is under way to identify and endorse several more measurement sets for a variety of topics, including coronary artery disease, asthma, population health status, arthritis, pediatrics, geriatrics, end of life, and alcohol use.

Table 2. Nontechnical Summary of Diabetes Measures

11 Measures	*What Each Measure Tells You*	*How Each Is Measured*
	STEPS TO GOOD CARE	
1. Checking For Foot Problems Regularly	Whether patients have their feet checked to avoid losing a foot to disease.	Patients complete a questionnaire yearly.
2. Checking Blood Sugar Regularly	Whether patients have their blood sugar checked to avoid more serious illness.	Laboratory billing or claims records.
3. Getting Regular Eye Exams	Whether patients have their eyes checked to detect problems that lead to blindness.	Claims records.
4. Advise To Quit Smoking	Whether patients who smoke are advised to quit smoking.	Patients complete a questionnaire yearly.
	SATISFACTION	
5. Getting Needed Services	How satisfied patients are with being able to access needed care and getting support services.	Patients complete a satisfaction questionnaire yearly.
	RESULTS	
6. Coping With Disease	How well patients continue their routine activities and cope with diabetes and its treatment.	Patients complete a questionnaire yearly.
7. Keeping Blood Sugar In Control	How many patients keep their blood sugar at levels that help avoid more serious illness.	Laboratory test results obtained from the laboratory or the patient's medical record.
8. Keeping Cholesterol At Safe Levels	How many patients keep their cholesterol at levels that help avoid heart disease.	Laboratory test results obtained from the laboratory or the patient's medical record.
9. Avoiding Hospital Stays	How many patients can manage their diabetes at home, with their doctor's help, and avoid being hospitalized.	Hospital billing or claim records.
10. Quit Smoking	How many patients who smoke quit smoking.	Patients complete a questionnaire yearly.
11. Ability To Maintain Daily Activities	How many patients who work lose time from work due to their illness.	Patients complete a questionnaire yearly.

Status of Measurement Set Adoption

Publications: FACCT's publication, called "Accountability!," provides information about its activities and the details of each measurement set for those who wish to adopt the FACCT measures. "Accountability!" is organized as a semi-annual publication, with two updates provided in between each new edition. Each new edition will contain information about new measurement sets that are endorsed and information to facilitate the implementation and use of existing and new measures. FACCT's "Accountability!" series is designed to be continuously expanded as lessons learned through the adoption of the measures allow FACCT to refine measurement specifications or recommend successful data collection and strategies that are being used in the field. Table 3 provides a sample of the specifications that are provided in "Accountability!" for a measure endorsed by FACCT. More detail about the specifications provided for FACCT measures is provided later in this chapter.

Table 3. Diabetes Mellitus Accountability Measure

Title
Glycated Hemoglobin Levels

Measurement Domain
Clinical Outcomes

Rationale for Performance Evaluation
Control of blood sugar levels has been proven to prevent complications in Type I diabetes and is thought to do the same in Type II diabetes. The HbA1c level of a patient is the best measure of overall glycemia over the previous 8-12 weeks. Levels correlate closely with the rate of appearance and progression of several microvascular and neuropathic diabetic complications (2). This is a valid intermediate endpoint and can be related to many other data elements. National practice based norms are available (17). Hyperglycemia (high blood sugar) is a characteristic of all forms of diabetes. Normalizing blood sugar levels reduces many symptoms and risks for many complications of diabetes, including decompensation due to diabetic ketoacidosis or hypersmolar hyperglycemic nonketotic syndrome, diabetic retinopathy, nephropathy and neuropathy. Normalization of blood sugar level requires frequent self-monitoring of blood glucose, careful attention to diet and exercise, appropriate insulin regimens and ongoing education and support of patients.

Target Population
A stratified random sample of patients should be drawn. Stratify sample according to age (18-44, 45-64, over 65) and whether or not patients are insulin treated. Persons who have had one or more hospitalizations related to their diabetes within two years or who have had at least two outpatient/physician visits within two years where diabetes was listed as the reason for the visit qualify for inclusion in the sample. In addition, patients may be identified by looking for persons listed in pharmacy records who receive insulin on a regular basis. Relevant ICD-9 codes are: 250-250.93, 357.2x, 362.0x, 362.02, 366.41. (Additional case-finding and sampling specifications provided elsewhere.)

Measure Type
Proportion of cases above threshold values

Community-Based Activities: In addition to the provision of written materials, FACCT is involved in a number of community-based activities to ensure the successful adoption of FACCT measures. For 1997, FACCT foresees that measures will be collected and reported to purchasers to help them understand plans' and systems' current competencies and practice styles and patients' experiences of their care, to point providers and plans towards important health improvement objectives, to compare systems of care (i.e., FFS vs. HMO), and to assist in the continuing education of consumers about important dimensions of quality.

Status of Work Supporting Consumer Use Of Information

FACCT is engaged in addressing many core issues regarding how best to present information to consumers. At the core of FACCT's

Constructing and Reporting the Measure
The most recent HbA1c level for each patient in the sample should be used to construct this measure. Values may be obtained through automated laboratory records or the medical record of the patient. Numbers of patients in each stratified group that have an HbA1c level above threshold values should be reported along with the total number of patients in each group. The number of persons in the entire sample who did not have an HbA1c level recorded should also be noted.

Threshold values are set for three age groups

18-44:	8%
45-64:	9.5%
Over 65:	10%

While there is substantial empirical evidence to support the use of this measure, some uncertainty exists regarding what the appropriate threshold values should be for each risk group. Because levels for insulin treated patients may be systematically higher than for non-insulin treated patients, proportion exceeding indicated threshold should be reported for each of the three age groups and according to whether or not patients are treated with insulin.

Testing and Use History
Major national studies have validated this measure as an indicator of performance in managing the primary risk factor for diabetics. In particular, the Diabetes Control and Complications Trial tested the proposition that the complications of diabetes mellitus in insulin-dependent diabetics are related to elevation of the plasma glucose concentration as measured by HbA1c levels. It was shown that proper control of blood sugar levels results in a substantial delay, slowing and reduction of complications of diabetes regardless of the age or sex of the patient or duration of diabetes. National laboratory standards for the HbA1c test are still forthcoming. Until standards are in place, the normal ranges and intra and inter-assay coefficient of variation used by each lab will need to be reported. Where patients in the sample used different laboratories with different normal ranges, values will need to be translated to correspond with the standards selected for the performance measurement system.

work is the consideration of how variations in consumer characteristics and circumstances influence their need for information and how that information should be presented. For example, information needs may vary according to an individual's or family's health state, insurance situation, family structure, the health care market in which they live, and so on. These differences may have important implications for the content, scope, context, sequencing, timing, and mode of communication of information about quality.

FACCT has begun to involve consumers in addressing these issues through a number of processes, such as key informant interviews, focus groups, and surveys. In addition, the measure identification process anticipates the context in which the information will be used, making the consumer-input steps in the measure identification process also important to FACCT's efforts to support the effective consumer use of quality information. FACCT and its sponsors are committed to providing accountability information to consumers as soon as possible.

FACCT's Origins And Structure

FACCT was founded in late 1995 by a consortium of purchaser and consumer organizations committed to establishing accountability for quality as a cornerstone of the evolving American health care system. FACCT's board of trustees is comprised of one-third consumer organizations, one-third private-sector payers, and one-third public-sector payers. The board oversees the strategic direction and activities of FACCT and approves of all measures prior to endorsement.

FACCT was founded on the notion that the need to examine and make available information on quality to those who use and pay for health care is essential, regardless of the organizational or financial construction of the health care system. The public-sector failure to secure major health care reform combined with the increase of managed care fueled the founding of FACCT as a voice for consumers and purchasers. FACCT believes the continued evolution of the health care system needs to be disciplined through direct accountability in order to ensure that the systems of care that are successful in the marketplace produce the best results.

Three councils comprised of both FACCT board members and individuals from other organizations oversee FACCT's activities: the FACCT Measures Council, Consumer Advisory Council, and Health Plans and Providers Advisory Committee.

1. Measures Council: The Foundation for Accountability Measures Council provides technical oversight to the FACCT measurement endorsement process. It reviews proposals and recommends accountability measures to the FACCT board for endorsement. It meets at least three times per year and members are active in advising FACCT throughout the process. The Measures Council makes recommendations to the FACCT board regarding which measures to endorse.

The Measures Council advises FACCT in the following areas:

- Proposed conceptual framework and philosophy underlying the FACCT measurement strategy;
- Proposed topics for measurement and specific measurement proposals;
- Proposed methodologies for data collection and casemix adjustment; and
- The use of measures by the health care system and the reporting of measures to consumers and purchasers.

2. Consumer Advisory Council: The Consumer Advisory Council (CAC) enables key consumer organizations to articulate the interests of consumers in improving health care system quality. FACCT recognizes several legitimate consumer interests, represented by diverse organizations. For purposes of the CAC, "consumer" means: (a) individuals selecting health care plans and services for themselves and their families and (b) patients experiencing the health system directly. The CAC helps FACCT draw upon the rich experience and knowledge of consumers to identify measures that accurately reflect aspects of care important to consumers. The CAC also helps FACCT communicate with existing organizations to provide consumers with relevant FACCT information for health care decisionmaking. The CAC includes members that represent general consumers as well as those with expertise in addressing a particular disorder or population. The activities of the CAC are in addition to the consumer-input activities undertaken when identifying and endorsing specific measurement sets.

3. Health Plans and Providers Advisory Committee: The Health Plans and Providers Advisory Committee (HPPC) involves representatives of health plans and providers in the selection and evaluation of performance measures, their implementation, and the use of performance data by health care organizations.

SUMMARY OF FACCT'S OPERATING PRINCIPLES AND PROCESSES

FACCT's Operating Assumptions

Today's health care system is undergoing constant change. While the role of accountability is critical to ensuring these changes benefit the health of people, neither consumers nor the health system are accustomed to the accountability model FACCT promotes. Many of the technical building blocks required to support an accountability system are also not in place in many health systems. At least three basic operating assumptions are identified that guide FACCT's work during this time of constant change, uncertainty, and new learning.

1. **It will take some time before the commitment, knowledge, standardization, and competencies are in place to ensure the creation of an accountable health care system.**
   - **Commitment:** For an accountability system to work purchasers and consumers need to be committed to obtaining information about quality, and health care organizations need to be committed to providing this information. In turn, both need to be committed to acting on this information in ways that improve system performance.
   - **Purchasers and Consumers:** While health care purchasers and consumers are growing in their commitment to measure and hold the health system accountable for quality, doing so is not yet a norm in all markets. In addition, patients often are not accustomed to requesting or using such information. This is a major barrier that recent advances in consumer education and stronger patient-provider partnership models of care may help remedy.
   - **Health Care Organizations:** While many health care organizations are currently able and willing to provide the information accountability requires, in the absence of a regulatory mechanism to enforce participation, many purchasers and health care organizations will need to rely on formal or informal contracts to secure participation in producing accountability information.
   - **Knowledge:** A great deal is known about how to obtain much of the data required to produce accountability information. However, data do not mean knowledge. How to best translate these data into information and knowledge for consumers is not

well understood. Significant learning will occur in the next couple of years as efforts to implement an accountability system in many health care markets across the country continue.

- **Standardization:** Both a standard set of measures and standardized tools for developing these measures are desirable—especially within any given health care market. There are important barriers to achieving standardization. It is hoped that FACCT's work will help overcome some of these barriers.
- **Standard Set of Measures:** Currently, no well-articulated consensus on what should be measured to meet needs of key users exists. Additional work is required to ensure that proposed measures will produce information that is meaningful to consumers and purchasers or that new measures are developed that achieve this goal.
- **Standardized Tools:** Many tools for developing quality measures currently are available. Work should continue to resolve the multitude of methodological and practical issues so that the tools used for purposes of accountability within and across many health care markets and nationally may be standardized using the best available knowledge.
- **Competencies:** Accountability requires the health care system to possess strong data collection and processing competencies. Ironically, the most difficult challenges for accountability are those posed by a health system not accustomed to collecting or using the data accountability requires. As health systems continue to improve their ability to assess and manage the health of populations, many of the data collection and processing competencies relevant to accountability will emerge. Problems related to the reliability and consistency of diagnosis coding, the accessibility and compatibility of electronic data systems, and quality in conducting patient surveys are essential to address. Keeping in mind that the information communicated to consumers is only as good as the data that went into the development of that information, many strategies to improve and monitor health system competencies in these areas will need to be developed.

2. **An accountability system should be structured to accommodate the variety of health care organization and financing arrangements that exist.** Accountability is essential, regardless of the organization or financing of the health care system. Consumers and purchasers are faced with a continuously changing and complex array of health systems. To meet the needs of consumers and purchasers, efforts should be made to hold accountable the variety of health systems that exist. Within any topical area, accountability measures

should be designed to be relevant regardless of the type of health care system setting they are applied to. While the specific methodology for implementing measures may need to vary when applied to one setting versus another, the underlying measurement concepts and essential technical elements should remain the same.

3. **The context in which information about quality will be presented as well as consumer preferences need to be considered carefully when determining appropriate standards of evidence.** It is important that consumers have confidence in claims that observed differences across health systems are real and meaningful. Deciding on what is real and meaningful requires that many assumptions about the standards of evidence be made. FACCT considers this to be a legitimate and very complex issue, worthy of serious debate on a global and measure-by-measure basis. Traditional standards of evidence are not necessarily transferable to the consumer marketplace. Any measurement system will involve many different types and magnitudes of data biases and many options for how to define a meaningful and real difference—some of which may be more or less tolerable to consumers. FACCT keeps these issues at the forefront of the measure specification process.

Process and Principles That Guide the Measure Identification and Specification Process

FACCT's Initial Framework

A two-tiered measurement topic selection framework guided FACCT's first year of work. Specifically, FACCT sought to identify sets of measures that focus on issues of relevance to the entire population as well as those more relevant to individuals with specific health conditions.

FACCT's population-wide measures provide information on how well the health system provides services to the entire population—both ill and healthy individuals—for which it is responsible.

FACCT's condition-specific measures provide information on how effectively the health system provides care for a population who is ill or at risk for an illness.

Table 4. Three Core Dimensions of Quality: Framework for Accountability

Results
How does the condition affect people's lives—their ability to function? Has the disease progressed or abated?

Satisfaction
How satisfied are people with the care and services received?

Steps to Good Care
How well is the health system delivering needed screening, diagnostic, and treatment services?

As outlined earlier, within each condition FACCT seeks to identify measures in three broad areas: results, satisfaction, and steps to good care (see Table 4).

The selection of specific topics within the population-wide and condition-specific areas was guided by a set of six criteria. FACCT convened an advisory panel of public- and private-sector purchasers, consumer representatives, and health services researchers to develop a means of prioritizing a target set of topics/conditions. This work resulted in the selection criteria listed in Table 5. The topics that FACCT focused on in 1996 reflect many of these criteria and represent a balance of people of different ages and sexes; primary, acute, and chronic care settings; prevention, diagnostic, and treatment services; and areas having a special impact on disadvantaged populations.

Table 5. Criteria Used To Select Initial Group Of FACCT Measurement Topics

Consumer interest
Is this condition of general interest to the public? Would information about performance in this area help consumers increase their understanding of health care quality and accountability?

Prevalence
Does this condition affect a large number of people?

Cost
Does it consume a disproportionate share of health care resources? Does it carry with it an unusually high financial burden for patients and families? What about the personal costs, such as lost productivity and diminished quality of life?

Opportunity to improve care
Can increased attention to outcomes help providers develop better treatment methods and services?

Opportunity to affect outcomes
Can the accountable organization improve outcomes for this condition through a change in access, diagnostic, treatment, or other services?

Opportunity to improve decisionmaking
Could patients affected with this condition use quality information to make more informed choices about providers and plans that would have a positive impact on their health?

FACCT's Evolving Framework

FACCT's framework is evolving to consider other approaches to selecting topics for measurement. Specifically, FACCT recognizes many different potential starting points for selecting measurement topics. As presented in Figure 1, topics may be selected according to the health experiences of individuals, their family and insurance status, the original selection criteria outlined above, and/or the preferred use of the resulting information. FACCT is reworking its measurement topic selection and measure identification process to consider each of these issues. The overarching framework will start with the goal of identifying measures that are relevant for persons in different life stages and health states. For example, as noted earlier, FACCT has begun to identify measurement sets for three major life stages—pediatrics, geriatrics, and end-of-life. Many existing FACCT measures may be incorporated within the broader rubric of life stages and

Figure 1. Alternative Starting Points for Selecting Measurement Topics

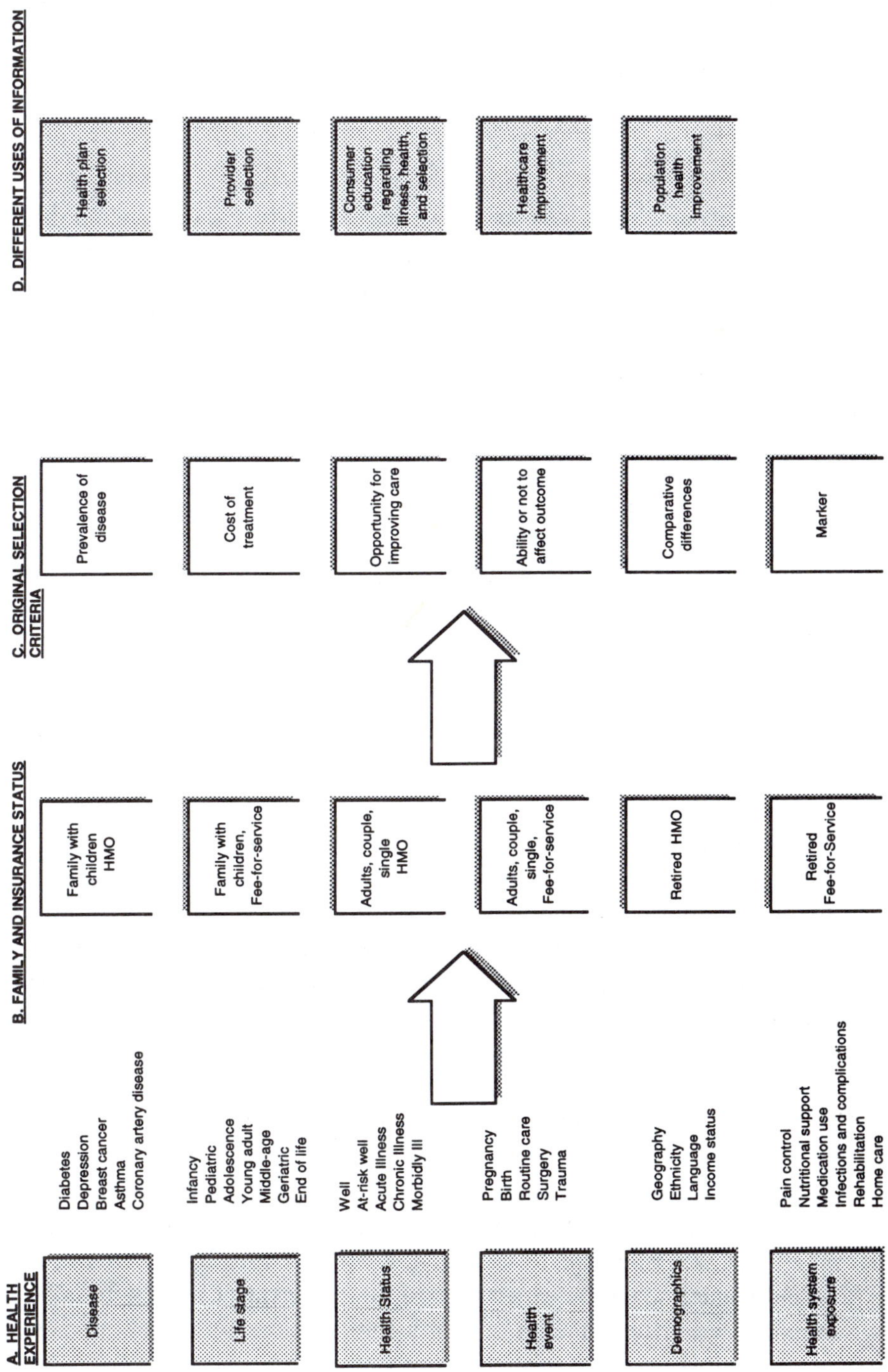

health states. In addition, when information about FACCT measures are communicated to consumers, many options for grouping and presenting information within and across measurement sets should be considered, some of which will be more relevant for some consumers. FACCT's evolving framework is influenced by the Consumer Advisory Council and results from consumer research that FACCT and other organizations have conducted.

Selecting Measures

FACCT's accountability measures have been identified and endorsed through an eight-step process. This process is briefly outlined below. While this process is presented in a linear fashion, in fact, many of the steps overlap and some are revisited as necessary.

Figure 2. Identifying the Measures: FACCT's Process

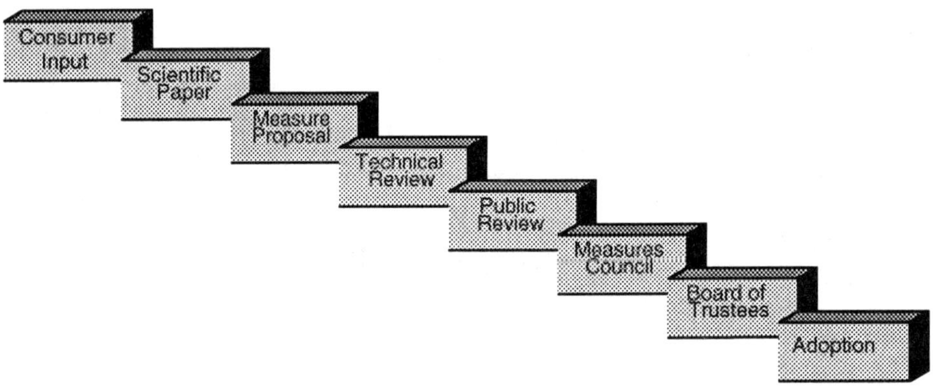

Step One: Obtain patient and consumer input regarding what attributes of quality are important to them. FACCT is committed to involving patients and other consumers throughout each measurement set identification process. Currently, FACCT has a standard of no fewer than four consumer focus groups per topical area, two of which are to be conducted at the beginning of the process. In addition to focus groups, FACCT will conduct key informant interviews with consumer representatives, conduct surveys with patient and consumers, and review existing literature regarding consumer interests. The Consumer Advisory Council will be an ongoing source of consumer input throughout the measurement set identification process.

Step Two: Commission scientific paper experts in the field. During its first year of operation, the U.S. Department of Health and Human Services' Agency for Health Care Policy and Research (AHCPR) and FACCT collaborated to identify and engage scientific experts in the development of a background paper to summarize the state of the art of health care accountability measurement for all topics initially selected. These papers provided the basis for further developing a set of measures for each topic. Scientific authors are expected to consider the information gained during the consumer-input process in the development of their paper. Each paper developed for each new topical area is distributed for review by both scientific and consumer audiences. Comments received are considered by FACCT staff and technical advisers and incorporated into subsequent steps of the process. Most of the papers completed to date are available from AHCPR by calling 800/358-9295.

Step Three: Draft measurement proposal. Using the scientific paper as a starting point, FACCT staff and other individuals with expertise in health care performance measurement develop a draft measurement proposal. This step involves a series of small meetings with expert advisers; additional primary or secondary research may be conducted to clarify unresolved issues essential to the measurement specification process.

Step Four: Conduct a roundtable meeting with experts and consumer groups. The paper and draft measures are sent out for review to several researchers, clinicians, providers in community practice, health plan and health system professionals, and professional societies. A meeting is convened to engage these experts in an assessment of the potential measures. Consideration is given to each individual measure. The relevance, scientific merits, and feasibility of each measure is discussed and recommendations are considered for the further development of the measures. During its first year of operation, AHCPR and FACCT collaborated to organize and conduct these meetings for each measurement topic.

Step Five: Illicit public review and consumer feedback. FACCT makes each measurement set available to interested parties and receives and considers comments from those who choose to submit formal comments about the measures. A request for review is sent to a discrete number of people whose interest in the measurement topic is clear. Review materials are sent to others who request them directly.

Step Six: Conduct technical review and reconsideration. FACCT assembles a group of technical experts to review and reconsider the draft measures based upon information gained during the scientific meetings and public review process. The measurement sets once again are refined and revised based on the deliberations of this group. FACCT's Measures Council then is convened to examine the final draft set of measures and make recommendations for further refinements that need to be made before the measurement set is sent to FACCT's board for endorsement. Additional consultation with field experts also takes place during this stage of the process. Criteria used to evaluate individual measures are outlined in the Appendix at the end of the chapter.

Step Seven: Board considers and endorses measures. FACCT's board of directors considers measurement sets recommended for endorsement by the Measures Council. The board assigns one of three levels of endorsement to each individual measure. These levels are:

- Level One Endorsement: Endorse for immediate use as defined.
- Level Two: Endorse for testing as defined.
- Level Three: Endorse for further refinement.

Step Eight: Adopt and implement measures. Even in the cases where full endorsement is given, it is understood that each of the measures will require further refinement for purposes of implementation in different health care organization, financing, and delivery settings and by different purchasers of care.

Specifying Measures

Three levels of specification are provided for each FACCT measurement set. The first level of specification describes the general approach to measurement, provides a summary of all data required for the entire measurement set, and details the case-finding and sampling methodology required. The second level of specification provides specific information about each individual measure. The attributes listed in Table 6 are included in each individual measure specification. The third level of specification provides additional guidance for implementing the measures. These specifications are being developed for FACCT measures that have been endorsed and are being implemented in many markets.

Table 6. Attributes Specified for Each Measure

Rationale for performance evaluation
The motivation for including the measure is discussed.

Target population
The criteria for including individuals in the numerator and denominator of the measure are described and the methodology for identifying these individuals is detailed.

Measure type
Most measures represent one of three types: a rate, a distribution, or a score. A rate reflects the incidence of an event for a defined number of people; a distribution reflects the proportion of persons falling into one or more categories; a score is simply a number. Whether the measure is a rate, a distribution, or a score is noted here.

Constructing and reporting the measure
Basic information regarding the construction of the measure is outlined here. Method for collecting the data is described. How the measure should be reported is summarized, including factors for stratifying and/or adjusting measures.

Testing and use history
A brief review of the testing and use history of each measure is provided.

Sampling and Casemix Adjustment

The successful specification of FACCT measures in large part hinges on the resolution of two important and interrelated issues: (1) sampling and (2) casemix adjustment. In order to compare the performance of health systems on FACCT measures, issues regarding sampling and casemix adjustment must be resolved. Many of the core assumptions that need to be made to determine appropriate sample sizes and casemix adjustment strategies require further research and/or implementation of the measures. This is true for all performance measurement systems.

These issues will not be discussed in detail here. However, several important assumptions regarding these issues may be considered.

Sampling. There are two primary tasks for sampling populations of patients for purposes of accountability measurement:

Sampling Task #1: Maximize generalizability.

1. Samples should be drawn such that the resulting measures provide information that is representative of the population for which they are developed. This goal is important for all FACCT measures and whether the measures are used for descriptive and/or comparative purposes.
2. If measures are meant to reliably indicate what the likely experience will be for future enrollees, even when measures are based upon the entire population of patients, the measures still might be considered to be unreliable if this underlying population is exceptionally small. This assumption will have the greatest impact on FACCT measures directed at conditions for which there are not large numbers of patients in all health systems. Sampling error should be evaluated as one of many potential types of error in all measures.

Sampling Task #2: Maximize ability to detect meaningful differences.

If a measure is to be used to make comparisons among health systems, FACCT recognizes that assumptions regarding the following five issues must be addressed in order to determine the sample/population size needed to detect meaningful differences among these health systems.

1. The reporting context (e.g. measures reported as one of a much larger set of measures, reported as part of a summary score, interpretive context accompanying the measure, etc.).
2. The comparative base (e.g. standard norm, mean of groups compared, etc.).
3. Definition of a meaningful difference from this base (e.g. 10 percent difference from the norm, .2 standard deviation units from mean, etc.).
4. Degree of variation in measure across health systems or other units of analysis anticipated.
5. Acceptable levels of power and significance for identifying meaningful differences across health systems.

Casemix adjustment. Comparing health systems on many FACCT measures requires adjusting for meaningful variations in the mix of patients affiliated with these health systems. FACCT has identified criteria for determining whether to adjust a measure for a certain factor. Evaluating whether a factor meets these criteria is strongly influenced by the underlying assumptions held regarding:

- the accountability of the health system—its responsibility and ability to influence factors that contribute to the attribute of quality measured,

- the specific unit of analysis to which the measures are applied, and
- the interpretation of relevant research literature about which there is often not a consensus.

For a factor to be seriously considered as an adjustment variable, FACCT evaluates whether it meets the following criteria.

- The probability of either a good or bad outcome on the measure is expected to be systematically and meaningfully different for patients who vary on this factor even if health systems are of equal quality.
- The health care system should not be expected to be held accountable for the presence or distribution of this factor.
- Significant variation in the distribution of the population on this factor is expected across health systems being compared.
- The factor is not already largely controlled through other means (e.g. case finding, other adjustment factors, etc.).

In addition to the criteria outlined above, FACCT has identified two principles related specifically to adjustment for socioeconomic variables:

1. A significant effort should be made not to use socioeconomic variables as proxy variables for other, more relevant variables.
2. When adjustment for socioeconomic variables is recommended, stratification versus direct adjustment is preferred.

Finally, FACCT recognizes that alternative methods for accounting for casemix variables can lead to different results. Care should be taken when recommending a specific approach (e.g. multivariate regression, direct adjustment, stratification, etc.)

Concepts That Guide the Adoption of Measures

FACCT recognizes that the nature of the private market—both its inherent characteristics and those magnified by the rapid changes now occurring—makes the construction and use of quality information complex. Absent regulation or industry standards, FACCT will continue to observe fluid formulations of health care delivery systems, financing arrangements, purchasing strategies, and even conceptualizations of "health care" itself.

In this context, FACCT understands that different users, facing different circumstances, will apply quality measures and the resulting data in different ways. From an analytical perspective, FACCT encourages users to recognize that their application of quality data is influenced by their approach to several issues, which are briefly described below:

- Quality theory and goals,
- Measurement purpose,
- Delivery model,
- Accountability model,

- Purchasing model, and
- Insurance model.

Quality theory and goals: As purchasers and consumers work with providers to define performance expectations, an implicit theory of quality is at work. Difficulty in making that theory explicit can create tension between consumers, patients, purchasers, providers, and insurers. FACCT encourages accountability relationships that involve measuring performance to be based upon an explicit theory of quality and an articulated set of quality goals. These goals can reflect multiple perspectives, including:

- Quality as correct and efficacious performance of medical services,
- Quality as achievement of desired health outcomes for personal care,
- Quality as achievement of favorable health status for individuals,
- Quality as satisfying consumer and patient expectations,
- Quality as achieving optimal population health status, and
- Quality as delivery of services efficiently and appropriately.

Measurement purpose: FACCT recognizes that any performance measurement system can serve multiple goals:

- Provide information to individual consumers to help in plan or provider choice,
- Provide information to purchasers to help in plan choice or setting shared goals with plan and health systems,
- Provide information to plans and providers to assist in quality improvement and clarifying and articulating organizational mission,
- Facilitate the continued testing and refinement of measurement science, and
- Provide information to consumers to educate them about what they should expect from their health care and their role in ensuring quality.

Delivery model: While consumers, purchasers, and policymakers often think in terms of traditional health care providers (e.g. doctors and hospitals), many alternative mechanisms for delivering care are achieving success, and health plans are increasingly obliged to provide reimbursement or fully incorporate these alternatives. Quality measurement needs to promote, not stifle, innovation and should encourage the use of new and successful alternative delivery mechanisms and processes, such as telephonic advice, electronic health assessment, monitoring, education, community-based (e.g., retail pharmacy, school) chronic disease management, and carveout disease management. When selecting quality measures to base an accountability system on, users should keep in mind that a focus on outcomes and the experience of the patient—versus specific mechanisms and processes of care—may do more to encourage such innovative approaches.

Accountability model: Individual communities may make different decisions regarding which health care entity is to be held accountable for specific health goals. Many parties may be held individually or jointly accountable for some aspect of community or individual health:

- Entire community,
- Health plans,
- Integrated health systems,
- Medical groups,
- Individual providers, and
- Patients and consumers.

FACCT encourages local sponsors to be explicit about the expectations they have for each of these "layers" of the health system and discourages a narrow and punitive model of accountability that does not appreciate the inherent, joint accountability of several parties for many important attributes of quality, such as health outcomes.

Purchasing model: The existence of different purchasing models requires that quality information be relevant and understandable to both individual consumers and different types of group purchasers of health care that serve as "brokers" of quality information for these individuals. Clearly, the recent emphasis on quality and value is being driven by organized purchasers representing large numbers of covered lives. Consumer organizations, lacking consolidated economic power, are less able to translate their quality objectives into enforceable, contractual terms. Yet the purchasing environment varies in each market. Government purchasers in Medicare, Medicaid, and for public employees are generally not permitted to select which plans or systems of care to offer based on quality standards. In those markets, the individual consumer is often the decisionmaker. National corporate purchasers are often the most sophisticated users of quality data and need to find ways to influence the behavior of providers or plans in local markets, perhaps by empowering individual consumers to select specific providers based on quality. Large local purchasers, often participating in coalitions, are best able to articulate and execute a set of quality standards. Each of the major purchasing models outlined may influence how accountability information is constructed and communicated.

Insurance model: The insurance model through which care is provided has implications for the construction and use of quality information. Different purchasers and markets take different approaches to health insurance—to the question of "what is being insured against?" For most of this century, health insurance applied to individual medical encounters and payment was based on reimbursement of fees for services individuals selected and received. This model has been modified in most major markets to address only covered benefits often identified as medically necessary by third parties. In the past 20 years, the managed care models have provided insurance for the "covered enrollee," receiving services from numerous providers organized under one financing structure. Most recently, purchasers are narrowing the managed care model to provide comprehensive services to each covered life, provided by or controlled through a designated "care system," which could be a medical group or an integrated delivery system.

Concepts That Guide the Presentation and Use Of Measures by Consumers and Purchasers

FACCT supports three interrelated areas of work to ensure effective consumer use of quality information: (1) identifying discrete consumer audiences, (2) preparing consumer education products and strategies, and (3) preparing data presentation formats.

As noted earlier, FACCT recognizes that many features of information communicated to consumers may need to be shaped according to the discrete characteristics and circumstances of consumers, including:

- the scope and content of that information,
- the context in which it is communicated,
- the interpretation and use of guidelines provided,
- the sequencing of content within materials developed,
- the timing for disseminating different types of information,
- the mode or vehicles for communication (written, interactive), and
- the tools and opportunities provided for consumers to seek additional information and assistance.

In particular, relevant distinctions among consumers may be based upon a variety of characteristics and circumstances:

- Distinct due to the relevance of measurement topics (e.g. has or does not have conditions, health risks represented by the measures),
- Distinct due to the degree of health need (e.g. well, at-risk, chronic, disabled),
- Distinct due to current choice position (e.g. extensive vs. limited choice; FFS vs. HMO/PPO choices),
- Distinct due to current degree of interest and/or sophistication about health care quality and accountability,
- Distinct due to differences in the most relevant and meaningful use of the information (select a plan, a physician, a lifestyle, a treatment), and
- Distinct due to unique language, socioeconomic, and cultural characteristics and needs.

As such, in order to ensure the successful use of quality information, FACCT is working to identify these distinct audiences and support the development of educational materials, decision tools, and vehicles for dissemination that are sensitive to the unique attributes of these audiences. FACCT also recognizes that consumer audiences for quality information are not static—they will evolve with exposure to quality information. As consumers become more aware of the opportunities they have to request and use information about quality to choose their health care providers and their health care treatments, as well as to make personal decisions about their own health behavior and use of the system, the scope, content, context, and vehicles for accessing this information available to them also should evolve. Understanding the way consumers evolve in their desire for and use of information about quality is also important to the design and use of educational materials, decision tools, and vehicles of dissemination. In particular, assumptions about how consumers evolve in their desire and use of quality information will have important implications for the staging and targeting of information made available to consumers over time.

Consumer audience segmentation strategies also may vary depending upon the mode of communication used. In particular, consideration should be given to whether information is given to consumers in static formats (e.g. mailed, written materials) or interactive formats (e.g. decision kiosks or Internet). In short, if interactive communications tools are used (e.g. decision kiosks, computers, etc.), "real-time" segmentation approaches are possible that will allow consumers to self-tailor the information they receive according to their specific characteristics and circumstances. On the contrary, for noninteractive settings (e.g. provision of written materials), prospective segmentation and tailoring of information will be required and should be sufficiently tailored to optimize the use and usefulness of quality information and draw the consumer into a more active, information-seeking stance.

CONCLUSION

FACCT's approach to accountability—to measuring and reporting on quality—is grounded in two principles: (1) the measures are a device for the public to express its goals for the health system, and (2) for the measures to be adaptable to the rapidly changing health care system, they must be grounded in individuals' experience of care.

Turning these principles into an operating measurement system is challenging and depends upon the good will and collaboration of stakeholders from throughout U.S. society. An effective accountability system requires ongoing appreciation of the need to continuously learn, collaborate, experiment, and pursue innovation. FACCT believes in "action research"—taking controlled, incremental steps toward supporting informed decisionmaking while evaluating and integrating the learning from each step as it occurs. With the partnership of patients, purchasers, providers, and colleagues, we can create a health system that can demonstrate accountability and continuously improve its ability to meet public needs.

APPENDIX: CRITERIA FOR ENDORSEMENT OF PERFORMANCE MEASURES

Background

A. FACCT will endorse selected measures of health system performance.

B. FACCT measures must satisfy two kinds of criteria:

- Each measure must meet criteria of consumer relevance, feasibility, and scientific merit; and
- Each set of measures must meet criteria of comprehensiveness, parsimony, and balance.

C. FACCT measures are intended to be applied to a diverse set of environments.

I. Criteria for Acceptance of an Individual Measure

A. Meaningful

- Relevance to consumers, patients, or purchasers
- Reflects (a) health outcome experienced by consumer or patient or, if sound measure is not available, (b) care or service process with demonstrated link to health outcome
- Encourages use of cost-effective services
- Definition is independent of financing or delivery structure in which care is provided; can be reasonably applied to variety of settings

B. Actionable

- Changes in measure can be influenced by activities of the health system
- Consumers are empowered by having information from the measured domain

C. Sound

- Reliable
    1. Reproducible
    2. Sensitive
    3. Specific
- Valid
    1. Face validity
    2. Logical validity
    3. Content and construct validity
    4. Convergent and divergent validity

D. Respectful
- Confidential
- Minimizes burden

E. Feasible
- Required data elements can be reasonably and reliably captured
- Has been used with known results in suitable settings

F. Communicable
- Unit of analysis and reporting
- Risk-adjustable
- Context-rich

II. Criteria for Inclusion in a Battery of Measures

A. Domain balance
- addresses one of five FACCT domains
- is parsimonious in addressing domain goals (i.e., inclusion of new measures into domain should supersede previous measure)

B. Continuum of care
- inclusion will lead to balanced view of entire experience of care when viewed with other measures in battery

Chapter 3

Joint Commission on Accreditation Of Healthcare Organizations

Performance Measurement and Accreditation

Jerod M. Loeb, PhD, and Deborah M. Nadzam, PhD, RN

The Joint Commission on Accreditation of Healthcare Organizations (JCAHO) was founded nearly 50 years ago, but its origins date back to the early part of the 20th Century with the formation of the Hospital Standardization Program of the American College of Surgeons. Today, the Joint Commission is the nation's oldest and largest health care accrediting body, providing evaluation and accreditation services for general, psychiatric, children's, and rehabilitation hospitals; health plans; integrated delivery systems; provider-sponsored networks; home care organizations (including those that provide home health services, personal care and support services, home infusion and other pharmacy services, durable medical equipment services, and hospice services); nursing homes and other long term care facilities (including subacute care and dementia programs); behavioral health care organizations (including those that provide mental health, chemical dependency, and mental retardation/developmental disabilities services for patients of various ages in various organized service settings); ambulatory care providers (including outpatient surgery facilities, rehabilitation centers, infusion centers, group practices, and others); and clinical laboratories.

To support the accreditation process, the Joint Commission develops and maintains contemporary, performance-based standards that are applicable to the organizations and systems that constitute the major sources of health care delivery in the United States. The Joint Commission then applies these standards in comprehensive onsite evaluations of organizations, the results of which form the basis for subsequent accreditation decisions. The Joint Commission's standards address the organization's level of performance in key functional areas such as patient rights, and the standards focus not simply on what the organization *has*, but what it actually *does*. Standards set forth performance expectations for activities that affect the quality of patient care—if an organization does the right things and does them well, there is a strong likelihood that its patients will experience good outcomes. The Joint Commission's standards are developed in consultation with health care and measurement experts, providers, purchasers, and consumers. Standards development is an ongoing, dynamic process that continually incorporates the experience and perspective of health care professionals and other individuals and organizations from throughout the country. The standards that result from this process focus on the essential elements of providing quality health care and are nationally recognized for the significant contributions they make to improving the quality of care delivered to patients. In recent years, several important changes in standards have been prompted by various needs, including:

1. Strategic issues such as a change in all standards to focus on performance and important functions in order to improve the accreditation process and foster continuous improvement in surveyed organizations.
2. Specific quality-of-patient-care issues that may require standards, such as the need for a more patient-centered approach to restraint and seclusion.
3. New and emerging organizational configurations or structures of delivery systems that may result in the need to add, delete, or change standards. For example, this may be desirable to facilitate—and even foster—the transition of individual organizations to integrated health delivery systems.
4. Changes in technology, practice, or other issues in the environment that may require the updating or deletion of specific standards, intent statements, scoring guidelines, or examples.
5. Research-based information that may make standards modifications desirable.
6. Legislation or regulation that may require new standards or modifications in existing ones.
7. The need to support improved efficiency in health care organizations that may result in reevaluation of existing standards with respect to the ratio of their benefits to their costs.

In managed care, the Joint Commission accredits networks that provide, or provide for, integrated health care services to a defined population of individuals; offer either comprehensive or specialty services (e.g. behavioral health); and include both a centralized integrating structure and the actual care delivery sites, which include components (e.g. hospitals, long term care facilities) and practitioner sites. Health care networks include health plans (e.g. health maintenance organizations, physician hospital organizations, independent practice associations), preferred provider organizations, and integrated delivery systems such as provider-sponsored networks. Network components may include hospitals, outpatient facilities, long term care facilities, home care programs, behavioral health care facilities, and other kinds of health-related services. The network accreditation program offers comprehensive evaluation of all important aspects of the network's performance. This includes evaluation of the principal administrative location from which the network is managed, a significant number of components of the network that deliver care to network members, and a sample of the offices of the practitioners who are members of the network's medical staff. The standards for health care networks specifically address issues related to systemwide integration, coordination, and accountability that are vital to integrated delivery systems and health plans. Standards cover the following areas: rights, responsibilities, and ethics; continuum of care; patient education and communication; health promotion and disease prevention; network leadership; human resource management; information management; performance improvement; patient assessment; patient care; environmental management; and infection control.

WHY SEEK ACCREDITATION?

Organizations seek to be accredited for many reasons. Among the most often-cited benefits of accreditation are improvement in the quality of patient care, strengthening of community confidence, enhancement of staff recruitment, the ability to substitute for Medicare and Medicaid certification (in-hospital, home health care, and clinical laboratory settings), fulfillment of licensure requirements in many states, recognition by insurers and other third-party payers, and the ability to attract managed care contracts. Underlying these perceived benefits of accreditation are several caveats regarding the basic purposes of accreditation itself. Accreditation has been assumed to offer *discernment* of the level of quality of an organization's provision of health care, *prediction* that the organization is likely to provide health care of at least acceptable quality in the future, *improvement* in the organization's provision of health care, and *recognition*—both within the organization and publicly—that the organization provides health care of at least acceptable quality and is continuously improving the quality of care it provides.[1]

Over the past decade, the Joint Commission has been engaged in a complete reengineering—The Agenda for Change—of the entire accreditation process. The Agenda for Change was designed to revise existing standards to focus more appropriately on performance; update the survey process to become more performance focused and educational; and develop, implement, and, ultimately, integrate the measurement of actual performance into the survey and accreditation process. Also included in this reengineering process is the introduction of laptop technology to increase the objectivity, efficiency, and consistency of evaluation. In the aggregate, the modifications associated with the Agenda for Change allow the Joint Commission to move from an accreditation process based exclusively on proxies for outcomes to a more contemporary process in which actual performance is measured in addition to the integrity of the processes that underlie particular outcomes.[2] Most health care accrediting bodies today use both performance measurement and standards compliance as integral but separate parts of the quality evaluation process.

PERFORMANCE MEASUREMENT

Performance in health care represents the totality of what is done coupled with how well it is done. For decades, the evaluation of compliance with expert-based, contemporary standards has represented by itself the sine qua non of quality assessment of health care organizations. This general approach is based on the premise that health care organizations that consistently "do the right things right" are likely to achieve good clinical outcomes. Indeed, compliance with standards is intended to create a prejudicial bias in favor of good outcomes.[3] On the other hand, performance measurement is designed to look more directly toward actual outcomes. Obviously, performance measurement requires the use of specific tools or measures designed to assess particular facets of care. A performance measurement system is defined by the Joint Commission as an interrelated set of process or outcome measures that, when used together, provide a meaningful performance profile of the organization to which the measures are applied.[4] In the current health care environment, a virtual mandate for measurement exists; nevertheless, a number of barriers to measurement have been identified. Measurement is by no means a neutral activity—it evokes considerable anxiety and frustration, particularly among those being measured. Although significant progress has been made, performance measurement in health care suffers from a distinct lack of concordant focus or philosophy. No standardized data dictionary exists—yet. It is clear that data collection itself is not without significant expense; in fact, the costs of data collection often can be prohibitive. In terms of reducing or eliminating the confounding influences of patient factors (i.e., adjusting for severity or risk), a similar lack of concordant focus exists. This extends to whether to adjust at all, and, if so, what technique(s) to use. Finally, the level at which measurement is undertaken—plan, organization, or individual provider or practitioner—each has its proponents and detractors.[5]

MEASURING PERFORMANCE IN HEALTH CARE NETWORKS

Recently, the Joint Commission, working with benefits managers from several major corporations, representatives from provider organizations, and individuals from the payer and health services research communities, elucidated a group of explicit principles to help guide the development of performance measures relevant to health care networks.[6] These general tenets include:

1. Measurement of health status and health care quality are essential to the improvement of health care.
2. The design of any meaningful measurement system must involve all key stakeholders, including purchasers, providers, evaluators, consumers, and government.
3. A basic prerequisite to the creation of a measurement system is the establishment of a rational framework within which measurement priorities can be determined and measures developed.
4. The measurement framework must be applicable to networks and components of networks, useful to purchasers and consumers in evaluating the quality of networks and their components, useful to government in formulating and assessing public health policy, and useful to providers in improving care.
5. The measurement framework must promote efficient and concise measurement that minimizes the associated administrative burden.
6. The measurement process must promote the accountability of both the network and the stakeholders of the network.
7. The measurement process should include definition of the individual or unit accountable for each specific measure.
8. The measurement system should be able to describe the health benefits achieved both by individuals and the population served by the network.
9. Data systems used for quality measurement and comparison must be built on relevant measures that meet established criteria for reliability, validity, and ease of data collection.
10. Data collection must focus on those data necessary for the measures, rather than those data most readily available.
11. The measurement system must constantly anticipate its own improvement.

From these basic general tenets, a framework for measurement was established for specific use in measuring the performance of health care networks.[7] Three categories involve the measurement of outcomes or processes of care that relate to various clinical conditions, while the remaining two are measured via compliance with established accreditation standards for health care networks:

1. clinical performance (prevention, early detection, appropriateness of treatment, effectiveness of treatment);
2. health status (general well-being of population served, measures for specific clinical populations served);
3. satisfaction (patient/enrollee, practitioner, purchaser);
4. process effectiveness (human resource management, management and deployment of other resources, management of information, patients' rights, efficiency of processes, performance improvement, coordination of care); and
5. communication and education (patient/enrollee education, communication to providers and patients/enrollees, public access to useful and understandable information).

NATIONAL LIBRARY OF HEALTHCARE INDICATORS

Using this framework as a basis, the Joint Commission has created a comprehensive indicator catalog known as the National Library of Healthcare Indicators™ (NLHI). The first edition of NLHI, released in 1996, covers measures specific to health plans and health care networks. NLHI is an effort to organize available and credible performance measures into a practical format that can be used easily by health care organizations, purchasers, providers, practitioners, etc. NLHI is an immediate resource of measures judged by content experts to have face validity; supports performance measurement and quality improvement efforts; provides applications for various types of health care organizations, including networks; makes available a standardized profile for each measure; allows exploration of available and credible measures to best meet unique measurement needs; and recognizes the wide array of measures developed.

Performance measures may originate from a variety of sources including academic institutions, consumers, database developers, government or government-funded projects, providers, health services researchers, insurers, performance measurement systems, professional associations, purchasers, and provider organizations. To identify measures for potential inclusion in NLHI, the Joint Commission developed the Request for Indicators (RFI) process. In the past, the Joint Commission has periodically issued RFIs seeking performance measures targeted to specific areas of health care represented by the Joint Commission's accreditation programs. In 1995, the first RFI was issued for networks and health plans, and in 1996, additional RFIs were issued for ambulatory care, long term care, home health care, and behavioral health care. The first edition of NLHI, arranged around the framework for performance described above, includes 225 performance-based measures judged to have face validity and applicability to networks and to the full range of health care delivery settings. With a user-friendly format, NLHI profiles each indicator, identifies which measure(s) are appropriate for different health care settings, and identifies which domains of performance, conditions, or procedures are covered by the measures. The publication includes an extensive, comprehensive index that permits users access to measures via multiple directions.

THE JOINT COMMISSION'S INDICATOR MEASUREMENT SYSTEM

From its inception, the Joint Commission's Agenda for Change has included plans for a state-of-the-art system to collect, compare, and analyze data on the performance of health care organizations. The goal for this system has been, and still is, to support the internal efforts of health care organizations to continuously improve their performance and, in so doing, to meet the need for ongoing measurement of health care processes and outcomes as part of the accreditation process.

The Indicator Measurement System (IMSystem) is a comparative performance measurement system, developed by the Joint Commission and launched for voluntary participation by hospitals in 1994. The IMSystem indicators measure actual clinical performance and have been tested for reliability and validity. Built according to industry (ANSI) standards and X12 specifications, the IMSystem is a sophisiticated measurement system that electronically collects and stores select patient-level data that are used to uniquely risk adjust the indicators and provide timely comparative reports to participants. Reports also can be uniquely tailored for specific audiences with specific data requirements.

IMSystem Performance Measures

The implementation of the IMSystem followed an unprecedented five years of performance measurement development and rigorous onsite reliability and validity testing. The research identified reliable and valid measures, as well as effective processes for the design of the IMSystem and its database. The IMSystem now includes performance measures for five patient populations including those receiving perioperative, obstetrics, trauma, oncology, or cardiovascular care, which together address well over half of all current inpatient admissions. In 1996, measures focusing on clinical functions of medication use and infection control were added. (All indicators are listed in Table 1.) These focus areas were identified to address high-risk, high-volume, high-cost, and problem-prone processes of care.

Table 1. IMSystem Performance Measures

Perioperative*

1. Patients developing a central nervous system (CNS) complication within two postprocedure days of procedures involving anesthesia administration.

2. Patients developing a peripheral neurological deficit within two postprocedure days of procedures involving anesthesia administration.

3. Patients developing an acute myocardial infarction within two postprocedure days of procedures involving anesthesia administration.

4. Patients with a cardiac arrest within two postprocedure days of procedures involving anesthesia administration.

5. Intrahospital mortality of patients within two postprocedure days of procedures involving anesthesia administration.

* For the indicators related to perioperative care, the population of interest (denominator) includes all patients undergoing specified procedures involving anesthesia. Presently, only inpatients are included in the population. However, as of January 1, 1997 organizations may choose to include outpatients in the population.

Obstetrical

6. Patients delivered by cesarean section.

7. Patients with vaginal birth after cesarean section.

8. Live-born infants with a birthweight of less than 2,500 grams.

9. Live-born infants with a birthweight greater than or equal to 2,500 grams, who have at least one of the following: an Apgar score of less than 4 at five minutes, a requirement for admission to the neonatal intensive care unit within one day of delivery for greater than one day, a clinically apparent seizure, or significant birth trauma.

10. Live-born infants with a birthweight greater than 1,000 grams and less than 2,500 grams who have an Apgar score of less than 4 at five minutes.

Cardiovascular

11. Patients undergoing isolated coronary artery bypass graft (CABG) procedures: number of days from initial surgery to discharge.

12. Patients admitted through the emergency department with a principal discharge diagnosis of acute myocardial infarction (AMI) receiving thrombolytic therapy: time from emergency department arrival to administration of thrombolytic therapy.

13. Patients with a principal discharge diagnosis of congestive heart failure with documented etiology.

14. Patients undergoing a percutaneous transluminal coronary angioplasty (PTCA): number of days from procedure to discharge.

15a. Intrahospital mortality of patients undergoing an isolated CABG.

15b. Intrahospital mortality of patients undergoing a PTCA.

15c. Intrahospital mortality of patients with a principal discharge diagnosis of acute myocardial infarction.

Table 1. IMSystem Performance Measures (cont.)

Oncology

16. Patients undergoing resection for primary cancer of the lung, colon/rectum, or female breast for whom a surgical pathology consultation report is present in the medical record.

17. Patients undergoing resection for primary cancer of the lung, colon/rectum, or female breast with stage of tumor designated by a managing physician.

18. Female patients with Stage I or greater primary breast cancer who, after initial biopsy or resection, have estrogen receptor analysis results in the medical record.

19. Patients with non-small cell primary lung cancer undergoing thoracotomy with complete surgical resection of tumor.

20. Patients undergoing resection for primary cancer of the colon/rectum whose preoperative evaluation, by a managing physician, included examination of the entire colon.

Trauma**

21a. Trauma patients with systolic blood pressure, pulse rate, and respiratory rate documented on arrival to the emergency department (ED) and at least hourly for three hours or until ED disposition, whichever is earlier.

21b. Trauma patients with specified intracranial injuries with Glasgow coma scale (GCS) score documented on arrival to emergency department and at least hourly for three hours or until ED disposition, whichever is earlier.

22. Comatose trauma patients with specified intracranial injuries discharged from the emergency department prior to endotracheal intubation or cricothyrotomy.

23. Trauma patients with head computerized tomography (CT) scan performed: time from emergency department arrival to initial CT scan.

24a. Trauma patients undergoing specified neurosurgical procedures: time from emergency department arrival to procedure.

24b. Trauma patients undergoing specified orthopedic procedures: time from emergency department arrival to procedure.

24c. Trauma patients undergoing specified abdominal surgical procedures: time from emergency department arrival to procedure.

25a. Intrahospital mortality of trauma patients with a diagnosis of pneumothorax or hemothorax who did not undergo a thoracostomy or thoracotomy.

25b. Intrahospital mortality of trauma patients with a systolic blood pressure of less than 70 mm Hg within two hours of emergency department arrival who did not undergo a laparotomy or thoracotomy.

**Trauma patients: Patients undergoing emergency hospital care for at least one of the diagnoses listed on IMSystem ICD-9-CM Code Table 6, General Trauma Population Codes AND who were admitted, transferred, or expired.

Table 1. IMSystem Performance Measures (cont.)

Medication Use

26. Inpatients 65 years of age or older in whom creatinine clearance has been estimated or measured.

27. Selected surgical procedures for which prophylactic intravenous antibiotics were received: timing of prophylactic antibiotic administration.

28. Inpatients with a discharge diagnosis of insulin-dependent diabetes mellitus who demonstrate self blood glucose monitoring and self-administration of insulin before discharge, or are referred for post-discharge follow-up for diabetes management.

29a. Inpatients receiving digoxin who have no corresponding measured drug level or whose highest measured level exceeds a specific limit.

29b. Inpatients receiving theophylline who have no corresponding measured drug level or whose highest measured level exceeds a specific limit.

29c. Inpatients receiving phenytoin who have no corresponding measured drug level or whose highest measured level exceeds a specific limit.

29d. Inpatients receiving lithium who have no corresponding measured drug level or whose highest measured level exceeds a specific limit.

30. Inpatients: number of prescribed medications at discharge.

Infection Control

31. Selected inpatient and outpatient surgical procedures complicated by a surgical site infection.

32. Ventilated inpatients who develop pneumonia.

33. Inpatients with a central or umbilical line who develop primary blood stream infection.

The individual measures of interest were developed by expert panels who were asked to identify events of import for the particular patient population or function to be measured. The data elements necessary to compute and adjust the measures then were identified and evaluated for availability and reliability. The research identified data elements that could not be collected consistently across organizations, resulting in deletion of some data elements from future consideration; in some instances this also led to the deletion of the associated indicators. Revisions to definitions and allowable values were made to other data elements to increase their reliability. Although over 70 indicators were extensively tested, only 42 were considered sufficiently reliable and valid for inclusion in the comparative performance measurement system. As a result, the data collection effort for participating organizations also was reduced. With sampling options available for some indicators, the potential exists for calculating over 90 different primary indicator rates.

Data Collection Software

As a result of the same research activity, the Joint Commission also determined that requiring the use of one software application was inefficient and too restrictive for many hospitals, even contributing to missing and/or inaccurate data at times. Therefore, to provide greater flexibility for participating in the IMSystem, the Joint Commission developed and published data collection and submission functional (programming) requirements—the *IMSystem Software Specifications*. The specifications allow each participant to determine the most efficient software solution for its organizations and include:

- a data dictionary with semantic and electronic definitions,
- report formats,
- submission file requirements,
- indicator calculation algorithms, and
- test data with expected results.

Participating health care organizations have utilized three major approaches relative to software:

1. in-house development of a solution by hospital information services staff,
2. purchase of a stand-alone solution available in the marketplace, and
3. request of hospital's current information system vendor to incorporate IMSystem functionality.

All three approaches have been used successfully by current participants. A list of available vendor products is maintained to support new participants' implementation plans.

Data Submission

A defined cycle for data collection, submission, validation, and analysis exists for the IMSystem. Participants are expected to submit patient-level data for patients in the populations of interest (as defined in the specifications). For example, if a hospital is using the IMSystem's cesarean-section indicator, then data must be sent on all delivered mothers and associated newborns. On the other hand, if an organization selects the surgical site infection indicator, they also choose selected surgical procedure groups to monitor for infections (17 groups are defined as options); related data elements for the sampled population only must be submitted. Core data elements required for all indicators include: an episode-of-care number (a computer-generated number that is not the patient's medical record number), the admission date or emergency department (ED) arrival date, the discharge date or ED disposition date, and the ICD-9-CM discharge diagnosis code(s). Other IMSystem patient data elements are used either to determine patient populations and indicator occurrences or to risk adjust the indicator.

Data are submitted quarterly to the IMSystem database in electronic, machine-readable format (modems, diskettes, and tapes are accepted). Data for patients discharged in a quarter must be submitted within 60 days of the end of the quarter. A unique feature of the IMSystem is the database's front-end filter—a set of processes that monitor the quality of submitted data and adherence to published specifications. The filter process first checks for correct file formats and for provider organization identifiers to ensure correct attribution of data. Each episode of care then is reviewed against hundreds of data edits, resulting in (1) a filter report used by the submitting organization to correct and resubmit data and (2) a database of high integrity for generating comparable indicator rates. In essence, this filter is a dynamic testing process of the multitude of software solutions created by participants and vendors. The filter report is provided back to the participating organization electronically (via the IMSystem bulletin board) or on hard copy (U.S. mail).

Analysis and Risk Adjustment

Analysis of the data begins immediately after the 60-day end-of-quarter submission deadline has passed. Currently, quarterly comparative reports are being produced and distributed to participants within another 60 days. Comparative reports provide risk-adjusted information, allowing an organization to review its observed performance against its predicted performance and as compared to other IMSystem users. Throughout the research phase of development, statisticians reviewed various methods of risk-adjustment and patient factors contributing to indicator rates. As a result, specific IMSystem indicators are risk adjusted using logistic regression techniques. Patient characteristics presumably contributing to indicator variance are identified through the literature and expert panel advice. Each indicator is adjusted uniquely, initially including identified patient factors as potential independent variables in the model. Only those factors contributing particular weighted contributions are included in the final risk model. A variety of goodness-of-fit tests are utilized to evaluate the resulting model. Each model is reevaluated every quarter. Details of the models are provided as an appendix to every quarterly report.

An example of a prototype control chart and comparison chart for low birthweight is displayed in Figure 1. The control chart shows variation in a process within one organization over time. Particular patterns on control charts may reflect out-of-control processes that should be investigated. The comparison chart plots the organization's *observed* quarterly rate (the dot) on the 95 percent confidence interval of the *predicted* quarterly rate (the middle cross bar). In this example, the organization's performance would be interpreted as variable, although still within the 95 percent confidence interval most of the time. Examination of care processes could be conducted to gain understanding as to the reason(s) for fluctuating rates.

Figure 1. IMSystem Indicator: Live Born Infants With a Birthweight of Less Than 2,500 Grams

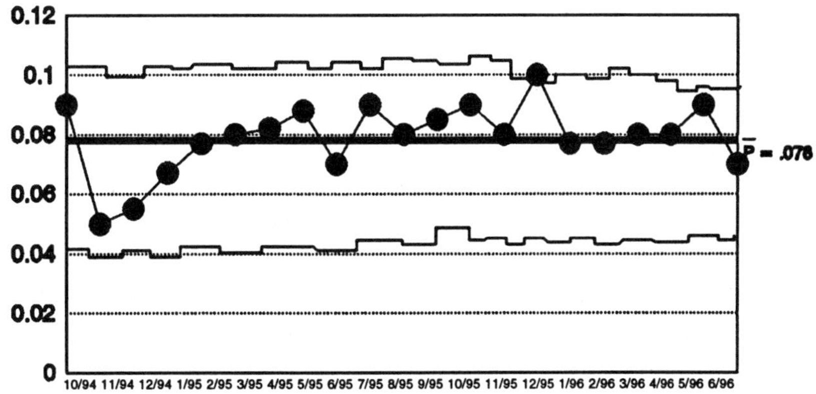

Subgroup Sizes: Min n=262 Max n=374

Comparison Chart

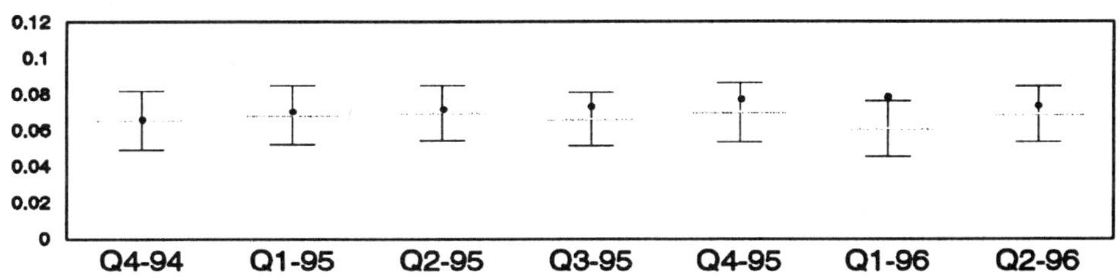

Evaluating Extant Measurement Systems

Accurate, fair, and consistent use of measurement data for accreditation purposes requires that there be representative indices of the health care services provided by each organization, including the use of appropriate methods to account and adjust for differences in their specific patient populations. Conversely, since organizations differ in size and other characteristics, a functional measurement strategy also must offer health care organizations flexibility and choices among the measures to be applied that are, or can be, tailored to their unique needs. Despite the practical challenges posed by the foregoing objectives, the Joint Commission remains committed to the integration of performance measures, including outcomes, into the future accreditation process. Inherent in this plan was the contemplated use of the Joint Commission's IMSystem as the standardized measurement tool in the accreditation process. This had the obvious advantage of allowing for reasonable comparisons among all health care organizations using the same system. During the course of development and testing of the IMSystem, considerable evolution had occurred in the health care environment.

In early 1995, recognizing the diversity of measurement systems now being used by health care organizations, the need to reduce duplicative measurement requirements, and the lack of flexibility inherent in mandating all organizations to use the same system, the Joint Commission's board of commissioners decided to permit accredited organizations to choose a measurement system from among a group of acceptable systems rather than require all accredited organizations to use the IMSystem. Obviously, this required a broader and more collaborative approach to the use of performance measures and measurement systems than that originally contemplated. To make this approach viable, several competing goals must be balanced appropriately. Successful incorporation into the accreditation process of multiple performance measurement systems depends on effectively balancing the potentially competing interests of utilizing a variety of potential measurement systems against the need to preserve the integrity of the accreditation process. Requiring each potential collaborating system to meet stringent participation requirements from the outset could effectively curtail the opportunity for some innovative systems to take part. On the other hand, incorporating performance measurement systems into the accreditation process without ensuring that they are capable of providing useful and relevant data might damage the credibility of the accreditation process itself. To help adjudicate this process, the Executive Committee of the Joint Commission's board of commissioners appointed an expert Council on Performance Measurement in 1995. The Council now serves as an advisory body to the Joint Commission for evaluating performance measurement systems with respect to their intrinsic qualities, and for the evaluation and selection of measurement systems that will be eligible for incorporation into the future accreditation process. The Council was charged with identifying the specific criteria against which candidate performance measurement systems would be evaluated, determining which systems meet the agreed-upon criteria, and reevaluating inclusion and exclusion criteria on a regular basis.

To build an effective and efficient measurement structure without imposing undue burden on accredited organizations, the Joint Commission now intends to integrate a group of acceptable existing measurement systems into its accreditation process under a single performance measurement umbrella. To successfully implement this initiative, performance measurement will be incorporated into the accreditation process in a way that upholds the integrity of the accreditation process by requiring all measurement data to be accurate, valid, comparable, and useful for performance improvement purposes; provides the opportunity for broad participation by existing measurement systems; allows reasonable time for measurement systems, the Joint Commission, and accredited organizations to adjust to the introduction of measurement data into the accreditation process (i.e., small incremental steps will be identified and implemented); and offers a flexible framework of expectations for health care organizations. A principal tenet of this plan is the opportunity for each accredited health care organization to select an appropriate measurement system from among a group of approved systems. Within each measurement system, further choice will be afforded to accredited organizations in the selection of indicators that are applicable to their specific services and best meet their needs.

FRAMEWORK FOR THE SELECTION OF PERFORMANCE MEASUREMENT SYSTEMS

The Joint Commission defines a performance measurement system as an interrelated set of process measures, outcome measures, or both that facilitates internal comparisons over time and external comparisons of an organization's performance. It is anticipated that performance measurement systems will meet the Joint Commission's needs by supplying comparative data from their participating organizations that can be incorporated into the survey and accreditation decision process and used to monitor an accredited organization's performance between onsite surveys. Obviously, to integrate disparate measurement systems into the accreditation process, a fair and effective method for identifying measurement systems that meets Joint Commission accreditation needs is required. That is, regardless of the purpose for which a measurement system might have been developed, it must be impartially assessed against established criteria by qualified evaluators for its potential usefulness in accreditation. As part of this process, each candidate measurement system is evaluated by the Council on Performance Measurement against designated "Attributes of Conformance" and related review criteria. As identified by the Council, these attributes relate to database capability, quality of performance measures, data quality, risk adjustment and stratification, performance measure-related feedback to participating organizations, and relevance to the accreditation process. The Council, however, recognizes that the art and science of performance measurement is a rapidly evolving field and innovation is the cornerstone of that evolution. In an effort to foster innovation, the Council evaluates candidate systems based on both the letter and spirit of the "Attributes of Conformance" and related criteria.

As recommended by the Council, the original draft of the "Attributes of Conformance" was released for public comment in early 1996. Public comment was solicited as an opportunity to inform candidate measurement systems about initial and long-term expectations of the Joint Commission and to assure all key stakeholders of the opportunity for input into the process. This call for comments included publication of the attributes in the *Journal of the American Medical Association*.[8] Although the majority of responses received from the field were supportive of the delineation established by the Council, responses reflected the obvious political, economic, and scientific realities of the barriers to performance measurement in health care noted earlier. While many were in agreement with the stated timeframes, some pointed to concerns related to stringency of the timeframes, dependency on automation, and issues related to resource requirements associated with the collection of measurement data. One common theme that emerged was the importance for any evaluation of extant performance measurement systems to be grounded in science and to be fair and defensible while not limiting innovation on the part of measurement systems.

Measurement systems are not expected to be fully prepared for integration into the accreditation process in the immediate future. However, systems with the eventual capability for meeting future accreditation requirements need to be identified quickly so that they can begin working with the Joint Commission to prepare for sharing measurement data that are accurate, valid, comparable, and useful in accreditation and performance improvement. With these needs in mind, a number of evaluation assumptions have been made by the Council on Performance Measurement. These include the understanding that the purpose of evaluation is to identify those systems having the potential to meet accreditation needs. Additional assumptions include the fact that the evaluation process will be based on compliance with current criteria; systems are evaluated against established criteria—not compared with each other; criteria are applied equally to all systems; initial evaluation is based on measurement system attributes rather than attributes of individual measures of performance; and future evaluation will be based on potential utility of specific measures of performance from within approved systems for use in accreditation. With these needs in mind, some criteria have been designated as requiring immediate compliance and are being used to identify early those systems with the potential to meet future accreditation needs. Other criteria have been slated for future compliance and will provide viable measurement systems with the direction and time necessary to meet the needs of accreditation as specified by the established criteria. Systems will retain their approval status as long as they continue to meet established criteria. Annual update information will be requested by the Joint Commission to assure systems' ongoing applicability to the accreditation process.

The "Attributes of Conformance" and associated review criteria are summarized as follows:

1. **Performance measures and data elements**: the system contains performance measures focusing on processes and/or outcomes related to patient care and/or organizational performance (immediate compliance); the system collects and stores (or has access to) data at the level of individuals (future compliance); procedures and/or algorthims are documented (future compliance).
2. **Database**: the system has a documented objective that describes its intent or purpose and one or more automated databases are present that are operational; are able to supply ongoing, longitudinal data; can link specific health care organizations with their respective data; and can support intraorganizational and intrasystem comparisons of performance measure data (immediate compliance).
3. **Data quality**: the measurement system regularly audits the accuracy and completeness of performance measurement data received from participating health care organizations (immediate compliance);

methods have been implemented for incorporating the results of data quality monitoring into continuous improvements in data quality (future compliance); mechanisms are available for the education/training of relevant staff at participating organizations (immediate compliance); data quality is monitored continuously at the individual participant level (future compliance).

4. **Risk adjustment/stratification for patient factors**: rationale is provided to account for those measures that are risk adjusted/stratified and for those measures that are not risk adjusted/stratified (immediate compliance); measures with denominators composed of individual-level data are risk adjusted/stratified with a unique model tailored to the specific measures (future compliance).
5. **Performance measure-related feedback**: actively participating health care organizations are provided access to comparative (interorganizational) performance measure-related feedback by the measurement system at least once per year (immediate compliance); education and data interpretation resources are made available by the measurement system to participating health care organizations (immediate compliance).
6. **Relevance for accreditation**: the measurement system demonstrates face validity of its measures including expert review and evidence of clinical and/or organizational relevance (immediate compliance); measures are reviewed by the system to ensure accurate and consistent identification of events they were designed to identify across multiple settings (immediate compliance); system is large enough to provide meaningful intrasystem comparative analysis (future compliance); system assists Joint Commission with conducting evaluative studies designed to demonstrate utility and relevance to accreditation (future compliance).

Development of a Data Collection Tool

Inherent in conducting an objective evaluation of extant measurement systems is the requirement to gather detailed information from candidate systems having varying levels of sophistication using a standardized data collection tool. Several important considerations were identified in devising survey tools to be pilot tested. These included the need for simplicity, obviating the perception of an undue data collection burden on measurement systems, identification of critical Joint Commission information needs, and assuring the ability to correlate the information received with anticipated evaluation requirements. Toward that end, the Council on Performance Measurement considered several alternative data collection strategies and approaches and derived several prototype data collection instruments, each of which was extensively field tested to assess utility. Tested were protocols for processing incoming information from measurement systems;

processes for communicating with systems in order to complete, clarify, or validate the accuracy of information submitted; the degree to which responses on the data collection forms enable evaluators to determine whether measurement systems meet compliance requirements; and the extent to which multiple evaluators come to the same conclusions regarding system compliance on individual components (i.e., interrater reliability).

Given the type and depth of information needed to evaluate each attribute and review criterion and the resource requirements of the various methods, the most reasonable data collection approach included a combination of mailed survey tools with telephone follow-up as needed. The final data collection tool includes separate sections reflecting demographic information and those data elements necessary to develop a robust system profile for use in assessing the potential utility of a given system to the accreditation process. At the currrent stage of evaluation, information bearing upon individual measures of performance within the system is collected only on the basis of the sampling of five measures.

As of late 1996, initial screening evaluations have been completed on 71 candidate measurement systems, the vast majority of which, on the basis of self-reported data, appear to meet the preliminary requirements. It is important to note that systems are being compared against established criteria and not against each other. Recommendations relative to which systems meet initial screening are made by the Council on Performance Measurement for transmission to the Joint Commission's board of commissioners for action. The first group of approved systems will be announced in early 1997.

ACCREDITATION AND PERFORMANCE MEASUREMENT INTEGRATION

The Joint Commission's evaluation of health care organizations has been grounded on the premise that the predictability of good outcomes can be based on the assessment of compliance with established performance-based standards. Thus, the current accreditation decision is based exclusively on compliance with existing standards. Standards typically describe structures and processes associated with important organizational and clinical functions. Compliance with standards is assessed at least triennially through an onsite survey conducted by intensively trained health care professionals. Additional surveys are conducted to either follow up on problems identified during the triennial survey or as a result of for-cause or random unannounced surveys. To date, measured results have not been included in evaluation activities.

Major reengineering described above has successfully improved the accreditation process—making it more objective and consistent across surveyors, more timely in terms of the accreditation decision, and more focused on performance. The next step in this reengineering project is to design and implement a more continuous accreditation process that includes both standards *and* performance measures (indicators and outcome measures) as complementary parts of the evaluation of health care organization performance. A continuous process inclusive of the results of care will more thoroughly assess an organization's current level of actual performance and more powerfully predict its future performance. To achieve this continuous accreditation process, the Joint Commission soon will require the periodic submission of performance measurement data by health care organizations seeking accreditation. Performance measurement data will be used to identify and assist the health care organization to improve care processes, to verify effectiveness of action and improvement initiatives, to shape the onsite triennial survey, and to improve and refine the standards.

As specific plans for integrating performance data were designed, key priorities for attaining the goal were outlined to include: (1) practicality and affordability for accredited organizations and the Joint Commission and (2) enhanced objectivity of the survey and accreditation process.

The inclusion of several approved systems, as described above, will provide the flexibility and choice to health care organizations, presumably building an effective measurement structure without imposing an undue burden on accredited organizations. Initially, accredited hospitals and long term care organizations will be expected to select a measurement system from among those listed as meeting the initial criteria and measures from within the selected system for use in the Joint Commission accreditation process. The measurement system selected by the organization will send the accredited organization's summary data, as well as system-level data, to the Joint Commission according to established frequencies and specifications. Maintaining system cohorts, the Joint Commission will review organization performance as compared to other organizations using the same measure from the same system. Trends and patterns of performance will prompt communication from the Joint Commission to the accredited organization, focusing primarily on the organization's understanding of its performance and plans for improvement.

Health care networks seeking Joint Commission accreditation already are expected to measure the performance of several functions. Performance improvement standards state that the network continuously measures important processes. Inherent within this overall standard are several specific standards that address areas in which performance measurement is particularly relevant. These include: the network continuously measures access to, and appropriateness of, care and services; continuing measurement of processes yields outcome data related to prevention, physiological function, functional status, and physical and psychological comfort of members; the network continuously measures member entry, assessment, and treatment processes; the network continuously measures processes related to the movement of members among network components and practitioner sites; the network continuously measures processes associated with important adverse clinical events; the network continuously measures preventive services and health promotion programs to evaluate their effectiveness; and the network continuously measures the use of clinical resources.

Health plans also are required to consider the performance of components. In the near future, all health plans accredited by the Joint Commission will be expected to use measures from a Joint Commission-approved set of measures. This is likely to include most of the measures contained within contemporary, consensus-driven measure sets such as those developed by the Foundation for Accountability (FACCT), the National Committee for Quality Assurance (HEDIS 3.0), the Joint Commission's Indicator Measurement System, the University of Wisconsin measures for long term care (MDS), and those developed at the University of Colorado for use in the home care environment (OASIS). In addition, increased review of component-level performance measurement data is anticipated.

CONCLUSIONS AND FUTURE PLANS

As the health care environment continues to mandate greater accountability, the importance of scientifically-based performance measurement activities will escalate. Practitioners, purchasers, providers, payers, and consumers all will depend on the availability of valid, useful information to make various decisions about the quality of care provided. Market forces are likely to be an important means by which greater standardization will occur within the performance measurement arena.

Since 1994, the Joint Commission has made performance reports based on standards compliance information available to the public. These reports include specific scores and national comparisons in areas relating each of the Joint Commission's standards. General information concerning accreditation and the accreditation process also is currently available to assist health care consumers through the Joint Commission's site on the World Wide Web (www.jcaho.org). Beginning in 1998, organization-specific performance reports also will be made available via the Web site.

Over the course of time, the performance measurement initiatives described here will coalesce to support a flexible process through which health care organizations seeking accreditation periodically will submit valid and reliable data to the Joint Commission. In turn, the Joint Commission will utilize the data to monitor the organization's actual level of performance and assist the organization in internal improvement activities. These same data, presented in a consumer-friendly format, also are likely to be an important means by which health care consumers can gain information bearing upon specific outcomes of interest to be used for decisionmaking purposes. It is important to realize that the "report card" movement in health care is still early in its evolution. However, the era of accountability is here, and perfection, while certainly a sound ideal, should not be viewed as the enemy of the good.

REFERENCES

1. Schyve P. "Models for relating performance measurement and accreditation," *International Journal of Health Planning and Management* 10: 231-241, 1995.
2. O'Leary DS. "Relating autopsy requirements to the contemporary accreditation process," *Archives of Pathology and Laboratory Medicine* 120: 763-766, 1996.
3. Loeb JM and O'Leary DS. "A call for collaboration in performance measurement," *Journal of the American Medical Association* 273: 1405, 1995.
4. *Ibid.*
5. Blumenthal D. "Quality of Care—What Is It?" *New England Journal of Medicine* 335: 891-894, 1996.
6. O'Leary DS, Nadzam DM, Loeb JM, and Jessee WF. "Framework for performance measurement of health care networks and health plans," *Managed Care Quarterly* 3: 48-53, 1995.
7. *Ibid.*
8. Loeb JM and Buck AS. "Framework for the evaluation of performance measurement systems: Attributes of conformance," *Journal of the American Medical Association* 275: 508, 1996.

Chapter 4

The Medical Outcomes Trust

Advancing the Science And Practice of Health Outcomes Measurement

Lyn Paget and Alvin Tarlov, MD

The Medical Outcomes Trust is a not-for-profit public service organization whose central mission is to advance the science and use of instruments for measuring health and the outcomes of health care from the patient's perspective. The Trust strives to accomplish this mission by promoting the use of standardized questionnaires completed by patients on one's health status, satisfaction with health care, and health-related quality of life. By serving as a clearinghouse for information about health outcomes and providing resources and education to promote the appropriate use of the questionnaires, the Trust supports the efforts taking place in all sectors of the health care delivery system. Researchers, clinicians, quality professionals, and managers who are involved in initiatives that include patient-based measures of health outcomes seek services through the Trust and form professional collaborations through the Trust's membership program. Principal services provided by the Trust include the distribution of instruments and publications, member services, conferences, and education.

The Trust, based in the United States and headquartered in Boston MA, is freestanding and not affiliated with any other organization. It commenced operations in June 1994 following receipt of a three-year grant for operations provided by the Henry J. Kaiser Family Foundation. The Trust is governed by a board of trustees and has a current staff of four full-time employees.

The goal of the Medical Outcomes Trust is to foster widespread adoption of health outcomes assessment in health care to improve the value of health care services. Its objectives are based on the following underlying principle: adoption of health outcomes measurement, monitoring, and management strategies and integration of these strategies into quality improvement systems offer the best opportunity to enhance health care services and to achieve the full value of those services. The Trust has five objectives:

1. Assure the development of high-quality **instruments** to measure health outcomes;
2. Assure the widespread **availability** of a comprehensive library of instruments to measure health outcomes;
3. Facilitate **standardization** of health outcomes measures;
4. Advance **applications technology** for ease of use and interpretation and for greater practical value in everyday medical practice; and

5. **Integrate** outcomes measurement with appropriateness, practice guidelines, and utility information (patient preferences) in systems of quality improvement.

The nine-member board of trustees (see box previous page) is chaired by Walter J. McNerney, former president of Blue Cross Blue Shield and current professor of health policy, J.L. Kellogg Graduate School of Management, Northwestern University.

SCIENTIFIC STANDARDS AND INSTRUMENT DISTRIBUTION

In the Trust's first year of operation, the board of trustees appointed an international Scientific Advisory Committee (SAC) to serve as an independent advisory group to the board and staff of the Medical Outcomes Trust. This six-member committee is responsible for the review of each instrument that is under consideration for placement in the Trust. Members of the Scientific Advisory Committee represent a cadre of esteemed professionals in outcomes measurement, health care quality, psychometrics, and measurement research (see box). The Committee's chairman is Edward B. Perrin, PhD, former director of the U.S. National Center for Health Statistics.

Scientific Advisory Committee

Edward B. Perrin, PhD
Chairman, Professor in the Department of Health Services, University of Washington

Neil K. Aaronson, PhD
Head, Division of Psychosocial Research and Epidemiology, the Netherlands Cancer Institute

Jordi Alonso, MD, PhD
Scientist, Health Services Research Unit, Institut Municipal d'Investigacio Medica, Barcelona

Audrey Burnam, PhD
Senior Behavioral Scientist, the RAND Corporation

Kathleen N. Lohr, PhD
Program Director, Health Services and Policy Research, Research Triangle Institute

Donald Patrick, PhD, MSPH
Professor, Department of Health Services, University of Washington

The SAC's initial task was to develop criteria by which this review could take place. These criteria were developed in 1995 through a group consensus process; before release by the Trust, the draft criteria were disseminated to 12 peer reviewers to solicit input for clarification and improvement.

EVALUATION OF HEALTH OUTCOMES INSTRUMENTS

The SAC of the Medical Outcomes Trust identified eight instrument attributes to serve as the principal bases of their review. The relative importance of criteria for instrument review may differ depending on the intended use(s) and application(s) of the instrument. For instance, instruments may be intended to distinguish between two or more groups of patients or populations, to assess change over time on an individual basis or at a group level, or to predict future health-related events. Also, instruments may be intended to be used in research (i.e., clinical trials) or in health care delivery.

The properties of an instrument are context specific. An instrument that works well for one purpose or in one setting or population may not do so well when applied for another purpose or in another setting or population. Ideally, one would want to have evidence of the measurement properties of an instrument for each of its intended applications.

CONCEPTUAL AND MEASUREMENT MODEL

Definition

A conceptual model is a rationale for and description of the concept(s) that the measure is intended to assess and the relationship between those concepts. A measurement model is defined as an instrument's scale and subscale structure and the procedures followed to create scale and subscale scores. The adequacy of the measurement model can be evaluated by examining evidence that: (1) a scale measures a single conceptual domain or construct; (2) multiple scales measure distinct domains; (3) variability in the domain is adequately represented by the scale; and (4) the intended level of measurement of the scale and its scoring procedures are well-justified.

Review Criteria

1. The conceptual and empirical basis for combining multiple items into a single scale score and/or multiple scale scores should be provided. This might include information on factor structure, distinctiveness of multiple scales, and internal consistency of scales as generated by methods such as factor analysis and Rasch or structural equation modeling.
2. Descriptive statistics for each scale should be provided, including information on central tendency and dispersion, skewness, and frequency of missing data. Any other evidence that the scale demonstrates adequate variability in a range that is relevant to its intended use should be provided.
3. A description of the intended level of measurement—for example, ordinal, interval, or ratio scales—should be provided, along with available supportive evidence. For preference-weighted measures, a rationale and evidence supporting scaling assumptions should be provided.
4. Procedures for deriving scale scores from raw scores should be clearly specified and a clear description of and rationale for transformations (such as weighting and standardization) should be provided.

RELIABILITY

Definition

The principal definition of test reliability is the degree to which an instrument is free from random error. This succinct definition implies homogeneity of content on multi-item tests and internal consistency (i.e., high correlations) among test items. The two approaches recommended for examining test reliability are coefficient α (Cronbach's alpha) and alternative form correlations. Because the latter approach is seldom used in health status assessment, the coefficient α can be considered the most relevant approach to reliability estimation.

A second definition of reliability is reproducibility or stability of an instrument over time (test-retest) and interrater agreement at one point in time. The two definitions are largely independent of one another.

1. **Internal Consistency:** Coefficient α provides an estimate of reliability based on all possible correlations between two sets of items within a test. For instruments employing dichotomous response choices, an alternative formula, the Kuder-Richardson formula 20 (KR-20), is available.
2. **Reproducibility**

- Test-retest reproducibility: Test-retest reproducibility is the degree to which an instrument yields stable scores over time among respondents who are assumed not to have changed on the domains being assessed. The influence of test administration on the second administration may overestimate reliability. Conversely, variations in health, learning, reaction, or regression to the mean may yield test-retest data underestimating reliability. Despite these cautions, information on test-retest reproducibility data is important for the evaluation of the instrument.
    - Inter-observer (interviewer) reproducibility: For instruments administered by an interviewer, test-retest reproducibility may refer to both intra-observer and inter-observer agreement.

Review Criteria

1. Reliability estimates and standard errors should be reported for all elements of an instrument, including the total score and subscale scores, where appropriate.
2. A clear description should be provided of the methods employed to collect reliability data. This should include (a) methods of sample accrual and sample size; (b) characteristics of the sample (e.g., sociodemographics, clinical characteristics if drawn from a patient population, etc.); (c) the testing conditions (i.e., where and how the

instrument of interest was administered); and (d) descriptive statistics for the instrument under study (i.e., means, standard deviations, floor and ceiling effects, etc.).

3. Where there are reasons to believe that reliability estimates or standard errors of measurement will differ substantially for the various populations in which an instrument is to be used, these data should be presented for each major population of interest (e.g., different chronic disease populations, different language or cultural groups, etc.).
4. Test-retest reproducibility information should be provided as a complement to, not as a substitute for, internal consistency. Reproducibility is more important when repeated measures with the instrument are proposed.
5. A well-argued rationale should support the time elapsed between first and second administration as well as the design of the study to ensure that changes in health status were minimal, i.e., including transitional questions on general and specific health or functional status.
6. Information about test and retest scores should include the appropriate central tendency and dispersion measures of both test and retest administrations.
7. For instruments yielding interval-level data, information on test-retest reliability (reproducibility) and interrater reliability should include intraclass correlation coefficients (ICC). For nominal or ordinal scale values, kappa and weighted kappa, respectively, are recommended.
8. Commonly accepted minimal standards for reliability coefficients are 0.7 for group comparisons and 0.90-0.95 for individual comparisons.

VALIDITY

Definition

The validity of an instrument is defined as the degree to which the instrument measures what it purports to measure. There are three ways of accumulating evidence for the validity of an instrument:

1. **Content-related:** evidence that the content domain of an instrument is appropriate relative to its intended use. Methods commonly used to obtain evidence about content-related validity include the use of lay and expert panel judgments of the clarity, comprehensiveness, and redundancy of items and scales of an instrument.
2. **Construct-related:** evidence that supports a proposed interpretation of scores on the instrument based on theoretical implications associ-

ated with the constructs. Common methods to obtain construct-related validity include an examination of the logical relations that should exist with other measures and/or patterns of scores across groups of individuals.

3. **Criterion-related:** evidence that shows the extent to which scores of the instrument are related to a criterion measure. Criterion measures are measures of the target construct that are widely accepted, valid measures of that construct. In the area of health status assessment, criterion-related validity is rarely tested because of the absence of widely accepted criterion measures.

Review Criteria

1. Evidence of content validity should be presented for every major use proposed of the instrument. Information about the methods for developing the content of the instrument should be provided.
2. Evidence of construct validity should be presented for every major use proposed of the instrument. When data related to criterion validity are presented, a clear rationale and support for the choice of criteria measures should be stated. A rationale should be provided to support the particular mix of evidence presented for the intended uses.
3. A clear description should be provided of the methods employed to collect validity data. This should include (a) methods of sample accrual and sample size; (b) characteristics of the sample (e.g., sociodemographics, clinical characteristics if drawn from a patient population, etc.); (c) the testing conditions (i.e., where and how the instrument of interest was administered); and (d) descriptive statistics for the instrument under study (i.e., means, standard deviations, floor and ceiling effects, etc.).
4. The composition of the validation sample should be described in sufficient detail to make clear the population(s) to which it applies. Available data on selective factors that might reasonably be expected to influence validity, such as gender, age, ethnicity, and language, should be described.
5. Where there are reasons to believe that validity will differ substantially for the various populations in which an instrument is to be used, these data should be presented for each major population of interest (e.g., different chronic disease populations, different language or cultural groups, etc.).

RESPONSIVENESS

Definition

Sometimes referred to as sensitivity to change, responsiveness is viewed as an important part of the construct validation process. Responsiveness refers to an instrument's ability to detect change, often defined as the minimal change considered to be important by the persons with the health condition, their significant others, or their providers. The criterion of responsiveness requires asking whether the measure can detect differences in outcomes that are important, even if those differences are small. Responsiveness also can be conceptualized as the ratio of a signal (the real change over time that has occurred) to the noise (the variability in scores seen over time, which is not associated with true change in status).

Common methods of evaluating responsiveness include comparing scale scores before and after an intervention that is expected to affect the construct, and comparing changes in scale scores with changes in other related measures that are assumed to move in the same direction as the target measure.

Assessment of responsiveness often involves estimation of the effect size. Effect size is an estimate of the magnitude of change in health status. Effect size translates the before-and-after changes into a standard unit of measurement. Different methods may be used to calculate effect size. Interpretation of effects is discussed in the next section.

Review Criteria

1. For any claim that an instrument is responsive, evidence should be provided on the change scores found in field tests of the instrument. These change scores should expressed ideally as effect sizes, with information provided on the methods used to calculate the effect size.
2. Claims for an instrument's responsiveness should be derived from longitudinal data, preferably comparing a group that is expected to change with a group that is expected to remain stable.
3. The population(s) on which responsiveness has been tested should be clearly identified including the time intervals of assessment, the interventions or measures involved in evaluating change, and the populations assumed to be stable.

INTERPRETABILITY

Definition

Interpretability is defined as the degree to which one can assign qualitative meaning to an instrument's quantitative scores. Interpretability of a measure is facilitated by information that translates a quantitative score or change in scores to a qualitative category that has clinical or commonly understood meaning.

There are several types of information that can aid in the interpretation of scores:

1. comparative data on the distribution of scores derived from a variety of defined population groups, including, when possible, a representative sample of the general population;
2. information on the relationship of scores to clinically-recognized conditions or need for specific treatments;
3. information on the relationship of scores or changes in scores to commonly recognized life events (such as the impact of losing a job); and
4. information on how well scores predict known relevant events (such as death or need for institutional care).

Review Criteria

1. A clear description should be provided of the rationale for selection of populations for purposes of comparison and interpretability of data. This should include (a) methods of sample accrual and sample size; (b) characteristics of the sample (e.g., sociodemographics, clinical characteristics if drawn from a patient population, etc.); (c) the testing conditions (i.e., where and how the instrument of interest was administered); and (d) descriptive statistics for the instrument under study (i.e., means, standard deviations, floor and ceiling effects, etc.).
2. Provide any information regarding various ways in which the data have been reported and displayed in order to facilitate interpretation.

BURDEN

Definition

Respondent burden is defined as the time, energy, and other demands placed on those to whom the instrument is administered. Administrative burden is defined as the demands placed on those who administer the instrument.

Review Criteria: Respondent Burden

1. Evidence should be provided that the instrument places no undue physical or emotional strain on the respondent. Developers should indicate when or under what circumstances their instrument is not suitable for respondents.

2. Information should be provided on the average and range of time needed to complete the instrument on a self-administered basis or as an interviewer-administered instrument for all population groups for which the instrument is intended.
3. Information should be provided about the reading and comprehension level assumed for all population groups for which the instrument is intended.
4. Information should be provided about any special requirements or requests that might be placed on respondents, such as the need to consult health care records or copy information about medications used.
5. Information should be provided on the acceptability of the instrument, for example, by indicating the level of missing data and refusal rates and the reasons for both.

Review Criteria: Administrative Burden

1. For interviewer-administered instruments, information should be provided on the average time and range of time required of a trained interviewer to administer the instrument. If appropriate (e.g., if the times differ significantly), the information should be given for face-to-face interview, telephone, and computer-assisted formats/applications.
2. Information should be provided on the amount of training and level of education or professional expertise and experience needed by administrative staff to administer, score, or otherwise use the instrument.
3. Information should be provided about any resources required for administration of the instrument, such as the need for special or specific computer hardware or software to administer, score, or analyze the instrument.

ALTERNATIVE FORMS

Definition

Alternative forms of an instrument include all modes of administration other than the original source instrument. Depending on the nature of the original source instrument, alternative forms can include self-administered self report, interviewer-administered self report, trained observer rating, computer-assisted self report, computer-assisted interviewer-administered, and performance-based measures. In addition, alternative forms may include proxy versions of the original source instrument such as self-administered proxy report and interviewer-administered proxy report.

Review Criteria

Alternative forms of an instrument will be evaluated employing the same criteria used for the original source instrument. This will include evidence of reliability, validity, responsiveness, interpretability, and burden. An additional criterion for evaluation of alternative forms will be comparability with the original instrument.

CULTURAL AND LANGUAGE ADAPTATIONS

Definition

The crosscultural adaptation of an instrument involves two primary steps: (1) assessment of conceptual and linguistic equivalence and (2) evaluation of measurement properties. Conceptual equivalence refers to equivalence in relevance and meaning of the same concepts being measured in different cultures and/or languages. Linguistic equivalence refers to equivalence of question wording and meaning in the formulation of items, response choices, and all aspects of the instrument and its applications. For evaluation of measurement properties, each cultural and/or language adaptation will be reviewed separately by the Scientific Advisory Committee for evidence of reliability, validity, responsiveness, interpretability, and burden.

Review Criteria

1. Information about methods to achieve conceptual equivalence should be provided. It is commonly recommended that the content validity of the instrument be assessed in each cultural or language group to which the instrument is to be applied.
2. Information about methods to achieve linguistic equivalence should be provided. It is commonly recommended that there should be: (a) at least two forward translations from the source language, preferably by persons experienced in translations and in health status research. This should result in a pooled forward translation; (b) at least one, preferably more, backward translations to the source language that results in another pooled translation; (c) a review of translated versions by lay and expert panels with revisions; and (d) field tests to provide evidence of comparability.
3. Any significant differences between the original and translated versions should be identified and explained.

INSTRUMENTS PLACED IN THE TRUST

Instrument submissions are reviewed by the SAC four times each year. Reports of the reviews are forwarded to officers of the Trust who report the recommendations to the board of trustees. The board grants final approval for all instruments to be distributed by the Trust.

Each instrument packet distributed by the Trust contains copies of the questionnaire(s), scoring instructions, a bibliography, interpretation guidelines, and several reprints of publications that describe the instrument's development and intended uses. The following section describes the instruments that have been recommended by the SAC and approved by the board for distribution by the Trust.

Descriptions of Instruments Available

London Handicap Scale

The London Handicap Scale is a six-item questionnaire developed to measure an aspect of health status in groups of patients with chronic, multiple, or progressive diseases. The term "handicap" is used in a technical sense, slightly different from its everyday meaning. Handicap is defined as the disadvantage experienced by an individual resulting from ill health compared with what is normal for someone of the same age, sex, and background. It takes into account the physical and psychological effects of disease or combinations of diseases and relevant nonhealth factors such as the physical and social environment. It also takes into account the effects of health service interventions acting at various levels: curing disease, relieving or palliating symptoms, reducing disabilities, and modifying the environment.

The instrument generates a profile of handicaps on six different dimensions as well as an overall handicap severity score. The dimensions are mobility (getting around), physical independence (looking after oneself), occupation (work or leisure), social integration, orientation (awareness of surroundings), and economic self-sufficiency. Each dimension has six levels, arranged in order of increasing disadvantage. A respondent chooses which level most closely fits his or her situation. Together this information forms a descriptive profile of the individual. This profile can be converted into an overall severity score using a table of scale weights. This score gives an estimate of the relative desirability or "utility" of the particular combination of disadvantages.

The weights were calculated from studies of the opinions of representative populations. Strictly, they should only be applied when comparing groups of patients, and scores for any one individual will be an approximation to that individual's handicap. In most applications, this distinction makes little difference since the intention will be to describe the overall experience of groups of patients (such as users of a service, arms of a comparative trial, residents of a particular area, or patients with a particular diagnosis). It must be emphasized, however, that the scale is not primarily intended for assessing or monitoring individual patients, although the descriptive profile may be found useful.

The London Handicap Scale was designed with the needs of the randomized controlled trial in mind and for comparisons between different interventions for health policy purposes. However, it also will be of use in cross-sectional surveys and longitudinal or cohort studies either as an explanatory variable or as an outcomes variable.

The scale is suitable for adults of all ages. The particular issues of chronic disease, multiple pathologies, and the importance of environmental and social factors arise most frequently with elderly people for whom the scale should be particularly appropriate. It was not designed for use with children.

The principal developer of the London Handicap Scale is Rowan Harwood, MD, Department of Health Care of the Elderly, University Hospital, Nottingham, England.

MOS-HIV

The MOS-HIV is a brief, comprehensive health status measure based on items from the Medical Outcomes Study that has been used extensively in studies of HIV/AIDS since its development in 1987. The MOS-HIV was one of the first disease-targeted measures available for this population and is widely used in clinical trials and other research and evaluation studies. It has been shown to discriminate among groups of patients that differ clinically from one another, to predict future outcomes, and to be responsive to differences among groups and clinically important changes over time.

Development of the MOS-HIV was prompted by the need for a brief instrument for use in multicenter AIDS clinical trials. The dimensions represented in the SF-20 assessment were the starting point of the instrument. Additional concepts important in HIV/AIDS (energy/fatigue, cognitive functioning, health distress, and quality of life) were added from the MOS item pool to create a 30-item form. In a subsequent version of the MOS-HIV, five additional items were added to better assess general health perceptions and pain, and response choices for physical functioning and role functioning items were altered to reflect extent rather than duration of limitation.

The questionnaire contains 35 questions that measure 10 dimensions of health: general health perceptions, pain, physical functioning, role functioning, social functioning, energy/fatigue, mental health, health distress, cognitive function, and quality of life. A single item also is included to assess health transition. Subscales of the MOS-HIV are scored as summated rating scales on a 0-100 scale; higher scores indicate better health. In addition to these subscales, two summary scores can be generated: Physical Health Summary and Mental Health Summary scores. The instrument takes approximately five minutes to complete and can be self-administered or given as a face-to-face or telephone interview.

The principal developer of the MOS-HIV is Albert W. Wu, MD, MPH, Health Services Research and Development Center, Johns Hopkins University.

Quality of Well-Being Scale

The Quality of Well-Being Scale (QWB) is a comprehensive measure of health-related quality of life that includes several components administered through an interview. First, it obtains observable levels of functioning at a point in time (usually the previous six days) from three separate scales: mobility, physical activity, and social activity. These scales each contain a variety of items. For example, an item on the social activity scale asks, "On which, if any, of the past 6 days, including weekends, holidays and so on, did (you . . .work on a job at all?)" Second, each patient identifies their most undesirable symptom or problem from a list of 27 items. Then, the observed level of function and the subjective symptomatic complaint are weighted by preference, or the utility for the state, on a scale ranging from 0 (for dead) to 1.0 (for optimum function). The weights were obtained from independent samples of 56 judges, randomly selected from the general population, who rated the desirability of the observable health status.

Several studies have shown that the weights do not vary as a function of demographic variables, including race, income, and gender. Most evidence has shown that the weights do not vary systematically as a function of prior experience of the rated health state. Using this system, it is possible to place the general health status of any individual on the continuum between death and optimal functioning for any point in time. Combining point in time scores with information on duration of stay in state yields estimates of Quality Adjusted Life Years (QALYs). The QWB has been used in a wide variety of clinical and population studies.

In addition, the QWB scale has been used in clinical trials and studies to evaluate therapeutic interventions in a wide range of medical and surgical conditions. These include chronic obstructive pulmonary disease, AIDS, cystic fibrosis, diabetes mellitus, atrial fibrillation, lung transplantation, arthritis, cancer, sinus disease, and a wide variety of other conditions. Specific validity and reliability data are available in each disease area. In cystic fibrosis patients, for example, QWB scores have been shown to be positively correlated with pulmonary function and exercise tolerance, and negatively correlated with age. Further, the QWB was able to track improvement over time in a two-week intervention for treatment of pulmonary exacerbation, with changes in QWB statistically significantly correlated with changes in pulmonary function. The properties of the QWB have been evaluated in over 100 scientific publications.

The principal developers of the Quality of Well-Being Scale are Robert M. Kaplan, John P. Anderson, and Ted Ganiats from the University of California at San Diego.

The Seattle Angina Questionnaire

The Seattle Angina Questionnaire (SAQ) is a 19-item instrument developed to quantify five clinically relevant domains of coronary artery disease. Nine items define the limitations in patients' physical capacity due to symptoms of angina pectoris. Two items assess the frequency of anginal symptoms and an additional item defines whether a change in the precipitants of angina has occurred over the past month. Four items describe patients' satisfaction with the treatment of their coronary artery disease and three items explore how much patients' coronary artery disease has impacted their quality of life.

The SAQ has been used as an outcome measure in several ongoing clinical investigations. The Quality of Life in Angina Research Trial is a randomized study of once-daily vs. multidosing antianginal medications that has successfully employed serial administration of the SAQ to define the quality-of-life differences between these two strategies for treating patients with chronic stable angina. Similarly, the OPUS trial is comparing optimal angioplasty with intracoronary stenting to define the quality-of-life differences between these two strategies of percutaneous coronary revascularization.

A quality improvement initiative based in Washington state is using the SAQ to gain improved insight into the functional status outcomes of coronary bypass surgery. The CABG Outcomes Assessment Team is a physician-led effort in which a pilot project, representing almost all cardiothoracic surgery groups in Washington (12), prospectively enrolled up to 130 patients each into a study to quantify the baseline, six-month, and one-year functional status of their patients. In addition to describing the process of post-surgical recovery, the SAQ will be used to define differences in the patient selection and outcomes of each group in the state. This information then will be presented blindly to the entire surgical community and allow a process of reflection and discussion to better define how to select and manage patients with advanced coronary artery disease.

Another such project involves a "natural history" experiment in a Veterans' Affairs general internal medicine clinic. In this project a sample of 100 patients with stable coronary artery disease were enrolled in an angina clinic run by a nurse practitioner with telephone support from a cardiologist. The SAQ was able to document substantial improvements in symptom relief and quality of life in the patients enrolled in the angina clinic compared with the hundreds of patients in the general internal medicine clinic who did not receive additional management assistance from the nurse practitioner.

Since self-administered questionnaires can accurately describe important clinical information, they can be scored and tracked over time to plot the course of a patients' condition. In coronary artery disease, the progression of symptoms can often be insidious since patients modify their activities to minimize the frequency and severity of their symptoms. In general internal medicine clinics, when physicians need to attend to a wide variety of comorbid conditions, both the doctor and the patient may fail to recognize that the symptoms of coronary artery disease have worsened. A description of the clinical status of patients' coronary artery disease, as provided by the SAQ, may prove to be a valuable aid to generalist physicians who manage patients with coronary disease. An eight-center Veterans' Affairs trial has recently begun to test this hypothesis in 16 general internal medicine units.

The principal developer of the Seattle Angina Questionnaire is John Spertus, MD, MPH.

SF-36 Health Survey

The SF-36 Health Survey is a 36-item multipurpose, short-form (SF) survey of general health status. It was constructed to satisfy minimum psychometric standards necessary for group comparisons involving generic health concepts. The eight health concepts were selected from 40 included in the Medical Outcomes Study to represent those hypothesized to be most frequently measured in widely used health surveys and those most affected by disease and treatment.

The SF-36 is suitable for self-administration, computerized administration, or administration by a trained interviewer in person or by telephone, to persons age 14 and older. The SF-36 has been administered successfully in general population surveys in the United States and other countries as well as to young and old adult patients with specific diseases. It can be administered in five to 10 minutes with a high degree of acceptability and data quality.

The SF-36 includes one multidimensional scale measuring eight health concepts:

1. **Concept:** Physical functioning (10 items, 21 levels). **Low score**: limited a lot in performing all physical activities including bathing or dressing due to health. **High score**: performs all types of physical activities including the most vigorous without limitations due to health.
2. **Concept:** Role Functioning—Physical (4 items, 5 levels). **Low score**: problems with work or other daily activities as a result of physical health. **High score**: no problems with work or other daily activities as a result of physical health.
3. **Concept:** Bodily Pain (2 items, 11 levels). **Low score**: very severe and extremely limiting pain. **High score**: no pain or limitations due to pain.
4. **Concept:** General Health (5 items, 21 levels). **Low score**: evaluates personal health as poor and believes it is likely to get worse. **High score**: evaluates personal health as excellent.
5. **Concept:** Vitality (4 items, 21 levels). **Low score**: feels tired and worn out all the time. **High score**: feels full of pep and energy all of the time.
6. **Concept:** Social Functioning (2 items, 9 levels). **Low score**: extreme and frequent interference with normal social activities due to physical or emotional problems. **High score**: performs normal social activities without interference due to physical or emotional problems.
7. **Concept:** Role—Emotional (3 items, 4 levels). **Low score**: problems with work or other daily activities as a result of emotional problems. **High score**: no problems with work or other daily activities as a result of emotional problems.
8. **Concept:** Mental Health (5 items, 26 levels). **Low score**: feelings of nervousness and depression all of the time. **High score**: feels peaceful, happy, and calm all of the time.

An additional concept, measured by a single-item, also is included in the SF-36: Reported Health Transition (1 item, 5 levels). **Low score**: believes general health is much better now than one year ago. **High score**: believes general health is much worse now than one year ago.

The widespread use of the SF-36 in general population surveys, clinical trials, and clinical practice and standardization of measurement across studies is producing considerable information about norms and benchmarks useful in comparing "well" and "sick" populations and for estimating the burden of specific conditions.

Although many studies appear to rely on the SF-36 as the principal measure of health outcomes, it may be best to rely upon it as a "generic core" battery of measures serving the purpose of comparing results across studies and populations. Because it is short, the SF-36 can be reproduced in a questionnaire with ample room for other more precise general and specific measures.

The SF-36 Health Survey has been approved by the Trust in English (United States, Australia/New Zealand, Canada, and United Kingdom), German, Spanish, and Swedish.

The principal developer of the SF-36 Health Survey is John E. Ware, Jr., PhD, Senior Scientist, The Health Institute, New England Medical Center and Tufts University, Boston.

SF-12 Health Survey

The SF-12 is a multipurpose short-form generic measure of health status. It was developed to be a much shorter, yet valid, alternative to the SF-36 for use in large surveys of general and specific populations as well as large longitudinal studies of health outcomes.

The 12 items in the SF-12 are a subset of those in the SF-36; SF-12 includes one or two items from each of the eight health concepts. Thus, the SF-12 measures eight concepts commonly represented in widely used surveys: physical functioning, role limitations due to physical health problems, bodily pain, general health, vitality (energy/fatigue), social functioning, role limitations due to emotional problems, and mental health (psychological distress and psychological well being). Both standard (four-week) and acute (one-week) recall versions are available.

The goal for the SF-12 project was to develop a one-page, two-minute questionnaire module that would reproduce the SF-36 physical and mental health summary measures with at least 90 percent accuracy while representing all eight SF-36 health concepts with one or more questionnaire items.

The breakthrough discovery of the Physical Component Summary (PCS) and Mental Component Summary (MCS) scales based on the SF-36, which reduced the number of statistical comparisons required in analyzing SF-36 data from eight to two, paved the way for the SF-12. Ten items were identified from six of the eight SF-36 scales that reproduced at least 90 percent of the variance in both PCS and MCS, as defined using the SF-36 scales. The addition of two more items created a 12-item short form that yielded more than satisfactory estimates of the PCS and MCS and made it possible to reproduce the profile of eight SF-36 health concepts.

The SF-12 uses two items each to estimate scores for four of the eight health concepts (physical functioning, role-physical, role-emotional, and mental health). Scores for the remaining four health concepts (bodily pain, general health, vitality, and social functioning) are estimated using one item each. Results from empirical studies to date indicate that 12-item versions of PCS and MCS correlate very highly with the SF-36 versions.

The summary scales based on the SF-12 (PCS-12 and MCS-12) are based on fewer items, define fewer levels, and should be expected to yield less reliable assignments of individuals to those levels than the SF-36 based summary scales. For large group studies, these differences in precision are not as important because confidence intervals for group averages are largely determined by sample size.

The eight-concept profile based on SF-12 items (calibrated to reproduce the original SF-36 scales) appears to be very similar, on average, to the original SF-36 profile, although each score is estimated with less precision.

The SF-12 Health Survey represents another attempt to balance the number of questionnaire items against other important considerations that determine the usefulness of the resulting scores. The strategy of trying to predict summary measures for two clusters of substantially related SF-36 scales appears to have been successful with the SF-12. By pooling the reliable variance across physical and mental health measures, satisfactory reliability while reducing the number of items was achieved. By summarizing measures that previously have been shown to produce the same or very similar results, summary measures simplify the analysis of health outcomes while minimizing information loss.

The principal developer of the SF-12 Health Survey is John E. Ware Jr., PhD, Senior Scientist, The Health Institute, New England Medical Center and Tufts University, Boston.

Sickness Impact Profile

The Sickness Impact Profile (SIP) is a behaviorally based health status measure. It has been used extensively in clinical trials since its development in the 1970s. The SIP was one of the first measures of overall health available to researchers, and it continues to be widely applied as a health status measure that discriminates among groups with different levels of health and is sensitive to changes in health over time.

Development of the SIP was prompted by the observation that frequently used clinical measures were not always sensitive to patient reports of progress. It was hypothesized that individual behavior would be a more useful measure for assessing new treatments, evaluating health care programs, and measuring the health levels of a population. Thus, the SIP was developed to supplement clinical measures of health and may be used to:

- determine general health levels of a population;
- compare subgroups or populations;
- evaluate different treatments;
- measure changes over time related to specific diseases or disabling conditions; and
- evaluate alternative approaches to delivering services including interventions in organization, finance, manpower, and technology.

The instrument consists of 136 items that describe activities associated with everyday living. Each item is written in the first person and the present tense. The SIP can be either interview- or self-administered. Respondents are asked to endorse (i.e., reply "Yes" to an interviewer or place a check on a self-administered form) those items that they are sure describe them on that day and are related to their health. For example, a respondent is instructed to endorse the item "I sit during much of the day" if he sits for much of that day and if the reason for sitting so much is attributable to his health. If the respondent sits much of the day because he has a sedentary job, then the respondent would not endorse this item.

The SIP is scored according to the number and type of items that are endorsed. Each item is assigned a numeric scale value that reflects its degree of dysfunction. Higher scale values indicate greater dysfunction. An individual's total SIP score is computed by summing the scale values for the items that he endorses, dividing by the total possible score (if all items were endorsed), and multiplying by 100. The score is expressed as a percent and can range from 1 to 100 where 1 represents no dysfunction and 100 represents maximal dysfunction.

Table 1. Sample SIP Items

Category	Sample Item
Sleep and Rest	I sit during much of the day
Emotional Behavior	I act nervous or restless
Body Care and Movement	I change position frequently
Home Management	I am not doing any of the clothes washing that I usually do
Mobility	I am not going into town
Social Interaction	I am going out less to visit people
Ambulation	I walk more slowly
Alertness Behavior	I do not keep my attention on any activity for long
Communication	I don't write except to sign my name
Work	I am not working at all
Recreation and Pastimes	I am doing fewer community activities
Eating	I am eating much less than usual

Scoring is also possible at the level of categories and dimensions. The 136 items are aggregated into 12 categories that represent specific areas of activity. To score an individual category, the scale values for all endorsed items in that category are divided by the total possible score for the category and multiplied by 100. Four categories—emotional behavior, social interaction, alertness behavior, and communication—can be further aggregated into a psychosocial dimension. Three categories—body care and movement, mobility, and ambulation—define a physical dimension. Dimension scores are computed in the same manner as category and total scores.

The principal developers of the Sickness Impact Profile are the late Marilyn Bergner, PhD, and Betty Gilson, MD, Ruth Bobbit, PhD, and colleagues at the University of Washington.

FUTURE DIRECTIONS

The Trust is part of a very dynamic and exciting movement in health care. As it evolves as an organization, the Trust is committed to maintaining an open dialogue with researchers, clinicians, and managers in the field who help guide the services of the Trust and keep the focus on high-quality, high-value programs.

By keeping apprised and maintaining up-to-date information on major initiatives in the outcomes movement, such as those taking place at the American Medical Association, Foundation for Accountability, Health Care Financing Administration, Joint Commission on the Accreditation of Health Care Organizations, National Committee for Quality Assurance, and the several other institutions involved in moving the outcomes agenda forward, the Trust keeps individuals in the field connected with the bigger picture. The Trust extends an open invitation to all individuals and groups developing measures for health outcomes to submit these measures to the Scientific Advisory Committee for evaluation. Promoting standardization is an essential theme in the Trust's message.

In the months to come, the Trust plans to develop its educational agenda to encompass a broader array of customized courses for specific instruments and specific measurement objectives. The library of instruments will be expanded to include a greater selection of condition- or disease-specific instruments. Standards set forth by the Trust through the efforts of the Scientific Advisory Committee will evolve to include satisfaction instruments, instrument translations, and instruments that are developed using an item banking or item response technology. Publications and documents that provide well-organized and valuable information will continue to be a major focus for the Trust. In 1997, it is anticipated that over 1,000 professionals will be members of the Trust and these individuals and organizations will be an integral part of the future direction and evolution of the Medical Outcomes Trust.

Chapter 5

CONQUEST

In Search of a Few Good Performance Measures

Ann G. Lawthers and Heather Palmer

Performance measures increasingly are becoming important tools in the health care field, particularly for managed care organizations. Much of the interest in performance measurement stems from concerns that managed care may create incentives to undertreat in order to control costs.[1,2] Performance measures can help answer such questions as: "Are managed care plans restricting patient access to effective health care?"[3]

Interest in performance measurement also has received a boost from the activities of accrediting organizations such as the Joint Commission on Accreditation of Healthcare Organizations (JCAHO) and the National Committee for Quality Assurance (NCQA). In the late 1980s, the Joint Commission began an ambitious effort to design, test, and implement measures of quality that could be used in the hospital accrediting process.[4] The National Committee for Quality Assurance introduced its own set of performance measures, the Health Plan Employer Data and Information Set (HEDIS), Version 2.0, in late 1993.[5] By the end of 1996, Medicaid and Medicare had their own sets of HEDIS measures, HEDIS version 3.0 had been released,[6] and the Foundation for Accountability (FACCT) had issued the templates for five sets of measures.[7]

DEFINING PERFORMANCE MEASUREMENT

As interest in performance measurement has grown, so too has the linguistic confusion surrounding the term "performance measure." The authors define a performance measure as a tool to describe and evaluate the activities of a health care provider. Performance measures may be grouped by domains or aspects of performance. Some performance measures assess quality, others describe resources, and still others evaluate the financial performance of a health care provider. Outcomes are not a domain of performance; they are a type of data (e.g. structure, process, and outcome data).[8] Outcome data will be discussed in-depth later in the chapter. Figure 1 shows examples of domains of performance.

Figure 1. Examples of Domains of Performance With a Focus on the Domain of Quality

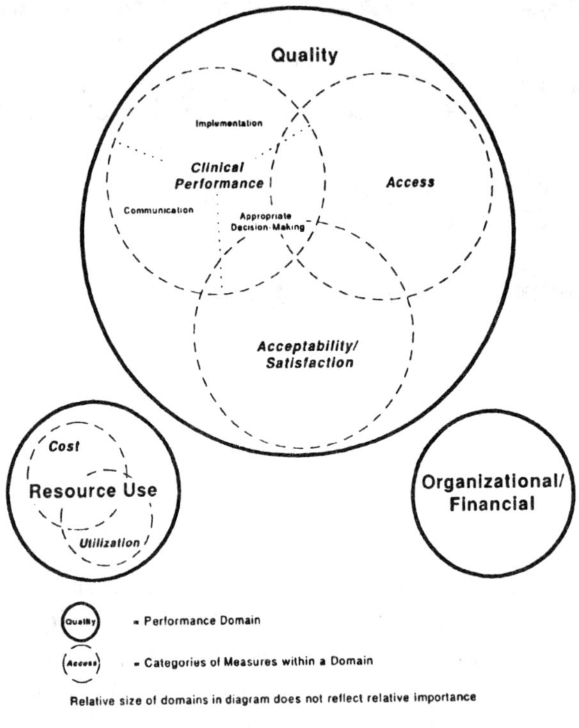

DEFINING QUALITY

This chapter is concerned only with measures from the performance domain of quality. But how do you define quality? The definition of quality varies according to who defines it—provider, patient, society, or government—but the definition also varies in its scope or breadth.[9] For example, the Institute of Medicine defines quality of care as:

> . . . the degree to which health services for individuals and populations increase the likelihood of desired health outcomes and are consistent with current professional knowledge.[10]

This definition links processes of care (health services) to outcomes of care, subject to consumer preferences (desired health outcomes) and current state-of-the art of medical practice.

To emphasize the importance of the patient perspective, another author adds "satisfaction" to the definition of quality: ". . .the production of improved health and satisfaction of a population."[11]

Others define quality by the areas it encompasses. For example, HEDIS 2.0 defines quality by the following aspects:[12]

- access to care,
- appropriateness,
- efficiency,
- technical outcome of care, and
- member satisfaction with services provided.

Quality measures are grouped into three categories: clinical performance, access, and acceptability/satisfaction, with some overlap between the categories. For example, clinical performance measures include measures of appropriate decisionmaking, implementation (including timeliness and safety), communication, and access. A measure of access—such as "When did the patient initiate prenatal care?"—also may be a clinical performance measure if the measure specifies a standard of what constitutes the appropriate timing of the first prenatal visit.

DEFINING CLINICAL PERFORMANCE MEASURES

Clinical performance measures, a type of quality measure, assess whether a health care provider delivers clinical services that are appropriate for each patient's condition; provides them safely, competently, and in an appropriate time frame; and achieves desired outcomes in terms of those aspects of patient health and patient satisfaction that can be affected by clinical services.[13]

Clinical performance measures must be distinguished from other types of quality measures such as satisfaction measures. Satisfaction measures assess the perceptions of the health care consumer vis-à-vis various aspects of the health care delivery system. Satisfaction measures, sometimes called patient ratings, are subjective measures that reflect patient preferences. A patient rating—such as "Did you wait too long for your appointment?"—asks the patient to evaluate the activity of waiting in light of his or her own preferences for waiting.

Infrequently, a satisfaction measure also may be a clinical performance measure, although typically, assessment of the clinical performance of a provider does not depend on a patient rating. The exceptions are measures assessing communication between provider and patient—such as "Were you satisfied with the amount of information supplied by your provider?" Giving patients information is an important clinical activity. Patients who feel they did not receive enough information have difficulty participating in their care.

Patient ratings must be distinguished from patient reports of facts—such as "How long did you wait for your appointment?" Patient reports are an important data source for clinical quality measurement and can be used to assess aspects of clinical performance such as patient/provider communication and the impact of clinical decisionmaking and implementation on the patient's perceived health status.

Measures of resource consumption, on the other hand, do not measure quality. Resource consumption measures fall into two categories: utilization and cost. A utilization measure may be transformed into a quality measure if it includes a standard of quality. For example, cesarean section rates are not quality measures. However, if a health plan or other agent undertaking measurement defines any rate higher than 20 percent as an example of poor quality care, then 20 percent becomes the standard of quality. The application of a standard of quality to a utilization rate transforms it into a quality measure.

WHY CLASSIFY CLINICAL PERFORMANCE MEASURES?

In recent years, the number of clinical performance measures has increased dramatically. For example, NCQA continues its major measure development efforts with HEDIS 3.0.[14] The Foundation for Accountability has introduced the template for its first set of measures.[15] As the number of measures grow, so does the potential confusion of the user. A user may ask: "How may I choose from among so many measures?" or "How do I know which measures are good measures?" Before the user can answer these questions and choose or compare measures, the user must understand the structure and characteristics of a clinical performance measure.

Understanding Clinical Performance Measures

Clinical performance measures most often are expressed as rates, although some measures may be expressed as averages, indices (e.g. health status index), or frequency distributions. The name of a clinical performance measure or the numerator and denominator description convey some initial information about a measure. However, a performance measure, any performance measure, is far more complex. To construct a typical clinical performance measure, the user must know the numerator criterion, detailed case selection and data collection procedures, detailed data specifications, and explicit analysis procedures.[16] An example is shown of some of the structural characteristics of a single measure: "Home blood glucose testing in a two-year interval" (Table 1).

In addition to understanding the structural complexity of a measure, a user also must understand the characteristics or attributes of measures. Consider the following examples:

Table 1. Structural Characteristics of a Measure

Measure Name	**Home blood glucose testing in a two-year interval**
Set Name	**QCare Diabetes - Records**
Numerator criterion:	Number of Medicare beneficiaries with any report of home blood glucose monitoring during the study period.
Case selection procedures:	Medicare beneficiaries who were continuously enrolled in a managed care plan for two years with a claim for diabetes in the first of those years AND a diabetes mellitus diagnosis confirmed by documentation in the patient's medical record.
Selected data specifications:	*Denominator* -- ICD9-CM code of diabetes mellitus (250.xx) at any ambulatory visit (CPT4 code of 99201-99205, etc.) in the first year of the reporting period. Diabetes diagnosis confirmed by the medical record. *Numerator* -- Any mention of home blood glucose testing in the patient's medical record.
Example of data collection procedures:	Acceptable synonyms for diabetes which may appear in the medical record include: anything with the word diabetes in it, IDDM, NIDDM, Type I, Type II, Dm, sugar diabetes, except *rule out diabetes or r/o diabetes.* Sample abstracting instructions: Any diagnosis of diabetes in visit notes; drug order for insulin or oral hypoglycemics; report of home blood glucose testing.
Example of analysis procedures:	Continuous enrollment: If enrollment date is before the beginning of the study interval and the disenrollment date is after the end of the study interval (or the patient is still enrolled in plan) then count the case as meeting the continuous enrollment provision.

- A measure constructed using implicit criteria (i.e. the judgment of an expert clinician) is very different from a measure constructed using explicit criteria (i.e. detailed written definitions of the criteria). Measures based on explicit criteria tend to be more reliable than measures based on implicit criteria.
- A process measure that evaluates communication between provider and patient is likely best assessed by data obtained from a patient survey. Users who have only computerized claims data available for measurement should focus on measuring those aspects of process that can be assessed with claims data, such as appropriate monitoring of an existing diagnosis or selecting tests for certain categories of patients.
- A measure based on an entire episode of illness may be difficult to implement if users have only a single source of data, e.g. inpatient hospitalizations or outpatient records. Measures of episodes often require data from multiple settings to provide the complete picture of the episode of illness.

Evaluating Clinical Performance Measures

Once the user understands both how a measure is constructed and its attributes, the user is ready to tackle the question: "What is a good measure?" The short answer: "It depends." The longer answer is that evaluating a measure requires knowing:

- measurement purpose and the intended use of the measure(s),
- characteristics of the clinical condition being measured, and
- characteristics of the measures being considered for use.

Begin With the End in Mind: Clarifying the Purpose of Measurement

Evaluating measures begins with defining the overall purpose of clinical performance measurement. What is the goal of the measurement activity? What questions will the measurement answer? While clarifying the objectives of measurement seems obvious, many users skip this step.

Clinical performance measurement may be done for many reasons—for accreditation, external comparison, internal quality improvement, provider contracting decisions, or consumer reporting. Measurement also may be done to answer more global policy and effectiveness questions, although measurement for these purposes is not considered performance measurement.

Examples of clinical performance measurement questions or objectives include:

- **For accountability and external comparison including accreditation, provider contracting, consumer choice.** Do these providers perform differently from one another? Do these providers perform satisfactorily? Are these providers improving their performance?
- **For internal quality improvement.** What is our current level of performance? What needs improving? Have we improved in response to an intervention?

Measures developed to answer internal quality improvement questions may have very different characteristics from measures developed to answer external comparison questions or to set provider payment. The measure described earlier (home blood glucose testing) was developed with Health Care Financing Administration funding to permit external comparison. HCFA, as the administrator of the Medicare program, wished to compare performance among managed care plans. The specifications for the home blood glucose testing measure include detailed allowances for patient factors. As discussed below, measures developed for internal quality improvement may require less detailed adjustments for patient factors.

Understand the Characteristics Of Clinical Conditions Being Measured

Conditions, like measures, have characteristics. For example, diabetes mellitus is a chronic condition that has a course of progressive disability. It is a low to moderate prevalence condition with prevalence increasing with age. The condition has a few potentially preventable outcomes (e.g. blindness), several risk factors (e.g. obesity or African-American race), and a number of comorbid conditions (e.g. hypertension). There are many services used in the prevention, diagnosis, and treatment of the condition.

The course of a condition, its prevalence, and other characteristics affect the decision of what is a good measure of clinical performance for individuals with that condition. Conditions with long and variable time courses may require data to be collected in multiple settings over time. Outcome data may be particularly difficult to collect for long time course conditions. Low-prevalence conditions typically yield small sample sizes and highly unstable measurement results. High-prevalence conditions that are vaguely defined (e.g. low back injury among workers or dementia among the frail elderly) make comparisons difficult because of potential variation in the way the denominator population is defined.

Ideally, the conditions chosen for measurement should be selected on the basis of the distribution of disease and the demographics of a defined population. Regardless of the purpose of clinical performance measurement, focusing measurement activities on a specific condition or constellation of conditions greatly enhances the usefulness and interpretability of the measurement.

Using Measure Characteristics To Evaluate the Suitability of a Measure

As with the characteristics of a condition, the characteristics of a measure affect the decision of what is a good measure. Some examples of important measure characteristics include:

Data requirements. Is the measurement activity limited to specific data sources? Sources of data for measurement can be grouped into three broad categories: medical record, administrative (e.g. claims, pharmacy, laboratory, operating room, or emergency room logs), and survey (e.g. patient survey or clinician survey). Our example, the home blood glucose testing measure, requires both medical records and administrative data for construction.

Intended use. Is the intended use of the measure internal or external? Measures that will be used within an organization may be less precise than those that will be used for external comparison of health plans or providers. Internal measures can benefit from insider knowledge of the circumstances and environment for care delivery. As noted earlier, the home blood glucose testing measure was intended for external comparisons. Hence the specifications were precise and detailed.

Process or outcome measures. A balanced measurement program includes measures of both process and outcome. Measuring process alone fails to answer the question of whether health care makes a difference in patient health. Likewise, measuring outcome alone offers no guidance about what or how to improve.

Rigor of development. How was the measure developed? Measures developed from clinical practice guidelines typically have more credibility than measures developed by consensus within a user group. Was the measure tested for reliability and validity? Measures that have undergone extensive testing for reliability and validity with refinements are more robust than measures with little or no testing. The home blood glucose testing measure was developed from clinical practice guidelines; however, it was not tested. Potential users need to test any new measure in their own setting.

Information Overload

With the large number of clinical performance measures and the variety of evaluation concerns, potential users of clinical performance measures face a bewildering array of issues. How can the user organize and make sense of the available information? The remainder of this chapter presents a framework for organizing and describing clinical performance measures and conditions and concludes with an overview of a prototype software interface to facilitate searching for and locating information about measures and conditions.

DERIVING THE TYPOLOGY OF CLINICAL PERFORMANCE MEASURES

The Typology of Clinical Performance Measures was born from a need to capture information about measures in a concise yet accessible fashion. The original goal of the Typology was to collect and analyze examples of the range of clinical performance measures with the aim of identifying the common properties or characteristics of measures.[17] It began as a six-month project funded by the Agency for Health Care Policy and Research (AHCPR) at the height of the 1994 federal health care reform movement. Subsequent funding lead to the development of the database and software interface known as CONQUEST (Computer Needs Oriented Quality Measurement System).

Iterative Development Process

The development of the Typology, and later the development of the CONQUEST database, was iterative. At the outset of the project, several government publications (Healthy People 2000,[18] Healthy United States 1992,[19] and the National Center for Health Statistics "Rainbow Series") were used to identify major health issues by population age group, e.g. infants, children, elderly, young adults.

Developers began with a population focus to help guide the search for clinical performance measures.

With the list of health issues in hand, a MEDLINE literature search was launched that quickly revealed two problems. First, clinical performance measures are not uniformly indexed. This means that a routine inquiry for measures of quality of care turned up thousands of possible articles. Second, clinical performance measures often are not described in detail in the peer-reviewed literature. The detailed specifications of most well-known measures are available only from the developers.

Therefore, to locate the measures currently in CONQUEST, a more focused networking search was initiated. First developers identified and telephoned individuals known to be engaged in performance measurement. Then developers asked these individuals for information about their measures and also requested referrals to others they knew to be pursuing performance measurement. In this manner, almost 1,200 examples of measures were collected.

The next step involved reviewing the measures and identifying characteristics and attributes common to all measures. Many concepts were suggested by previous work in the measure development field. This phase was iterative; a conceptual framework was proposed, a few measures were coded, and the framework was revised, if needed.

It was found that measures may be grouped into:

- Sets: A set is a group of measures developed and/or used together.
- Subsets: Subsets are groupings of measures within a set. Subsets may include measures of similar clinical content (e.g. diabetes, heart failure), similar data type (e.g. process/outcome), or similar setting (inpatient/outpatient).

In CONQUEST, version 1.0, sets of measures range in size from one to over 300. Well-known measure sets include HEDIS 2.5 and the JCAHO's IMSystem measures.

The characteristics of measures naturally group themselves into three categories: characteristics describing the measure content, characteristics describing the data required to construct the measure, and characteristics related to evaluating the measure.

Describing Measure Content

The content of each measure is captured by five categories in the CONQUEST database:

- Clinical rationale,
- Description of numerator and denominator,
- Type of data: outcome, process, or proxy outcome,
- Relevant age groups, and
- Care needs.

Table 2. Describing Measure Content

Measure Name	**Home blood glucose testing in a two-year interval**
Set Name	**QCare Diabetes - Records**
Clinical Rationale	The American Diabetes Association recommends that patients be actively involved in their care. Patients should be involved in home monitoring of blood glucose. Self monitoring allows patients to participate in evaluation of their goals of therapy and adjustment of their regimens. Records of self-monitoring can be important aids for the physician in adjusting the regimen to accommodate the diurnal fluctuations of blood glucose levels.
Numerator Description	Number of patients with any report of home blood glucose monitoring during the study period.
Denominator Description	Health plan beneficiaries over 65 year old, continuously enrolled for two years with specified diabetes mellitus diagnoses associated with specified service codes in the first of these years AND a diabetes mellitus diagnosis confirmed by medical record documentation.
Type of Data	Process Aspects of process: ▪ Selecting treatments and immunizations ▪ Frequency and periodicity
Relevant Age Groups	Ages 65 and older
Care Needs	Treatment/management of an established disease

Each of these categories is described briefly below. Table 2 shows the application of these concepts to the coding of a single measure—the QCaRE home blood glucose testing measure described earlier. For more details about the Typology categories and how measures are coded, refer to the CONQUEST 1.0 User's Guide.[20]

Clinical Rationale

For measures to be useful to clinicians and relevant to policymakers, they must relate to good medical practice. Good is defined, preferably, by scientific proof of efficacy or effectiveness. The clinical rationale of a measure describes the burden of illness of a condition and the benefit to patients of the treatment, management, or outcome assessed by the measure. The rationale may include citations of clinical practice guidelines or outcomes research. The rationale is supplied by the developer of the measure.

Description of Numerator and Denominator

The database includes text descriptions of each measure's numerator and denominator. These descriptions summarize key points of the actual measure specifications. Specifications, including algorithms (where applicable), must be obtained from the developer.

Type of Data: Outcome, Process, or Proxy Outcome

Three types of data may be used for clinical performance measurement: process, outcome, and proxy outcome.

An outcome is a patient's health status, i.e. medical and physiologic (biological, pathological, behavioral states), functional status and well-being (quality of life, productivity, disability), and habits or health risk states. Examples of outcome data include death, infections, ability to perform activities, or involvement in risky behavior.

A proxy outcome is a provider action from which patient states may be inferred, e.g., discharges and readmissions (within certain time frames) as proxies for complications of care. Common proxy outcome measures include admission, readmission, or emergency room visit.

A process of care is what is done to, for, or by patients in the delivery of health care, e.g., taking a history, ordering a test, prescribing medication, educating patients. The data answer the questions: Were the health services provided appropriate for this type of patient and were they provided safely, effectively, in the appropriate time frame, and with appropriate communication about the care with the patient and other clinicians?

Relevant Age Groups

This category is intended to capture all the patient age groupings for which a measure was designed and tested. With further testing, users may expand the application of a measure to other age groups.

Care Needs

Care needs correspond to primary, secondary, and tertiary prevention. Primary prevention includes activities to prevent the occurrence of a disease, such as influenza immunization. Secondary prevention includes screening (e.g. mammography) and other early detection activities. Tertiary prevention involves treating an established condition to ameliorate its symptoms and prevent secondary complications.

Describing the Data Required To Construct a Measure

The data required to construct a measure fall into two categories:

- Constructing the numerator and
- Constructing the denominator.

Each category may be further divided into discrete measure attributes. Table 3 shows the coding of the home blood glucose testing measure for these attributes.

Table 3. Describing Data To Construct the Measure

Measure Name	**Home blood glucose testing in a two-year interval**
Set Name	**QCare Diabetes - Records**
Constructing the Denominator	
Data Source	Medical records and administrative data
Sampling Frame	Users
Inclusions/Exclusions	Selection by diagnosis (independently verified) and selection by enrollment status
Sampling	No sampling done
Constructing the Numerator	
Data Source	Medical record
Time Window	Defined time period: Two years, user-specified
Type of Criteria	Explicit criteria applied at the level of the individual case

Constructing the Denominator

The denominator of a performance rate defines the population that will be observed to determine conformance with the medical review criterion. Four attributes capture key characteristics of the denominator: data source, sampling frame, inclusions and exclusions, and sampling.

The first attribute includes the data sources used to construct the denominator, such as medical records, pharmacy, or other administrative data. The second attribute identifies the universe or population from which the patients (denominator) are drawn, either enrollees or users. The third attribute describes any exclusions or inclusions to the denominator such as inclusions by patient age, inclusions by diagnosis, or exclusions by site of care (e.g. nursing home). The inclusion/exclusion criteria are applied to the sampling frame to make the denominator as homogeneous as possible prior to creating the performance measure. The final attribute captures any sampling conducted to reduce the number of cases in the denominator.

Constructing the Numerator

The numerator of a clinical performance rate is the subset of the denominator population that experiences the event specified in the review criterion. The Typology describes a numerator with three attributes: data source, type of numerator specifications, and time window reviewed for the occurrence of the numerator event.

One or more data sources may be used to define the numerator, although typically only a single data source is used. An example of using two sources is using administrative data to identify patients who have had a type of procedure and using the medical record to identify whether they had general anesthesia.

The time window is the time period during which the denominator population is examined for the occurrence of the numerator event. It may be categorized as follows:

- **Episode of care:** the course of an illness or condition, often including care delivered in multiple settings and by multiple clinicians.
- **Institutionalization:** includes all care delivered in a hospital, rehabilitation hospital, nursing home, or other institution, from admission to discharge, regardless of length of stay.
- **Defined time period:** an explicit time frame for the receipt of care, e.g., January 1, 1992 through December 31, 1993; within 21 days of abnormal test result; or within 24 hours of admission.
- **Visit or point in time**: A single event, e.g., a patient visit or cesarean section.

Type of criteria describes the attributes of a measure's numerator. For example, the numerator may be specified using either explicit or implicit criteria.

Describing Issues for Evaluating a Measure

As described earlier, a measure may be evaluated many ways. The CONQUEST database includes categories that are useful for evaluating the suitability of a measure for a particular purpose. These include:

- Measure purpose,
- Allowance for patient factors,
- Standards of quality,
- Reliability and validity testing,
- Procedure used to develop measure,
- Extent of testing,
- Extent of use, and
- Current use.

Each of these categories is briefly described below. Table 4 presents the coding of the home blood glucose testing measure.

Measure Purpose

Two attributes summarize the measure purpose: organizational setting and type of review for which the measure was developed.

Measures are classified by the setting(s) for which they are designed, even though they might apply to other settings. Knowing the care setting for which measures were designed is important to users since existing data sources vary among settings. It can be difficult to collect truly comparable data in different care settings, even from apparently similar data sources.

Table 4. Describing Issues for Evaluating a Measure

Measure Name	**Home blood glucose testing in a two-year interval**
Set Name	**QCare Diabetes - Records**
Measure Purpose	
Developed for Use in or by	Managed care
Setting	Ambulatory care setting.
Type of Review Developed for	Internal quality improvement and external quality improvement by a government program.
Other Evaluation Issues	
Allowance for Patient Factors	Subgroup analysis
Standard of Quality	External comparison
Reliability and Validity Testing	Never tested
Procedure Used to Develop Measure	Clinician panels using formal methods and published clinical practice guidelines.
Extent of Testing	Never tested
Extent of Use	Never used
Current Use	Not in use

The type of review category captures the original reason the measure was developed. For example, clinical performance measure sets may be developed for internal quality improvement; decisionmaking by businesses, consumers, or health plans; or government agency review. Measures developed to manage patient outcomes on a case-by-case basis or to assess the efficacy of treatment on a case-by-case basis are not clinical performance measures (they are not intended to assess average performance). However, such measures are included in the database because they may be adapted for clinical performance measurement.

Allowance for Patient Factors

This category captures five types of allowances for patient factors. First is paired data at the patient level, where measurements are typically made at two different time periods. Next is risk adjustment devised specifically for the particular measure. Third is risk adjustment devised for wide application, such as those that are in the public domain or can be purchased (e.g., APACHE or MedisGroups). Fourth is risk adjustment applied to patients with specific diseases. Last is analysis by subgroup where performance rates are stratified and reported by subgroups based on relevant patient factors (clinical and demographic) collected along with denominator and numerator data.

Allowance for patient factors is an important evaluation criterion, particularly for measures of outcomes. Unless outcome data are adjusted for differences in patient risk for the outcome, comparisons of outcome data merely illustrate differences in casemix rather than differences in the quality of care.

Standards of Quality

Performance measurement presumes comparing the results of measurement to a standard. Standards of quality are external to the measure itself. Up to three types of standards may be used for comparisons. The types of standards captured in CONQUEST are external comparison, prescriptive standards, or internal standards with comparisons of performance within a provider group over time.

Validity and Reliability Testing

Validity describes how well a performance measure assesses what it is supposed to measure—quality. The language describing types of validity testing often varies by discipline (e.g., psychology, sociology). Validity testing is grouped into several categories: comparisons with the results of other methods, criterion or gold standard validity testing, and criterion validity testing.

Reliability is the degree to which a measurement is reproducible. A measure cannot be valid unless it is also reliable. For administrative data, reliability relates to consistency in coding. For medical records data, reliability means achieving the same review results for a case using different reviewers or the same reviewer at another time. Developers may undertake one or more tests of reliability for all or some of the measures in a set. Types of reliability testing captured in the CONQUEST database include test-retest reliability, interrater reliability, data accuracy checks, and internal consistency analyses.

Validity and reliability testing is an essential component of performance measure development. Invalid and/or unreliable measures are uninterpretable and may undermine the credibility of the organization using them.

Procedure Used To Develop Measure Criteria

Measures may be developed using a variety of procedures. Perhaps the simplest method is consensus within a user group. This may range from informal meetings to iterative feedback methods. Another development procedure involves clinical panels using formal methods such as modified-Delphi processes. Evidence searching, the application or revision of preexisting instruments (such as the SF-36), and published guidelines often provide the material for performance measures.

The procedure used to develop criteria may affect the validity of a measure and therefore is an important evaluation consideration.

Extent of Testing

Performance measures are usually tested in stages with extensive communication between developers and users resulting in revised and refined measurement instruments. Testing is captured by several categories. The conceptual category is used for measures that are specified but not yet implemented. Limited testing describes a measure's initial use, usually with a limited sample. Beta testing and post-beta testing describe measures undergoing further testing by other investigators and/or for different settings or populations.

Knowledge of the extent of testing helps potential users of a measure assess whether it is ready for use or requires further examination and revision.

Extent of Use

Extent of use is coded in three categories: single site, single organization (many sites), and multiple organizations. Regardless of whether or not a measure has been formally tested for reliability and validity, wide use provides evidence that it is valued, at least by its users.

Current Use

The current CONQUEST database contains many measures no longer in use. Some users may wish to restrict their search for measures to those currently in use. However, simply because a measure is no longer used does not automatically mean it is worthless. Measures no longer in use or never used are included in CONQUEST as examples of innovative measure logic or structure and are intended to stimulate measure developers to consider creating similar measures with updated clinical content.

DERIVING A TYPOLOGY OF CONDITIONS

The Typology of Conditions was a natural outgrowth of the effort to develop a Typology of Clinical Performance Measures. The term condition means a diagnosis (such as cerebrovascular hemorrhage) or a patient state that may be associated with more than one diagnosis (such as paraplegia) or that may be as yet undiagnosed (such as low back pain). The Typology of Conditions and the resulting Condition database seek to identify attributes of conditions that affect the choice of clinical performance measures for that condition.

Iterative Development Process

As described above, the developers began by identifying the major health issues for the U.S. population by age group. For the Typology of Conditions, they supplemented the initial list of health issues with conditions linked to the measures included in the Typology of Performance Measures.

Next, developers sought to identify the types of information about conditions that would be of use to individuals and organizations undertaking clinical performance measurement. Through an iterative process of coding information about conditions, review of the coded information, and revision of the classification form, the framework for the Typology of Conditions emerged.

The characteristics of conditions fall into two broad categories: characteristics describing the condition and characteristics associated with the treatment and management of the condition.

Characteristics Describing the Condition

A condition may be described by:

- Age groupings applicable to the primary condition,
- Forms of the primary condition,
- Prevalence of the primary condition,
- Cost and utilization associated with the primary condition,
- Potentially preventable adverse events associated with the primary condition,
- Comorbidities of the primary condition, and
- Risk factors for the primary condition.

Each of these categories is described briefly below and the importance of the category for understanding performance measurement is explained. The principles discussed are illustrated by showing the coding for the condition "unstable angina" (see Tables 5-7). The data are from the AHCPR Clinical Practice Guideline for Unstable Angina.[21]

Ages Affected by the Condition

This category captures the age groups affected by the condition. Users of clinical performance measures often are interested in particular populations and may wish to learn more about characteristics of conditions afflicting a specific age group.

Describing the Forms of a Condition

The form of the primary condition refers to a variant of the condition. Examples of forms include stress incontinence and urge incontinence for the condition of urinary incontinence, or emphysema and chronic bronchitis for chronic obstructive pulmonary disease. Phases or stages of a condition are not considered variants.

Each form of the condition has one or more possible time courses. The time course is coded as follows:

- acute: having a rapid onset, severe symptoms, and a short course;
- acute recurrent: recurring acute conditions;
- chronic stable: a condition of long duration showing little change over time;
- chronic cyclic: chronic conditions showing patterns of cycling; and
- chronic progressive: long duration conditions showing a slow progression.

Understanding the time course of a form of a condition is essential to understanding what outcome measurement is useful for the condition. Acute conditions can be readily assessed using outcome measures because their course is of short duration. Chronic conditions, on the other hand, are more difficult to assess with outcome measures because changes in health status tend to be small, incremental,

Table 5. Describing Clinical Conditions

Condition: **Unstable Angina**				
Age Groups	Ages 25 and up			
Form of the Condition	Form	Time Course	Frequency of Occurrence	Disability Associated with Form
	Increasing angina	Acute	Usually	Ranging from minimal impairment to permanent impairment, even death
	New onset angina	Acute	Usually	Ranging from minimal impairment to permanent impairment, even death
	Non Q-wave angina	Acute	Sometimes	Ranging from minimal impairment to permanent impairment, even death
	Post MI-angina	Acute	Sometimes	Ranging from minimal impairment to permanent impairment, even death
	Rest angina	Acute	Usually	Ranging from minimal impairment to permanent impairment, even death
	Variant angina	Acute recurrent	Rarely	Ranging from minimal impairment to permanent impairment, even death
Prevalence	Data not available			
Utilization	3.1 million hospital days per year 570,000 hospitalizations per year			
Cost	Unknown			

and variably related in time to the delivery of care. For example, it is very difficult to link a stroke occurring today to poorly treated hypertension 10 years ago. Also, functional status in a condition like rheumatoid arthritis varies over time so that detecting the contribution made by clinical performance is hard to assess.

The forms of a condition also can be described by the frequency with which each form occurs and the type of disability associated with each. In the current version of CONQUEST, data describing forms of the condition are limited. The goal was to create a framework of categories for the Typology of Conditions as a shell to be filled in as data become available.

Capturing Information About Prevalence

Information about the prevalence of a condition and its impact on health care costs and utilization provides a sense of the impact of the condition on the health of a population. Prevalence refers to the number of cases of the condition present in

Table 6. Potentially Preventable Adverse Outcomes

***Condition:* Unstable Angina**

Outcome	Time Course	Prevalence	Disability
Acute ischemic pulmonary edema	Acute	Unknown	Moderate impairment, recovery 1-6 months
Acute myocardial ischemia	Acute	Unknown	Permanent impairment 1-50% disability
Advanced AV block	Acute	Unknown	Permanent impairment 1-50% disability
Cardiogenic shock	Acute	Unknown	Permanent impairment 1-50% disability
Death	Not applicable	5 - < 10%	Death
Malignant ventricular arrhythmia	Acute	Unknown	Permanent impairment 1-50% disability
Mitral valve regurgitation	Chronic progressive	Unknown	Permanent impairment 1-50% disability
Recurrent ischemic episodes	Acute	Unknown	Moderate impairment, recovery 1-6 months

Table 7. Comorbidities and Risk Factors

***Condition:* Unstable Angina**

Comorbidities	Acute congenital heart failure Cerebrovascular disease Chronic obstructive pulmonary disease (COPD) Chronic systemic disease Malignancy Mitral regurgitation murmur Renal failure Systemic hypotension
Risk Factors	Anemia Cigarette smoking Cocaine use Coronary thrombus Diabetes mellitus Environmental temperature extremes Family history of premature (age <50) coronary artery disease Females > 69 years History of resuscitation from sudden cardiac death Hypercholesterolemia Hypertension Males > 59 years Noncompliance with medical therapy Prior MI Severe psychological stress

the population at a specified time. The Typology is structured to capture age- and gender-specific prevalence data as well as ethnic or other population group data, if available.

Prevalence information helps users decide where to focus their performance measurement efforts. High-prevalence conditions typically make good measurement topics. On the other hand, users will need compelling reasons to invest scarce measurement resources in low-prevalence conditions as the number of cases will be small and the measurement results subject to substantial variation.

Impact of a Condition on Health Care Costs and Utilization

The utilization data captured by the database are intended to provide a broad overview of the burden of illness for the specified condition. The types of data included (where available) include hospital days, office visits, and the frequency of certain tests commonly associated with the condition. A condition with substantial financial impact may weigh heavily in favor of including the condition in a program of measurement and quality improvement.

Potentially Preventable Outcomes of a Condition

Potentially preventable adverse outcomes are the natural sequelae of a condition that may be modified or prevented with appropriate treatment. Retinopathy and nephropathy are examples of potentially preventable adverse outcomes of diabetes mellitus. Some clinical performance measures track the incidence of potentially preventable adverse outcomes, subject to two caveats. First, many adverse outcomes are rare events, which means that few cases will occur in any given population. Second, many potentially preventable adverse outcomes occur only years after medical care is given, making it extremely difficult to infer a link between a particular provider of care and the outcome.

Comorbidities of a Condition

Comorbidities are conditions that exist at the same time as the primary condition. Forms of the primary condition are not considered comorbidities. Comorbidities may include conditions that also are classified as potentially preventable adverse outcomes or risk factors. An example of a comorbidity is hypertension, which is associated with many conditions such as diabetes and ischemic heart disease.

Comorbidities influence a patient's course of illness and outcomes. Knowledge of a condition's comorbidities allows measure users to design appropriate subgroup analyses or other adjustments for patient factors.

Risk Factors of a Condition

Risk factors are chemical, environmental, genetic, psychological, or physiological states that predispose an individual to the development of a disease. Users of performance measurement may wish to focus measurement activities on strategies designed to modify risk factors and thereby influence long-term patient outcomes. In addition, if performance measurement is based on comparing providers on outcomes, allowances must be made for differences in risk factors within the population served by different providers.

Characteristics Associated With Prevention, Detection, and Management of a Condition

Characteristics associated with the prevention, detection, and management of a condition are limited only by the current state of medical knowledge and science. Two categories of characteristics include:

- Clinical services used in the diagnosis and treatment of the primary condition, and
- Provider settings and health care professionals associated with the primary condition.

The concepts presented are illustrated in Tables 8 and 9. These tables show the coding for the condition "unstable angina."

Table 8. Selected Clinical Services

Condition: **Unstable Angina**	
Service	**Recommendation**
Intravenous thrombolytic therapy	Explicitly classified as 'not recommended' by the guideline
Telephone evaluation	Explicitly classified as 'not recommended' by the guideline
Pain scales	Optional for all patients with condition according to guideline
Serum lipid levels	Optional for all patients with condition according to guideline
Calcium channel blockers	Optional for certain patient groups according to guideline
Exercise stress testing	Optional for certain patient groups according to guideline
Standard balloon angioplasty	Optional for certain patient groups according to guideline
Aspirin	Recommended by guideline for all patients with the condition
Beta blockers	Recommended by guideline for all patients with the condition
Left ventricular ejection fraction evaluation	Recommended by guideline for all patients with the condition
Risk factor modification - smoking cessation	Recommended by guideline for all patients with the condition
Antiarrhythmics	Recommended by guideline for certain patient groups
Cardiac catheterization	Recommended by guideline for certain patient groups
Coronary artery bypass graft (CABG)	Recommended by guideline for certain patient groups
Intra-aortic balloon pump (IABP)	Recommended by guideline for certain patient groups
Intravenous heparin	Recommended by guideline for certain patient groups
Telemetry monitoring	Recommended by guideline for certain patient groups

Table 9. Provider Settings and Health Care Professionals

Condition: **Unstable Angina**	
Provider Settings	Inpatient - acute care Inpatient - subacute care Ambulatory care - generalist Ambulatory care - specialist Home and community setting ER
Health Care Professionals	Physician Nurse practitioner, Physician's assistant Nurse Pharmacist Occupational therapist Physical therapist

Clinical Services Used in the Prevention, Detection, And Management of a Condition

Clinical services are provided to the patient in the course of diagnosis and treatment of the condition. Examples of clinical services include history taking, physician examination, preventive care, tests, procedures, drugs, self-care education, and advice. Using information in clinical practice guidelines and the scientific literature, categories were created describing whether a service should or should not be used for specified categories of patients. Our coding of the services contained in the AHCPR clinical practice guidelines was verified by members of the guideline panel. Guideline-related services were classified as:

- Recommended for all patients with the condition,
- Optional for all patients with the condition,
- Recommended for a subset (certain patient groups) of the condition,
- Optional for a subset of the condition,
- No recommendation for or against because of lack of evidence,
- Explicitly classified as "not recommended" by the guideline, and
- Noted as "contraindicated" by the guideline.

The Condition Typology organizes information about clinical services to help users identify important clinical activities to monitor as part of a measurement program. Recommendations from clinical practice guidelines are summarized and presented to users in the Condition database. Practice guideline-related performance measurement becomes increasingly important as the rapid pace of scientific development in the field of medicine makes keeping current an important aspect of clinical performance for health care providers.

Provider Settings and Health Care Professionals Associated With the Primary Condition

The Condition Typology captures additional information about a condition. For example, the types of settings typically used for the diagnosis, treatment, and/or management of the primary condition are classified as are the types of health care professionals involved in the treatment/management of the condition. These data assist users practicing in specific settings or occupations to search CONQUEST for appropriate measures.

CONQUEST: INFORMATION ABOUT CLINICAL PERFORMANCE MEASURES AND CONDITIONS

In the process of developing the Typology of Clinical Performance Measures and the Typology of Clinical Conditions, almost 1,200 clinical performance measures and over 50 clinical conditions were collected and coded (see Table 10). The data were originally coded on paper forms and later transferred to a relational database. Measure coding was verified by the measure developers. Condition coding was verified by an AHCPR guideline panel member for the AHCPR guideline conditions.

Table 10. CONQUEST Fact Sheet

Number of Measures:	1,185 measures Measure data validated by measure developer
Number of Measure Sets:	53 sets
Number of Conditions:	52 clinical conditions AHCPR Guideline condition data validated by Guideline Panel member
Development Funded by:	Agency for Health Care Policy and Research

To make the information in the database more accessible, a software interface was developed—together they make CONQUEST, a prototype database and interface designed to assist users with the process of identifying and selecting clinical performance measures suited to their purposes. CONQUEST is menu driven, allowing users to select the type of search or report from among several options. For example, the main menu offers the viewer the choice of searching for information, printing reports, adding/editing information in the measure and condition databases, and viewing the on-line help screens. With this interface, the user can locate information about clinical conditions and clinical performance measures and evaluate any measures found.

CONQUEST's three main uses are as a:

- source of information about clinical performance measures,
- source of information about clinical conditions, and
- tool to evaluate clinical performance measures.

These uses are described below.

Using CONQUEST As a Source of Information About Measures

The first use of CONQUEST is as a source of information about measures. For example, a corporate purchaser of health care may wish to locate outcome measures explicitly designed for managed care settings, or a state Medicaid director may be interested in measures of processes of care for children that use administrative data. A hospital quality assurance committee may wish to assess the quality of care given to patients with cardiac conditions such as acute myocardial infarction, unstable angina, or congestive heart failure.

With the CONQUEST main menu's "Search for Information" function, the user can easily search for measures explicitly designed for specific conditions or for measures that may be adapted to the condition. Choosing the "Other Searches" function of the software, users may design their own searches, selecting search parameters from among the measure attributes described earlier. For example, one user may choose to search for measures designed for "managed care," "medical records data," and "processes of care," while another chooses to search on "outcome measures" and "inpatient setting." Selecting "Print Reports" from the main menu allows the user to print out all the information in the database about a single measure or a measure set.

Using CONQUEST As a Source of Information About Conditions

CONQUEST is also a source of information about clinical conditions. With the "Print Reports" function, the user may print all or only some of the information in the database about a condition. For example, a managed care organization may be planning to contract out mental health services and wishes to establish criteria for monitoring the quality of the contracted services. With information from CONQUEST, the managed care organization can select conditions to monitor based on information about the prevalence, utilization, and cost of various mental health diagnoses. Next, the organization can identify key aspects of the diagnosis and treatment of the selected diagnoses that represent current "best practices" according to clinical practice guidelines. Finally, using information about the comorbidities and risk factors of the selected conditions, the organization can design performance measurement analyses that take into account issues of casemix.

Using CONQUEST To Compare and Evaluate Measures

Earlier, the authors described how the determination of a "good measure" depends on the reasons for measurement, the characteristics of the clinical condition being measured, and the characteristics of the measure under consideration. In the following paragraphs, the authors specify some of the specific measure and condition characteristics suited to two common measurement purposes: external accountability and comparison and internal quality improvement. How CONQUEST may be used to identify measures with these characteristics is outlined.

Characteristics of Measures To Be Used Externally By Purchasers, Consumers, and Regulators

Measures for accountability and external comparisons must address issues of variation in performance (do providers perform differently from one another?), minimum levels of acceptable performance (do providers perform satisfactorily?), and improvement (is performance improving?). Measures used for accountability and external comparison should have the following characteristics:

- **High reliability and validity.** Measures to be used for external comparisons or for decisions about reimbursement or contracting must be highly reliable and valid. Using poorly validated measures merely damages the credibility of an agency or group. The CONQUEST software includes two standard reports—one comparing measures on the types of testing for reliability and one comparing measures on types of validity testing. These reports permit users to specify multiple measures for comparison and view relevant information on a single page (see Figures 2 and 3).
- **Risk adjustment for outcome measures.** Outcome measures used for quality comparisons must be risk adjusted. Otherwise, outcome comparisons between providers reveal primarily differences in casemix, not quality. The CONQUEST software interface allows users to determine whether the measure employs risk-adjustment strategies. Both the standard and custom measure reports print the coding of this category for viewer review.
- **Allowances for patient factors for process measures.** Assessments of the quality of the process of care also benefit from consideration of patient factors. For example, subgroup analyses may be used to create more homogeneous populations for analysis. Using the CONQUEST software, users may determine whether a measure incorporates allowances for differences in patient factors.

Figure 2. Comparison of Measures by Reliability Testing

Set Name	Measure Name	Measure Code	Test-Retest Reliability	Inter-Rater Reliability	Data Accuracy	Internal Consistency
Complications Screening Program BIH	Postoperative acute myocardial infarction	SCRE1A09	no	no	no	yes
HCUP-3	Postoperative acute myocardial infarction	HCUP1C03	no	no	no	no

These measures may have been modified since the date they were coded. (Date may be found on the standard measure report.) Measures may be adaptable to other clinical conditions, patient populations, care settings, or uses. Once adapted, they should be retested for reliability and validity.

Figure 3. Comparison of Measures by Validity Testing

Set Name	Measure Name	Measure Code	Face Validity	Comparison with the Results of Other Methods or Measures	Criterion or Gold Standard Validity Testing
Complications Screening Program BIH	Postoperative acute myocardial infarction	SCRE1A09	yes	yes	yes
HCUP-3	Postoperative acute myocardial infarction	HCUP1C03	yes	no	no

These measures may have been modified since the date they were coded. (Date may be found on the standard measure report.) Measures may be adaptable to other clinical conditions, patient populations, care settings, or uses. Once adapted, they should be retested for reliability and validity.

- **Sufficient numbers of cases to make comparisons (conditions with moderate to high prevalence).** It is nearly impossible to compare providers whose measurement results are based on a small number of cases because the results vary greatly on the basis of chance. The CONQUEST Condition database provides information about the prevalence of conditions and can assist users to make a determination of which measures are likely to suffer from the small numbers problem.

Characteristics of Measures To Be Used for Internal Quality Improvement

Measures to be used for internal quality improvement must answer the questions: "What is our current level of performance?" "What needs improving?" and "Have we improved in response to the intervention?" Measures used internally for quality improvement have the following characteristics:

- **Measure is clinically relevant.** To be credible to clinicians, what is being measured must be viewed as important to patient care and health outcomes. In other words, a measure must be clinically relevant. The CONQUEST database provides a short clinical rationale to assist users in determining the clinical relevance of a measure. While the rationale is typically abbreviated, it may contain references to the scientific literature for users who wish to further explore the importance of a measure.

- **Measure covers important processes or outcomes.** One test of clinical relevance is whether a measure captures important processes of care and patient health outcomes. The CONQUEST database captures 10 attributes of process measures, which are grouped into decisionmaking (five attributes), implementation (three attributes), and communication (two attributes). CONQUEST also includes six attributes of outcome measures (generic/condition specific, global/single, subjective/objective, data format, functional/clinical/health risk state, and processes assessed by outcome).

Two of the standard reports available in CONQUEST permit comparisons of multiple measures on dimensions of outcome and process. These reports allow users to quickly identify measures that assess the aspect of process or outcome of interest. For example, Figure 4 (next page) shows six different measures about blood pressure, each one assessing different aspects of process.

- **Measures, particularly outcome measures, should be sensitive to changes in performance.** Performance measures used for internal quality improvement should be able to detect clinically important changes in performance. Achieving this objective may be difficult for certain types of measures. For example, some outcome measures, specifically those constructed from multiple outcomes or that represent global assessments of outcome, may be difficult to interpret as showing change. Others, such as measures based on outcomes that occur only over long periods of time, demonstrate change very slowly.
- **Measure is easily interpretable. It points the way toward improvement.** Sometimes the user's reaction to performance measurement results is: "That is interesting but what can I do about it?" For example, measuring the rate of in-hospital deaths may reveal a higher than expected death rate but tells a hospital or external regulatory agency very little about what needs to be done to reduce the death rate. Measures chosen to drive internal quality improvement should be actionable.

FUTURE DIRECTIONS

Where do we go from here? The present version of the CONQUEST database is incomplete. As of April 1996, the database contained 1,185 measures in 53 measure sets and 52 conditions. Since the database was delivered to the Agency for Health Care Policy and Research, HEDIS 3.0 has been released, FACCT has announced its recommendations for measure, and the Joint Commission has revised their measures. Many other measure sets exist that are not yet in CONQUEST.

In September 1996, the Agency granted a contract to evaluate and update CONQUEST to MEDSTAT Inc., with the Harvard School of Public Health and

Figure 4. Comparison of Process Measures

Measure Name	Measure Code	Set Name	Selecting Information to Collect About the Patient	Selecting Treatments and Immunizations	Selecting Site of Care	Making Appropiate Diagnosis	Responding To Information About the Patient	Timeliness	Frequency and Periodicity	Technical Proficiency	Communication with Patients	Communication with Other Clinicians
Appropriate evidence for a new diagnosis of hypertension	DEMR1A01	DEMPAQ Records	no	no	no	yes	no	no	no	no	no	no
Appropriate indications for blood pressure test	DEMR2A01	DEMPAQ Records	no	no	no	no	no	no	no	no	no	no
Appropriate response to an abnormal blood pressure test	DEMR2B01	DEMPAQ Records	no	no	no	no	yes	yes	no	no	no	no
Blood pressure in documentes record by nurse if congestive heart failure	RPPS1B01	RAND Prospective Payment System	yes	no	no	no	no	no	yes	no	no	no
Blood pressure measurement at each visit	RPRE2E01	RAND Prenatal Care	yes	no	no	no	no	no	yes	no	no	no
Blood pressure within one monthof new prescription of ACE	DEMR3C03	DEMPAQ Records	yes	ni	ni	ni	no	yes	no	no	no	no

These measures may have been modified since the date they were coded. (Date may be found on the standard measure report.) Measures may be adaptable to other clinical conditions, patient populations, care settings, or uses. Once adapted, they should be retested for reliability and validity.

Mikalix as subcontractors. This three-year contract will add new measures and conditions to the database. It also will evaluate the Typology and the software interface. Ultimately the feasibility of making CONQUEST a self-supporting enterprise will be tested.

REFERENCES

1. Gottlieb M. "Republican Bills on Health Bow to Wishes of Doctors." *New York Times*; October 31, 1995: Section A, Page 1, Column 1.
2. Kilborn PT. "Tucson HMO's May Offer Model for Medicare's Future." *New York Times*; March 26, 1996: Section A, Page 1, Column 1.
3. Stocker MA. "The Ticket to Better Managed Care." *New York Times*; 1995; October 28: Section 1, Page 21, Column 2.
4. Nadzam DM, Turpin R, Hanold LS, and White RE. "Data-driven performance improvement in healthcare: The Joint Commission's Indicator Measurement System (IMSystem)." *Joint Commission Journal on Quality Improvement*; 1993; 19(11): 492-500.
5. National Committee for Quality Assurance. Health Plan Employer Data and Information Set and Users' Manual. Version 2.0. Washington DC: NCQA, 1993.
6. National Committee for Quality Assurance. HEDIS 3.0. Washington DC: NCQA, 1996.
7. Foundation for Accountability. Personal communication, David Lansky, June 21, 1996.
8. Donabedian A. *The Definition of Quality and Approaches to Its Assessment.* Ann Arbor MI: Health Administration Press, 1980.
9. Donabedian A. "Reflections on the Effectiveness of Quality Assurance." In RH Palmer, A Donabedian, GJ Povar. *Striving for Quality in Health Care.* Ann Arbor MI: Health Administration Press, 1991.
10. Lohr KN, ed. *Medicare: A Strategy for Quality Assurance, Vol. I.* Washington DC: National Academy Press, 1990, p. 4.
11. Palmer RH. "Considerations in Defining Quality of Health Care." In Palmer RH, Donabedian A, Povar GJ. *Striving for Quality in Health Care.* Ann Arbor MI: Health Administration Press, 1991.
12. NCQA. HEDIS 2.0. *Ibid.*
13. Agency for Health Care Policy and Research. "Using Clinical Practice Guidelines to Evaluate Quality of Care. Vol 2." Rockville MD: AHCPR, AHCPR Publication # 95-0046, March 1995.
14. NCQA. HEDIS 3.0. *Ibid.*
15. Lansky. *Ibid.*

16. AHCPR. "Using Clinical Practice Guidelines to Evaluate Quality of Care." *Ibid.*

17. Palmer RH, Lawthers AG. Center for Health Policy Studies/Center for Quality of Care Research and Education. "Understanding and Choosing Clinical Performance Measures for Quality Improvement: Development of a Typology." Rockville MD: AHCPR, Publication No. 95-N001, 95-N002, 1995.

18. HHS, PHS. Healthy People 2000. Washington DC:HHS, PHS, Publication No: 91-50212.

19. National Center for Healthy Statistics. Healthy United States, 1992. Hyattsville MD; Public Health Service, 1993, Publication No. 93-1232

20. Palmer RH, Lawthers AG, et al. *CONQUEST 1.0 Overview of Final Report and User's Guide*. Agency for Health Care Policy and Research: Rockville MD: Publication No. 96-N009.

21. Braunwald E, Mark DB, Jones RH et al. "Unstable Angina: Diagnosis and Management. Clinical Practice Guideline Number 10." AHCPR Publication No. 94-0602. Rockville MD: Agency for Health Care Policy and Research and the National Heart, Lung, and Blood Institute, Public Health Service, U.S. Department of Health and Human Services. March 1994.

ACKNOWLEDGMENTS

This research was supported by the Agency for Health Care Policy and Research under contract number 282-91-0070 and 282-92-0038, Delivery Order #3. The authors wish to thank Laura Peterson, RN, for her helpful suggestions. The contributions of the many individuals who made the development of CONQUEST possible are acknowledged in the CONQUEST 1.0 User's Guide.

Chapter 6

American Medical Association

Models for Assessing Physician and Health Plan Performance

Gail H. Thomason and William F. Jessee, MD

The growth of managed care in the United States this decade is now legendary. Enrollment in health maintenance organizations (HMOs) and preferred provider organizations (PPOs) has grown dramatically in just the last two years. At the end of 1993, 46 million Americans were enrolled in HMOs and 60 million Americans were enrolled in PPOs,[1] while the numbers grew by the end of 1995 to 58.2 million in HMOs and 91 million in PPOs.[2] This means that over 149 million Americans now receive their health care through these delivery systems. Moreover, 64 percent of all physicians had contracts with HMOs and 69 percent with PPOs in 1995[3]—with profound impact.

Managed care's emphasis on illness prevention, wellness counseling, and disease management holds great promise. Standards for analyzing and ensuring that this promise is realized remain critical. For the past 150 years, the American Medical Association (AMA) has engaged in standard setting and patient advocacy to ensure that medical professionals and health care systems deliver the highest quality medical care available in the world.

The AMA was founded in 1847 to set standards for allopathic physicians and to distinguish these professionals from the untrained and the quack.[4] Since that time, the AMA has been instrumental in the establishment of medical education standards. The AMA started the Accreditation Council for Graduate Medical Education, which accredits residency programs, the Accreditation Council for Continuing Medical Education, which accredits entities that can grant continuing medical education credit, and the Liaison Committee on Medical Education, which is the national body in charge of the accreditation of medical education programs granting the MD degree.[5] The AMA was a founding member of the Joint Commission on Accreditation of Healthcare Organizations, the original standard setter for hospitals, which now also accredits a variety of other health care organizations and ambulatory health care networks. Throughout the last 150 years, the AMA has been involved in every major quality standard-setting activity involving the medical profession and health care delivery.

This chapter focuses on three of the AMA's current quality initiatives that relate to managed care: the delineation of the essential characteristics of a quality health plan, evaluation of clinical practice guidelines, and the American Medical Accreditation Program (AMAP).

First, the AMA recently has defined characteristics essential to quality in health plans, defining what is necessary to provide "good" managed care. Second, the AMA, in conjunction with numerous national medical specialty societies, the federal government, and other interested parties, continues to promote the development and implementation of scientifically sound, clinically relevant clinical practice guidelines through its clinical guidelines (practice parameters) initiative. Finally, the American Medical Accreditation Program is a voluntary physician accreditation program that sets standards and evaluates the credentials, personal qualifications, environment of care, clinical performance, and patient care results of individual physicians. Designed to reduce duplicative physician review and the attendant cost to the health care delivery system, AMAP also will enhance continuous quality improvement for the medical professional.

ESSENTIAL CHARACTERISTICS OF A QUALITY HEALTH PLAN

Goals

Managed care, as it has become a dominant feature of health care delivery, also has become an increasingly visible target for allegations of abuse. Criticisms of gag clauses, drive-through deliveries, and possible withholding of needed services in capitated payment systems have become frequent fare in the lay press. Despite the potential for such abuses, however, managed care plans continue to hold real promise as mechanisms to improve patient care while enhancing cost effectiveness.

In this chapter, the American Medical Association sets forth its perspective on a set of health plan characteristics that are essential to the operation of a quality managed health care plan. The AMA intends to demonstrate that such characteristics can be and have been made operational through case studies of health plans that exemplify one or more of these essential characteristics.

The essential characteristics have been divided into six categories: patient rights, the patient-physician relationship, economic alignment, the physician credentialing process, continuous quality improvement (including both clinical and administrative performance), and accreditation. While many of these—and other—characteristics are implied in the standards for health plans and networks set by the National Committee for Quality Assurance (NCQA) and Joint Commission on Accreditation of Healthcare Organizations (JCAHO), respectively, the AMA believes that it is vital that they be set forth explicitly to guide physicians, policymakers, and purchasers in making decisions about managed care.

Defining Quality

Quality must be defined before essential characteristics of a quality health plan can be identified. The AMA's House of Delegates, which sets AMA policy, has defined "quality of care" as the degree to which health care services influence the probability of optimal patient outcomes.[6] AMA policy also defines medical care of high quality as care that:

- produces the optimal possible improvement in the patient's physiological status, physical function, emotional and intellectual performance, and comfort at the earliest time possible consistent with the best interests of the patient;
- emphasizes the promotion of health, the prevention of disease or disability, and the early detection and treatment of such conditions;
- is provided in a timely manner, without either undue delay in initiation of care, inappropriate curtailment or discontinuity, or unnecessary prolongation of such care;
- seeks to achieve the informed cooperation and participation of the patient in the care process and in decisions concerning that process;
- is based on accepted principles of medical science and the proficient use of appropriate technological and professional resources;
- is provided with sensitivity to the stress and anxiety that illness can generate, and with concern for the patient's overall welfare;
- makes efficient use of the technology and other health system resources needed to achieve the desired treatment goal; and
- is sufficiently documented in the patient's medical record to enable continuity of care and peer evaluation.[7]

Patient Rights

The AMA has engaged in a number of activities with other organizations that have examined the issue of patient rights. The AMA participated in the drafting of the National Health Council brochure "Putting Patients First: Patients' Rights and Responsibilities"; has commented on the National Committee for Quality Assurance's "Draft Standards for Accreditation 1997" and Health Plan Employer Data & Information Set (HEDIS) 3.0 draft standards for 1997 (which, for the first time, solicits a description of health plan efforts to orient and educate new members); and has developed its own "Principles of Managed Care," among other activities. The following are key quality characteristics from the perspective of patient interaction with the health plan.

Key characteristics include:

- **Patients and physicians have the right to open communication on treatment options, regardless of plan coverage decisions.** Trust is fundamental: patients must be comfortable that they have full information when making health care decisions. First, patients must know that they can fully discuss all treatment options with their physicians, weighing the pros and cons of each option. Otherwise, patients will lack confidence in the treatment they receive, which can be detrimental to positive clinical outcomes. Second, open communication is necessary for patients to give fully informed consent to treatment.
- **Patients have the right to informed consent in treatment decisions and timely access to specialty care.** While related to the patient right of open communication, this characteristic expands the issue to address access as well. Not only must a patient have confidence in the competency of the medical professionals treating him or her; the patient must be able to see and be treated by the appropriate professional. One central goal of managed care is to prevent acute illness. Timely access to specialty care is an effective way to prevent deterioration of a patient's health status.
- **Plan keeps patients' confidential information confidential.** Confidentiality is not only a legal requirement, but necessary for effective treatment. If patients do not have confidence that communications with medical professionals and their health plan will be kept confidential, they may not be willing to provide necessary information for diagnosis and treatment. Patient concerns range from impact on employment status if an employer learns confidential information, to societal opinion. Compelling examples include whether or not a patient is an intravenous drug user (risk of HIV), has ever been pregnant (disclosure of prior history of giving a baby up for adoption or having an abortion), or has a family history of certain cancers or socially stigmatized diseases.

- **Plan accepts responsibility for conveying concise and easily understood information to all enrollees on**:
  1. coverage (including eligibility, exclusions, out-of-area coverage and conditions under which emergency care outside of the plan will or will not be covered);[8]
  2. authorization requirements;
  3. payment decisions (including payment for experimental treatments);
  4. appeals and grievance processes;
  5. costs of coverage and care (including copayments and deductibles); and
  6. termination provisions and procedures.

For patients to make informed and effective health care decisions, they must understand when and how to access the plan. Misunderstandings between patients and the health plan will be minimized if patients understand exactly what is covered by their plan, how to ensure coverage by obtaining proper authorization, and how a plan arrives at payment decisions. Time-consuming, emotionally draining (to the patient), and publicly damaging (for the plan) arguments can be reduced or eliminated. Clear, objective, and accessible appeals and grievance processes also enhance patient confidence in a health plan. Disclosure of cost information (copayments and deductibles) permits patients to make informed choices when selecting a plan and when accessing care.

- **Treatment of emergency medical conditions must be covered whether or not the provider giving care is participating in the plan.**[9] If patients are afraid that their health plan will not cover an emergency room visit because they do not know whether chest pain is acute indigestion or a heart attack, they may not seek medical care when such care is critical and most effective. This patient right does not preclude educating the public so that emergency rooms are not overburdened with cases of indigestion or nonthreatening cases of colds or influenza. However, when an "emergency medical condition" exists in the mind of a prudent layperson, the patient's right to evaluation and treatment must trump a health plan's right to direct a patient to specific health care facilities or providers.
- **Patients have the right to know how providers are compensated, including any incentives or restrictions.** Patients must have confidence that they know and understand their medical condition and treatment options available and they must be comfortable that their health care providers are acting in the patient's best interest. They have the right to understand the incentives and restrictions their providers are operating under—whether the incentive is perceived as being toward overtreatment (as the fee-for-service system has been

described) or undertreatment (as the system of capitation has been described)—so that they have complete information when making health care decisions.

- **Patients have the right to appeal coverage decisions and to communicate with, and seek the assistance of, their physician regarding such appeals.** Patients arrive at treatment decisions after fully informed discussions with their physicians. If a health plan denies coverage of an agreed-upon treatment, the physician is likely to be in the best position to explain to the health plan why coverage is appropriate in this particular instance. Prohibiting physicians from communicating with or assisting patients under such circumstances puts the patient at an extreme disadvantage vis-à-vis the health plan.

Patient-Physician Relationship

Preservation of the unique patient-physician relationship has been fundamental to the AMA since its founding. This relationship remains fundamental to U.S. health care delivery. Patients today, raised on television shows from *Marcus Welby, MD,* to *Medical Center* to *ER* and *Chicago Hope*, assume and expect their physician to uphold this unique relationship. Managed care promises to improve disease management and enhance patient care through development and use of clinical practice guidelines, but effective use of these tools can be realized only through a partnership between physicians and the health plan.[10] In a quality health care plan, physicians and the health plan work together to optimize patient care. Issues are discussed and consensus achieved on the best approach to patient care, such as the review and usage of applicable clinical guidelines. Nevertheless, the ultimate decisions regarding care are made by the physician, in concert with the patient, while the ultimate decisions regarding payment coverage are left to the health plan. Attention to the following key characteristics of a quality health plan can enhance and preserve the patient-physician relationship.

Key characteristics include:[11]

- **Certain professional decisions are so integral and critical to quality patient care that they should always be the ultimate responsibility of the physicians practicing in the health plan (irrespective of plan characteristics or the market in which the plan operates).** These include:

  1. **What diagnostic tests are appropriate.** Ultimately, this is a decision that can be made only by a trained medical professional familiar with the patient.
  2. **Recommendations to patients regarding treatment options, including noncovered care.** In the Patient Rights section, the patient's right to open communication regarding all treatment options was discussed. The patient relies on the physician for

information and recommendations. This is so fundamental to the patient-physician relationship that ultimate responsibility must rest with the physician.

3. **When and what surgery is indicated.**
4. **Hospital length of stay.**
5. **When and to whom in-plan physician referral is indicated.**
6. **When and to whom out-of-plan physician referral is indicated.**
7. **When and with whom consultation is indicated.**
8. **When hospitalization from the emergency department is indicated.**
9. **When nonemergency hospitalization is indicated.**
10. **Choice of in-plan service sites for specific services (office, outpatient department, home care, etc.).**
11. **Frequency/length of office/outpatient visits or care.**
12. **Use of out-of-formulary medications.**
13. **When termination of extraordinary/heroic care is indicated.**
14. **Scheduling on-call coverage.**
15. **Terminating a patient-physician relationship**
16. **Whether to work with, and what responsibilities should be delegated to, a mid-level practitioner.**

Each of these items either is a medical decision that must be the ultimate responsibility of the physician or is integrally tied to the patient-physician relationship. This ranges from specific conversations regarding heroic treatment to knowledge of drug reactions for a specific patient.

- **Plan provisions should support physician behavior with respect to patient care decisions that uphold the "Principles of Medical Ethics."**
- **Physician payments that provide an incentive to limit the utilization of services should not link financial rewards with individual treatment decisions and should not be based on performance over short periods of time.**

Efficient use of resources is an important goal; however, it should not be tied to the medical decisions made in any one case. Such tying would not only damage the patient-physician relationship, but goes against the principles of medical ethics and risks undertreatment, and thus harm, to the patient. The danger in evaluating performance over short time periods is that "outlier" patients, requiring greater-than-anticipated treatment or intervention, may skew averages substantially. If financial rewards or incentives are applied in such a short period, physicians will be under great financial pressure to undertreat. If, however, the performance incentives are based on performance over a longer period of time, odds are that severity will be averaged. The incentive to undertreat any one patient is lessened if the financial risk is spread over a larger population.

Economic Alignment

This section identifies characteristics necessary for the plan to align the economic incentives that affect providers, patients, and the plan itself. The plan design should be such that maintaining patient health produces favorable economic consequences for all three parties. The plan is designed to accomplish this objective by building into plan design certain incentives and requirements.

Key characteristics include:

- **Including economic incentives patients to reduce health risks and modify health behaviors where necessary.** For example, no copayment is required when patients visit physicians for child immunizations, periodic health risk appraisals, or breast cancer screenings; the premium is reduced for individuals who successfully complete smoking cessation programs or who do not smoke; or discounts at fitness facilities are secured for individuals who sign up, and continue to use, such facilities.
- **Creation of mechanisms for patients to more effectively provide self-care for minor illnesses, while not delaying seeking care for conditions requiring medical care.** Examples of such mechanisms include demand management and patient education programs, with economic incentives for their use. New mothers who have been educated on early childhood colds and diseases will be better able to judge at what point a crying, sick infant should be seen by a physician or taken to the hospital emergency room.
- **Basing physician and other provider reimbursement at least in part on achieving measurable performance objectives in the areas of clinical performance (both process and outcome measures), patient satisfaction, and health status.** Each of these four items—process, outcome, patient satisfaction, and health status—is important. Reimbursement should balance all four and not be unduly weighted in favor of any one item.
- **Equitably sharing savings from improvements in cost-effectiveness (i.e., improved quality per unit cost) among providers, patients, and the plan.** Increased cost effectiveness requires the cooperation and participation of all parties involved in the system—providers, patients, and the health plan. Resultant savings should be shared among all such parties as a reward for past performance and as an incentive for future actions. The marketplace will, in turn, pass on a portion of these savings to purchasers through price competition among plans.

Credentialing Process

One of the keys to a quality plan is quality physicians and other health professionals. Each health plan engages in a process through which it researches and evaluates the credentials of the medical professionals who will be caring for patients. This section identifies key aspects of the credentialing process, including professional participation and objectivity in selection of criteria, timeliness of decisionmaking, and availability of information to plan participants.

Key characteristics include:

- **Physicians and other providers practicing in the network have been involved in the development of criteria for network participation.** Physicians know best what it takes to be an excellent physician. Therefore, practicing physicians should be involved in determining which criteria are important in choosing physician participants and how those criteria are to be applied. This does not, however, imply that physicians or other medical professionals in the plan should set plan policies regarding the aggregate number of physicians or numbers by specialty of physicians participating in a plan.
- **Physicians and other providers actively participating in the network review applicants for network participation and make recommendations, based upon approved criteria, regarding their initial acceptance and subsequent reappointment.** Once the plan, with input from participating providers, has set criteria, providers should be included in evaluating applicants. Providers are best able to evaluate their peer's capabilities and ability to meet the plan's objectives, especially in light of local practice and resource limitations.
- **Criteria for network participation and for continuation in the network are made readily available to all network members and applicants.** Providers should understand what the plan's criteria and objectives are in order to evaluate whether or not they wish to apply and participate. The "black box" mode is not conducive to strong provider-plan relations.
- **Criteria for network participation that relate to each of: (1) education and training; (2) clinical performance (including compliance with clinical guidelines and patient care outcomes); (3) patient satisfaction with care and service; (4) utilization behavior; and (5) cost-effectiveness of care are clearly identified, objectively measured, and equitably applied.** Providers strive to deliver quality care and are accustomed to evaluating scientific findings. In other words, they respond to objective information. Further, subjective decisionmaking is likely to be perceived as arbitrary and may actively impede provider-plan relations.
- **No provider is added to the network until basic credentials have been verified (licensure, DEA, malpractice insurance) and the**

full credentialing process is completed not later than 90 days after joining the network. Verification of basic credentials before a physician is added to the plan's provider network serves as a baseline patient protection, can be accomplished in relatively short order, and allows a provider to begin seeing plan participants relatively quickly. Providers should not have to wait for the full credentialing process to be completed before they can participate in the plan. Nevertheless, their participation should be conditional until the full process has been completed. This process should not take months to complete; the plan should be committed to a three-month timeframe. This is particularly important for physicians just starting practice or who have recently relocated.

Continuous Quality Improvement

The plan should actively engage in continuous quality improvement activities in both its clinical and administrative performance. With AMAP, described below, the AMA will provide several tools for physicians to engage in continuous quality improvement. It is imperative for all parties to encourage continuous quality improvement, for it is key to improving health status and enhancing cost effectiveness nationally. There should be a well-organized and comprehensive process for the medical management of patient care, developed and implemented with active participation by physicians and other providers in the network. All physicians and other providers in the network should receive frequent feedback from the plan comparing their clinical performance, adjusted for differences in patient mix, with that of others in the plan, plan averages, and "best practices" benchmarks.

Key Characteristics in Clinical Performance

The clinical quality improvement program should include:

- **Use of clinically valid guidelines or practice parameters to help manage the care of common patient conditions across the continuum from ambulatory, to inpatient, to post-hospital care.** These guidelines should be readily available to all providers and should be used as educational tools for providers. Guidelines should be used not only to manage individual patients, but also to develop compliance profiles for each physician. These profiles should be fed back to physicians on a regular basis. Compliance rates should be correlated with patient outcomes and satisfaction to assure that the guidelines are clinically valid and that following them produces measurably favorable impact on patient care.
- **Profiling the performance of individual practitioners, groups of practitioners, and institutions on a regular basis using well-defined and readily available measures of clinical performance,**

patient satisfaction, and health status. These profiles should compare individuals, groups, and institutions with others in the plan, with plan averages, and with "best practices" and should be regularly fed back to each individual, group, and institution in the network. Physicians have spent their educational and professional lives in a competitive, goal-oriented environment. They are scientists who respond to scientific information. Our current system does not provide them with objective, well-defined information regarding their performance compared to their peers caring for similar patients. Such information would enhance each individual provider's performance in terms of clinical performance and patient satisfaction. Hearing that patients are not happy with the amount of time they spend in the waiting room or are not comfortable asking questions and that they are comfortable with other physicians is a tremendous, nonpunitive behavior modification incentive.

- **Regular measurement of important aspects of clinical performance for major health care problems or conditions cared for by the plan; of patient and provider satisfaction with the plan and its providers; and of the health status of plan members.** These measurements should be used to create the profiles discussed above and to identify trends or patterns that may require changes in the operation, benefits, coverage, or delivery mechanisms in place in the plan itself.
- **The health plan provides a formal, substantial role for actively practicing physicians in setting guidelines and reviewing and adjudicating patient care quality issues.**[12] This may be accomplished through a variety of mechanisms. Patient care quality issues include, but are not limited to:
  1. utilization review and quality assurance activities;
  2. clinical guidelines;
  3. disease management programs and protocols;
  4. formulary development;
  5. development and review of compliance with corrective action plans;
  6. information (data) development and review;
  7. credentialing and renewal of participating agreements with physicians; and
  8. use of new technologies and procedures.

Many of these issues have been discussed earlier in other sections and require input and analysis from medical professionals actively participating in caring for the plan's participants.

Key Characteristics in Administrative Performance

There should be a similar program for evaluating and continuously improving the administrative performance of the plan itself. This must include systematic measurement of, and actions to improve, such aspects of the plans performance as:

- timeliness of claims payment or capitation payments and reconciliation;
- accuracy of claims payment;
- customer-service response times to patient inquiries, complaints, and grievances;
- customer-service satisfaction rates among patients and providers;
- accuracy and timeliness of membership enrollment; and
- provider satisfaction with the operation of plan medical management functions, such as:
  1. prior authorization;
  2. large case management;
  3. disease management processes; and
  4. patient education/demand management programs.

Accreditation

Systemic evaluation of the structures and processes of health plans by outside reviewers serves a useful function for both the plan and the public. Increasingly, such evaluations are being sought by employers and, in some cases, consumers, as reassurance that the plan has met basic quality standards. The plan receives feedback from a third party according to publicly available standards. To the extent these standards are established, evaluated, and modified with input from all interested parties (plans, providers, patients, and payers) they are particularly useful measures. To address similar issues with respect to physicians operating in health plans, the AMA has designed the American Medical Accreditation Program (AMAP), which is described later in this chapter.

Key characteristics include:

- The plan and its delivery network(s) should be in substantial compliance with relevant accreditation standards such as those established by the National Committee for Quality Assurance (health plan)[13] and the Joint Commission on Accreditation of Healthcare Organizations (network). Accreditation by one or both of these organizations may be a useful benchmark to be considered for evaluating the quality of a health plan or network.
- The utilization management program should be accredited by URAC.

CLINICAL GUIDELINES (PRACTICE PARAMETERS)

Goals

For a number of years the AMA has been working with national medical specialty societies, the federal government, and other interested parties to promote the development and implementation of scientifically sound, clinically relevant, clinical practice guidelines.[14] Clinical practice guidelines are in widespread use. A 1994 report revealed that 82 percent of HMOs used specific clinical practice guidelines, and that of those, 85 percent had dedicated staff for developing and implementing guidelines.[15]

Clinical guidelines hold significant promise for improving the quality and cost effectiveness of health care services. Some of these guidelines have been developed internally by HMOs, some have been adapted from those issued by the Agency for Health Care Policy and Research (AHCPR), and still others have been developed by third parties and may or may not have been adapted by the users.[16] While this adaptation is useful in addressing local variations in patient management, it unfortunately defeats the objectives of standardization and scientific validation of the cost effectiveness of care in compliance with such guidelines.

The AMA has undertaken several initiatives intended to facilitate the development of clinical practice guidelines; to evaluate and identify those clinical practice guidelines that are useful to physicians and managed care organizations and that can assist them to provide cost-effective care; and to act as an information resource by publishing and making available information on existing clinical practice guidelines. These AMA activities are accomplished through: the Practice Partnership; the Practice Parameters Forum; a new program to review and overtly recognize clinical practice guidelines based on assessment against criteria for scientific validity and on expert evaluations by peers; and publication of the *Outcomes Research Resource Guide*, the *Practice Parameters Directory*, and the *Practice Parameters Update*.

Practice Parameters Partnership And Practice Parameters Forum

In 1989 the AMA established the Practice Parameters Partnership and the Practice Parameters Forum. The Practice Parameters Partnership consists of 14 national medical specialty societies, the Agency for Health Care Policy and Research, the Joint Commission on Accreditation of Healthcare Organizations, and the American Hospital Association. The Partnership holds three meetings per year.

The Partnership plays a major information-sharing role in coordinating the clinical practice guidelines development and dissemination activities of the member organizations.

The Practice Parameters Forum includes more than 80 physician organizations and other participating groups and meets twice annually. The Forum brings together scientific and broad-based clinical expertise for two purposes: to promote development of scientifically sound, clinically relevant clinical practice guidelines and to provide an opportunity for the exchange of information and ideas between physicians, medical societies, insurers, government agencies, and other interested parties. These two groups have developed several publications, including *Attributes to Guide the Development of Practice Parameters/Guidelines*, *Principles of Practice Parameters*, and *Implementing Practice Parameters at the Local, State and Regional Levels.* In addition, the AMA annually publishes a listing of clinical practice guidelines, *Directory of Clinical Practice Guidelines*, and a related newsletter, *Practice Parameters Update*.

Clinical Practice Guidelines Recognition Program

Recently, the AMA has developed a detailed process for evaluating clinical practice guidelines and granting recognition to those that meet defined criteria.[17] Recognition of an evaluated guideline will last for five years, absent modifications or revisions to the guideline. Criteria for this evaluation address documentation for the guideline; involvement in the development of the guideline by physicians and physician organizations affected by the recommendations in the guideline; the importance of the issue that is the subject of the guideline; the process used to develop the guideline (including the use of scientific evidence and credentials of the developers of the guideline); the specificity of the guideline; its clinical soundness; currency (the guideline has been developed, reviewed, or revised in the last five years); availability (the guideline is easily available to physicians who may be affected by its recommendations); disclosure of any conflicts of interest involved in developing the guideline or in its recommendations; and the guideline's logical flow.

The process for evaluating a guideline includes several steps:

- Clinical practice guidelines are solicited for review from health plans, commercial vendors, and medical organizations.
- Preliminary methodological review of a submitted guideline is conducted by the AMA to determine if the guideline warrants more detailed review of clinical content by an expert panel of peer reviewers. In cases where it is unclear whether the guideline merits the detailed review, an outside advisory panel assists in the determination.
- A guideline that is not accepted for more detailed review is returned to the applicant with an explanation and request for additional information, where appropriate.

- A guideline that appears to meet all necessary criteria during the preliminary review is referred to no less than three content experts and a methodologist. Qualifications of these reviewers include relevant experience and expertise, availability, and lack of conflicts of interest. Accordingly, no individuals who participated in the development of the guideline may serve as its reviewers.
- The peer review panel conducts a guideline review and completes an evaluation. Depending on the length of the guideline, this process takes approximately three weeks. AMA staff then compile the evaluations, obtain outstanding information when necessary, and summarize the reviewers findings.
- The peer review panel agrees to final comments and recommendations; if consensus of the panel is not achieved, differing views are reflected in the summary.
- The review panel's recommendations are presented to the AMA's Council on Scientific Affairs (CSA) for review and approval, after which the sponsoring organization is notified of the CSA's decision.
- The recognized guideline then is published in the AMA's *Directory of Clinical Practice Guidelines* (formerly the *Directory of Practice Parameters*) and the owners of the guideline are authorized to use the AMA recognition (with a disclaimer statement).

To support this evaluation process, the AMA has created a database of potential peer reviewers either with specific knowledge of substantive scientific areas that are addressed by clinical practice guidelines or have experience and expertise in developing clinical practice guidelines. The database currently contains almost 500 potential peer reviewers who are willing to participate in this program.

AMERICAN MEDICAL ACCREDITATION PROGRAM

As an extension of its role in establishing and maintaining professional standards, the AMA began investigating methods by which it could assess physician performance in 1995. The study was motivated by the AMA's historic role in setting standards for the profession of medicine; by growing requests from patients and employers for more information about their physicians; the profession's increasing need for public accountability; and the fact that no professional organization comprehensively has evaluated and accredited individual physicians and their practices.

This program begins from an enviable position: the quality of medical care delivered by the physicians of America is excellent. However, it is also possible that we can improve the quality of that care by attempting to decrease inappropriate variation. Real differences—age, gender, socioeconomic condition, presence or absence of other diseases, nutritional status, heredity—exist among patients and these differences need to be recognized. Beyond that, there are variations among clinicians that can only be accounted for by differences in practice styles. To the extent possible, it is desirable to account for these clinical differences among patients and to limit or decrease other variations.

Managed care organizations have responded to patient and employer demands for quality evaluation by implementing credentialing and office and medical record reviews, and by profiling physician practice patterns. However, these processes are fragmented, duplicative, and inconsistent from one plan to the next, resulting in unnecessary confusion to physicians and expense to the health care system. In contrast, AMAP offers physicians and purchasers of health care a standardized accreditation program that reduces cost to the health care system and hassle to the individual physician, and that has the added benefit of providing meaningful feedback to physicians that can be used to improve the quality of care they provide their patients.

AMAP reviews and evaluates the credentials, personal qualifications, environment of care, clinical performance, and patient care outcomes of each individual physician who seeks accreditation. Those who meet the AMAP standards are designated as "AMAP accredited"—recognition that they have met stringent national standards for physician quality. AMAP strongly emphasizes continuing enhancement of physicians' clinical performance, providing them with information and practical assistance in improving the quality of patient care. No other organization currently conducts a program of this scope or depth.

Goals

The foundation of AMAP is a comprehensive set of standards that recognize physicians who meet (or surpass) professional and practice requirements in the areas of credentials, personal qualifications, environment of care, clinical performance, and patient care results. The program has three objectives:

1. To design and implement a widely accepted, accountable, publicly credible accreditation process that is directed and operated by the medical profession, replacing the fragmented and duplicative credentialing and review processes that have caused unnecessary confusion among patients, physicians, hospitals, and health plans—at significant cost to all parties.
2. To develop a standard portfolio of information about physician qualifications and performance for use by managed care organizations (MCOs) and hospitals, and to facilitate ready access by authorized parties to each accredited physician's portfolio, including information about clinical performance and patient care results.
3. To develop an effective, constructive operating partnership with the Federation of Medicine (state, local, and national medical specialty societies) to assure that the program effectively meets the interests of patients and physicians.

Five Components of AMAP

AMAP consists of five basic components: credentials, personal qualifications, environment of care, clinical performance, and patient care results.

Credentials: This component includes a review of basic physician credentials such as education, training, licensure, and specialty certification. Such information as professional work history, hospital privileges, professional liability experience, disciplinary actions, and other pertinent information that managed care organizations, hospitals, and government programs require for their credentialing, application, and selection processes also are included.

Personal Qualifications: This component addresses other qualifications of physicians that affect the quality of care they provide. First and foremost is the physician's agreement to abide by the AMA's "Principles of Medical Ethics," including its seven essential standards of conduct.

Participation in at least one organization that conducts peer review; completion of current and relevant continuing medical education; and completion of a self-assessment program covering both clinical performance and medical practice operations also is required under this component.

Environment of Care: This component entails a comprehensive on-site review of the clinical, operational, and management systems in a physician's office or other practice site. The AMAP review is similar to the "site visits" conducted by various managed care organizations and is designed to satisfy the requirements of each, as well as of organizations that accredit managed care organizations and networks (JCAHO, NCQA, URAC). Evaluators look at the physical facilities, documentation of medical records, diagnostic and treatment policies and procedures, and office management systems. AMAP has developed national standards and a defined methodology for the environment of care survey, but contracts with qualified local medical societies or external vendors to conduct the surveys according to AMAP specifications.

Clinical Performance: Once the program is fully operational, AMAP-accredited physicians will receive and review information about their clinical performance compared with norms and national benchmarks. This will provide educational feedback for physicians and help them improve the quality of care their patients receive. Eventually, accredited physicians will be required to achieve predefined levels of performance on these measures and demonstrate a pattern of improvement. The focus will be on enhancing physician performance by providing comparisons to other physicians, coupled with suggested methods of improvement.

Patient Care Results: Similarly, accredited physicians will participate in periodic, formal patient satisfaction surveys (addressing consumer assessment of the physician, office personnel and procedures, office appearance, and promptness of service), as well as an objective program of measurement of clinical outcomes and health status.

Pilot testing of these last two components will be conducted to develop specific recommendations for making the patient satisfaction component of AMAP operational by 1998, and the balance of the patient care results and clinical performance components are expected to be operational by 1999.

How AMAP Works

AMAP became operational in limited areas in 1997 and will be expanded and phased in over the next three to five years. Both the startup phase and the mature, operational phase have characteristics that reflect the program's acceptance in the marketplace. Basically, AMAP functions in this manner:

1. The physician applies for AMAP accreditation. Each physician who elects to apply completes an application and pays AMAP a small application fee. The physician applicant agrees to permit release of the results of the review and the accreditation decision to the plans and hospitals that he/she identifies on the application form (if these entities participate in AMAP).

   During AMAP's startup phase, it is expected that physicians primarily will choose to seek accreditation as a result of recruitment and retention decisions by major health plans and hospitals that have elected to utilize AMAP accreditation as a measure of quality. Notice is then sent by the health plans and hospitals to all participating physicians informing them of their option to seek accreditation from AMAP.

   In the mature phase of AMAP, invitations to apply for accreditation will be sent on an automatic basis, perhaps triggered initially when first starting practice in a new geographic region, and automatically thereafter (for renewal of accreditation); or in the case of young physicians, in the last few months of their residency or fellowship program.

2. Each health plan and hospital authorized by the physician receives his/her AMAP results. Hospitals and health plans that receive information about a physician will share the cost, paying a flat fee for each physician. The prices charged by AMAP to MCOs and hospitals are significantly less than their cost for collecting the same information themselves.

3. The accreditation process is completed and reports are shared with the individual physician and with each previously designated plan and hospital. The AMAP report sent to plans and hospitals will include the results of the assessment process, the portfolio of information on qualifications and performance, and the accreditation decision. To apply its accreditation standards, AMAP will assemble an extensive portfolio containing all information required by health plans, networks and hospitals accredited by NCQA, URAC, or JCAHO, as well as those data elements required for AMAP accreditation.

4. Additional plans or hospitals, at the request of the physician, may purchase a report. If the physician subsequently wishes to join another participating health plan, or apply for privileges at another hospital, he or she may authorize the release of his/her portfolio. The health plan or hospital pays a fee for the portfolio, but there is no additional charge to the physician.

5. Accreditation also is available to individual physicians who are either not involved in MCOs or who wish to go through the process without having to share the results with third parties. In such cases, the full accreditation fee is charged to the individual physician.

Standards for Accreditation

Accreditation standards have been developed through an open process, involving physicians, purchasers, health plans, hospitals, and consumers, and will evolve over time. Final responsibility for approving all standards resides with the AMAP Governing Body. The AMAP Governing Body (AGB) consists of 17 voting and five nonvoting members, appointed by the AMA board of trustees. Voting members of the AGB include representatives from managed care plans, hospitals, employers, consumers, voluntary health organizations, accreditation organizations, the AMA board of trustees, and members of the Federation. Nonvoting members include a representative from the Health Care Financing Administration and the chairs of the four advisory committees to the AGB: credentials and personal qualifications, environment of care, performance measures, and Federation.

Before the current standards were adopted, they underwent a stringent review process involving members of the Federation, accrediting bodies, purchaser groups, consumers, health plans, and voluntary health agencies. The initial standards address the credentials, personal qualifications, and environment of care components of AMAP. Standards for the clinical performance and patient care results components will be developed as pilot testing of potential measures is conducted. While the data collected in the pilot testing phase will not be included in the accreditation decision, they will be used to provide feedback to participating physicians and to build a database that permits development of statistically valid profiles and for norms. Pilot testing will be conducted to develop specific recommendations for making the patient satisfaction component of AMAP operational by 1998 and the balance of the patient care results and clinical performance components operational by 1999.

By 2001, there should be sufficient data to formulate recommendations for developing standards on using clinical performance and patient care results information in the accreditation process. This will include a method for weighing the various measures, calculating indices that reflect overall performance, adjusting for differences in patient mix, and determining the level(s) of performance necessary to maintain accreditation.

REFERENCES

1. The AMCRA Foundation, *1994-95 Managed Care Overview* 27 The AMCRA Foundation, 1995.
2. *The Business Word: Health Care Strategic Management*, Information Access Company, Sept. 1, 1996.

3. Emmons DW and Simon CJ, "Managed Care: Evolving Contractual Arrangements," in *Socioeconomic Characteristics of Medical Practice 1996* 15, 16 Martin L. Gonzalez, ed., AMA Center for Health Policy Research, 1996.
4. Starr P, *The Social Transformation of American Medicine*, 90-91 BasicBooks, 1982.
5. *The Health Care Almanac*, 416-418, Lorri A. Zipperer, ed, American Medical Association, 1995.
6. AMA Policy 450.975.
7. AMA Policy 450.995(1).
8. Citizens for the "Right to Know," *Choices: Good Health Care Depends on What you Know*, states: "Would you buy a car without looking under the hood, checking the gas mileage or taking it out for a test drive? Of course not. . . . It is difficult to find out exactly what a health plan covers, but educating yourself and asking the right questions before you sign up can help protect you and your family." Citizens for the "Right to Know," 1995.
9. "Emergency medical condition" is defined as a medical condition, the onset of which is sudden, that manifests itself by symptoms of sufficient severity, including severe pain, that the absence of immediate medical attention could reasonably be expected by a prudent layperson, who possesses an average knowledge of health and medicine, to result in: (1) placing the patient's health in serious jeopardy, (2) serious impairment to bodily functions, or (3) serious dysfunction of any bodily organ or part. AMA Policy 130.970.
10. Shortell, Gillies, and Anderson found it is simply not possible to achieve any measurable level of clinical integration for patients without a close relationship of physicians with an organization delivery system. *Health Affairs*, Winter 1994, p. 53. See also NCQA proposed 1997 standards, QI 2.
11. The following key quality characteristics have been taken from the AMA's "Principles of Managed Care" (a summary of AMA policy in 1994) and a 1996 report by the AMA's Council on Medical Service to the AMA's House of Delegates, "Physician Decisionmaking in Health Care Systems."
12. Shortell, Gillies, and Anderson. *Ibid.*
13. *Newsweek*, June 24, 1996, p. 58, included NCQA accreditation as one of its six criteria for rating HMOs.
14. "Clinical practice guidelines are strategies for patient management, developed to assist physicians in clinical decisionmaking. The term 'clinical practice guidelines'. . . includes practice parameters, and other patient management strategies such as clinical algorithms, defined in AMA Policy 410.971 as 'guidelines' established to aid a physician in the diagnosis and treatment of patients." AMA Report of the Board of Trustees, 4 - I-96.
15. *1994 HMO Performance Report,* Group Health Association of America, 1994.
16. *Ibid.*
17. AMA Report of the Board of Trustees, 4 - I-96.

Chapter 7

The American Academy of Family Physicians

The Physicians' Approach to Quality In Managed Care

Susan Black, MD, and David Massanari, MD

The evolving field of quality measurement and improvement offers new opportunities to help ensure the health care that patients receive is optimal, outcomes-based, and provided in the appropriate setting by a quality provider, as well as meets the expectations of the patient. The continuum of quality from the perspective of physician ranges from credentialing of the physician, to measuring physiologic outcomes of care, to determination of patient satisfaction. Unfortunately, to date, the cost pressures of managed care have focused narrowly on how to reduce expenditures in the provision of health care services—with less real emphasis on how to improve quality. Ironically, the two goals can be complementary, with quality care often being the more affordable option. Greater attention to quality improvement will result in better health care for all patients, regardless of the type of their insurance/health plan, and in an improved health care system in general.

The American Academy of Family Physicians (AAFP) is an international membership organization of practicing family physicians, family practice residents, and students and teachers of family medicine. The organization serves about 84,000 members whose practices include community health centers, solo private practices, hospitals, independent practice associations, multispecialty groups, and single specialty groups. The Academy, as an organization representing family physicians, strongly believes that quality improvement and measurement efforts above all must be patient-centered, evidence-based, and practicing-physician friendly. As a source of continuing medical education (CME), AAFP's central mission is to update its members continually on discoveries in medicine and teach them new techniques of delivering care—regardless of whether they practice fee-for-service medicine or managed care and regardless of where they practice. The Academy is convinced that practicing physicians must be involved in quality-focused activities and strives to engage practicing physicians in the process through the development of tools to assist members in this endeavor.

When managed care started to take hold in the United States, the AAFP considered what its role would be within the evolving system. The very definition of quality is changing every day, and the measurements used to determine the level of quality constantly are being tested by those who make the guidelines: managed care organizations, the National Committee for Quality Assurance, the government, and various medical specialty and subspecialty groups. The definition of quality depends on who is determining it: patient, employer/purchaser, physician group, or government. The AAFP seeks to assist its members in determining how they could best deliver cost-effective care while maintaining quality and the sanctity of the doctor-patient relationship.

AAFP's mission to educate its members and to help them keep current in all fields of health care now has expanded to include issues of assessing and improving quality in managed care. The Academy also must advocate for patients and members, provide members with the educational tools they need to provide quality care, and help develop patient-centered outcomes. In the current managed care system, it often seems that financial interests are the only concern of the managed care industry and that those interests can lead to compromises in quality, especially where standard treatments are not supported by definitive, outcomes-based research. Over the next several years, as we wait for the results of outcomes research, family physicians (and the Academy) will have to fight harder and harder to assure patients receive the health care they deserve.

ISSUES IN QUALITY MEASUREMENT

To the extent that patients define quality, they often base their definition on factors such as the availability of the physician, the ease of getting an appointment, the location of the office, the demeanor of the receptionist, whether they were able to get the referral they wanted, the physician's affability, and, as far as they can appraise them, the physician's clinical skills. When the employers who pay for most health care define quality, they consider cost, availability, practice, location, and outcome—not only in terms of morbidity and mortality but in terms of disability and absence from work. Physicians tend to define quality in terms having little to do with any of the above except for morbidity and mortality—that is, delivering a good outcome in the least invasive and dehumanizing manner. And where government defines quality, it has to look not only at cost and outcome but also at the political ramifications of care (see Table 1).

Where improvements in care prolong the lives of elderly, demented nursing-home patients, can a government-funded insurance program escape some hint of ambivalence about the quality of care that benefits the socially marginal and powerless at great expense to voting taxpayers?

Table 1. The Eye of the Beholder: Perspectives on Quality

Viewpoint	Criteria of Quality
Patient	Factors such as the availability of the physician, the ease of getting an appointment, the location of the office, the demeanor of the receptionist, whether they were able to get the referral they wanted, the physician's likeability, and, as far as they can appraise them, the physician's clinical skill.
Employer	Factors such as cost, availability, practice location, and outcomes (morbidity, mortality *and* disability, and absence from work)
Physician	Outcomes: morbidity and mortality
Government	Outcomes: cost, political ramifications

Under the fee-for-service system, patients who did not perceive that they were receiving superior service from their physician simply could seek care from another physician. Today, many patients are locked into an insurance system that denies them that luxury. Where the patient used to be the "customer," that role is being taken up more and more by the purchasers of health care. Employers and the government increasingly are demanding the power to determine what the services they are buying will include and who will deliver those services. This puts the family physician in the awkward position of serving several masters at the same time and having to balance views of quality constantly. In the current atmosphere our historic duty to deliver the best possible care often seems as if it is pushed and bullied by the overwhelming need to stop the continual escalation in the cost of health. As the family physician is often the first contact patients have with the health care system, he or she often is placed in the uncomfortable position of explaining to the patient what their employer actually bought for them and what they can expect from their new plan. This often means a lower level of benefit, and the deliverer of the news is often blamed for the news. This adversarial role of the family practitioner threatens the quality of care historically provided by the physician's role as patient advocate.

In the early and mid 1990s, at least in part because of the growth of managed care, three quality-related questions became crucial to primary care physicians.

The remainder of this chapter will discuss the Academy's response to these issues:

1. Which physicians are equipped to deliver quality care?
2. How can clinical "best practices" be identified?
3. How should organized medicine respond to the business community's growing interest in measuring the quality of the health care products being purchased?

IDENTIFYING HIGH-QUALITY PHYSICIANS

As managed care organizations began to select panels of physicians for their insurance products, they were faced with the challenge of identifying high-quality physicians with little or no data on which to make this determination. In the absence of anything more meaningful, many organizations seized upon board certification as a convenient surrogate for quality, thereby making it relatively difficult for nonboard-certified physicians to obtain managed care contracts.

The sudden importance of certification posed an acute problem for more than 9,000 family physicians, especially those who had started practice before family practice residency training became available (see Figure 1) and who chose not to take the American Board of Family Practice (ABFP) exam when they could. (A window of opportunity for nonresidency-trained family physicians to sit for the certification exam closed in 1976.)

To address this problem, the AAFP met with the ABFP to urge the reopening of the so-called "practice-eligible route" to certification. Furthermore, AAFP established a dialogue with managed care organizations to better understand their concerns and urge them to consider indicators of quality in addition to certification in their credentialing. It also aggressively worked with nonboard-certified members to help them understand their options.

Figure 1. Certification status of 43,022 active members

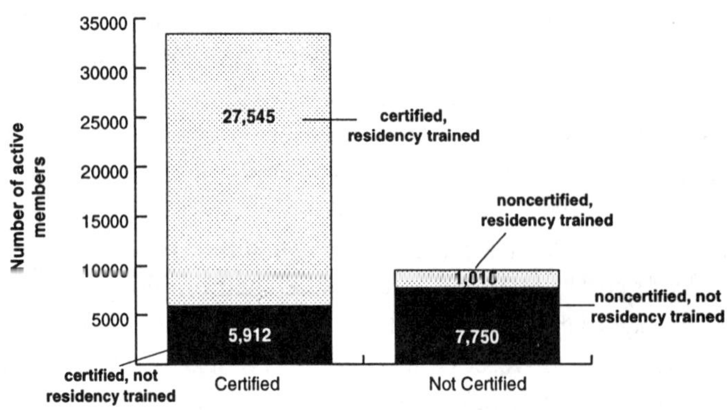

A graph of the certification status of active members of AAFP shows that in 1994, 33,457 (about 78 percent) were certified, while 9,565 (about 22 percent) were not. Just over 80 percent of noncertifi\ed active members (7,750) were not graduates of family practice residency programs.

[From AAFP membership data from Feb. 1994]

At the annual meeting of AAFP in Boston in 1994, the Academy held a forum for nonboard-certified physicians to allow them to express their concerns about privileging, credentialing, and decredentialing. Reports from physicians attending this forum suggested the range of problems nonboard-certified family physicians face. For instance, some managed care organizations starting up in a new area would allow the nonboard-certified doctors into the newly forming panel only to decredential them a year or two later. Such actions on the part of managed care organizations deprived physicians not only of future patients but of substantial numbers of current patients. AAFP members thus felt betrayed by the HMOs; it seems physicians had been manipulated for the sole purpose of enrolling their patient population. Given the rapidity of the credential/decredential cycle, it was not unreasonable to suspect the HMOs of using lack of certification to pursue an economic strategy.

To many, lack of board certification seemed to be an excuse that had nothing to do with quality. Many physicians reported that patient satisfaction, utilization, and outcomes measurements were as good as that of the physicians who were allowed to stay in the HMOs. Although some members requested reopening board certification to derail these managed care practices, the Academy and the ABFP refused to reopen the certifying exam to physicians who had not been "grandfathered" into certification by 1978. They felt that to do so would open up many legal issues. Additionally, it would devalue the residency training—and the certification—of all of the family physicians who had taken formal residency training on their way to board certification.

The ABFP and the AAFP sent a joint letter to managed care organizations stating clearly that board certification should not be used as the sole standard of quality in credentialing family physicians. In its meetings with executives of 14 of the country's largest HMOs, the AAFP leadership spoke candidly about the problems of nonboard-certified family physicians and asked the HMOs to cooperate in developing more meaningful ways to assess quality. The AAFP board of directors then reviewed suggestions made by Academy members, HMOs, and other organizations such as NCQA and the Washington Business Group on Health (WBGH) active in measuring quality in health care. As one outcome of its discussions, the AAFP board decided that the Academy should develop a set of practice-assessment tools that individual physicians could use to measure, improve, and demonstrate quality in their own practices. (This led to the development of the "Vital Signs" project discussed below.)

Despite the efforts of the AAFP on behalf of its nonboard-certified members, many of them still believe themselves to be financially discriminated against in the managed care industry, despite their delivery of quality health care. The Academy strongly urges that training, demonstrated competence, continuing medical education, experience, and other relevant information be used in making participation decisions.

DEFINING "BEST" CLINICAL PRACTICE

In the early 1990s, the AAFP recognized that the development of clinical guidelines based on sound scientific methodology would be crucial to improving the delivery of quality care. The Academy therefore embarked on a course to train a number of its members to develop guidelines. Initially through the AAFP Task Force on Clinical Policies for Patient Care and now through the Commission on Clinical Policies, Research and Scientific Affairs, the Academy is acting on three fronts.

First, it is analyzing and writing high-quality clinical policies for its membership. The three policies completed so far cover management of middle ear effusion in young children, administration of oxytocin, and vaginal birth after cesarean section. Currently, a policy on head trauma in children is nearing completion, a set of policies on managing type II diabetes is in process, and policies are planned in other areas. In order to increase the production of policies, the Academy has formed a unique partnership with the department of family medicine at the University of Washington to create a program in clinical policies.

Second, the Academy is working in conjunction with other bodies involved in policy creation and coordination, including the Council of Medical Specialty Societies, the AMA Practice Parameters Partnership and Forum, and the Institute of Medicine. Moreover, family physicians have been members of almost every guideline panel created by the Agency for Health Care Policy and Research. The Academy's policies on middle ear effusion and head trauma in children were developed in conjunction with other specialty societies. The Academy actively reviews policies being created by other organizations and has completed a set of criteria for working with other organizations in developing policies.

Third, the Academy has established a methodology of approved clinical practice guidelines as well as implemented a program to educate its membership about the nature and use of such clinical policies. It already has presented a number of courses across the country on how to develop guidelines that are scientifically based and patient-centered.

The methodology differs from that of traditional medicine in which clinical policies have represented the pooled opinions of experts. This traditional approach to policy development has been termed "global subjective judgment" to emphasize the fact that policies developed by such a route represent the judgment of the experts rather than a dispassionate analysis of the evidence. The authority of a policy developed by this approach rests on the expertise of the panel that developed it. Consequently, such policies don't devote a great deal of energy to analyzing the relationship between the policy and the available evidence, revealing the underlying biases of the expert panel, or justifying its recommendations.

Integral to the Academy's clinical policy initiatives is the belief that the best policies are based on careful evaluation of available evidence and include explicit descriptions of the process by which they were developed. Such policies may be more justifiable, and they certainly are more open to evaluation. Moreover, the

Academy believes that clinical policies need to be patient centered; they need to acknowledge how individual and cultural differences may affect patient preferences and the values patients place on various outcomes.

The fundamental shift from an implicit to an explicit approach mirrors the shift in medical research and practice. In the past, medical studies primarily have compared one treatment with no treatment or with a placebo. Today, the researcher, clinician, and policymaker must decide among multiple competing interventions that have varying effects on multiple outcomes. This decision requires the policymaker to provide explicit estimates of the magnitude of the different effects, not just determine whether there are statistically significant differences from placebo or inaction. At the practice level, the new policies should simplify, standardize, and improve clinical decisionmaking. In order to stimulate clinicians to modify their existing practices, the policies must be viewed as better than customary practice. At the societal level, clinical policies should reflect and resolve the competing values of patients, physicians, payers, and politicians. In order to be generally accepted, the policies must persuade all the parties involved that their needs and concerns have been acknowledged. An optimal clinical policy is one that explicitly addresses each of the following elements: evidence, outcomes, costs, preferences, and priorities.

The AAFP clinical guidelines program has been widely used by Academy members at their local hospitals, in their states, and on national policy development panels.

As an organization committed to outcomes-based medicine, it is difficult for the Academy to accept solutions that are not based on science but rather on emotion or consensus. AAFP is greatly concerned with congressional intervention into medical practice decisions stemming from newly federally mandated coverage requirements, such as those recently enacted for maternity length of stay. The Academy is aware of related questions now arising for length-of-stay restrictions for breast surgery and anticipate that similar concerns may arise in regard to other interventions. While decisions by the insurance industry that hurt patients are unacceptable, AAFP questions the appropriateness of a solution based on legislative mandates. All guidelines should be addressed by physicians, patients, insurers, and employers without congressional intervention.

TOWARD A BETTER DEFINITION OF QUALITY

As the business community became more interested in quality in health care over the past few years, many new organizations came to focus on questions of measurement of quality in health care. These included, among others, NCQA, WBGH, and the Group Health Association of America, recently renamed the American Association of Health Plans (AAHP). The AAFP sensed that while these organizations truly were concerned with quality, most approached the issue strictly from the point of view of the purchaser of health care and, in some instances, were perhaps more interested in the cost aspects of quality than in issues such as outcomes and patient satisfaction. Recognizing the important position these organizations would hold in the definition and assessment of quality, the AAFP sought to establish a working relationship with them in order to assure the inclusion of clinical and patient views of quality in what the industry eventually defined as quality in health care.

In 1995, Academy staff and volunteer members met with several of these organizations. Conversations with NCQA concerned the importance of including the physician community in the process of establishing quality standards as well as other areas of mutual interest. In part as an outcome of these meetings, the NCQA established a Practicing Physicians Advisory Council, on which medical specialty societies including the AAFP are represented. Other ongoing, mutually beneficial projects include the NCQA's providing input on the AAFP's "Vital Signs" project (the AAFP's evolving set of practice-quality self-assessment tools) and the AAFP's review of and input into NCQA's HEDIS 3.0 guidelines.

The AAFP has become an associate member of WBGH. In this role, AAFP has worked with other WBGH members to assess employer health insurance needs and has participated in the WBGH's rural health conference. WBGH staff members also have provided useful review of the AAFP's "Vital Signs" project. In addition to the Academy's ongoing work with NCQA and WBGH, it continues to interface with AAHP, the Foundation for Accountability (FACCT), and other organizations interested in defining and improving quality.

The following is an excerpt from the chapter titled, "How to Conduct a Self-Audit of Your Medical Records," of monograph 3 of the Academy's "Vital Signs" series, Medical Records Documentation.

The best way to prepare your practice for managed care audits is to perform self-audits. Conducting a self-audit is not as daunting as it might appear. You can keep it very simple and still gain valuable information. Get into the habit of performing self-audits on a regular basis and your records should be able to stand up to the most rigorous MCO documentation guidelines. Furthermore, being able to prove that you consistently score well on chart audits is a great marketing tool when you're negotiating new (or renegotiating existing) contracts with health plans. MCOs want to do business with physicians who adhere to good documentation standards.

How frequently self-audits should be conducted

Most health plans audit on a cycle that is in conjunction with their recredentialing process. In most cases that means every two years, although some plans audit more frequently. A good rule of thumb is to follow the pattern established by the majority of health plans your practice has contracted with. However, if the number of physicians in your group and/or the number of health plans your practice contracts with charges significantly, you may want to accelerate your audit cycle.

When to conduct the audit

Some practices find they are able to conduct self-audits during the course of regular office hours; others prefer to do this off-hours. The number of records and staff involved will dictate how long the audit will take, but on the average, plan on at least a half-day. You can make the process as formal, or as fun, as you would like. For example, if the staff is going to conduct the audit on a Saturday afternoon after the office is closed, invite everybody to change into casual attire, have lunch brought in, agree on a radio station, then get down to business. (You can be relaxed and still be professional!)

You shouldn't be concerned about the expense of having staff working extra hours, or putting off regular duties to conduct a practice audit. However, there are many good reasons why doing so is worth it, not the least of which is the chance of increasing the quality of patient care you provide. Conducting a self-audit is a waste of resources only if you fail to follow through with correcting any weaknesses the audit may uncover.

Choosing the sample of records to audit

Select records of patients seen during a specific time period, such as within the last 30 days. A good workable number is 10 records per provider. You can choose all 10 records of patients from the same health plan, or if, you contract with multiple plans, choose a cross-section of plan members. For example if you contract with two plans, choose five patient records per plan. If you contract with more than three health plans, you may want to increase the number of records per provider you look at.

In addition to developing productive relationships with other organizations, the AAFP continues to work within its membership to improve the quality of the care delivered and its ability to measure that quality. The Academy always has devoted a good deal of energy to improving care by providing clinical CME to its members through courses offered at the annual assembly and other venues and through publications—most notably *American Family Physician*, the Academy's clinical journal. With the growth of managed care and the increasing importance of demonstrating quality of care, these CME efforts have grown to include a good deal of nonclinical as well as clinical material, including:

- Several days' worth of CME at the annual assembly in the general areas of managed care and health care system integration, including presentations on clinical guidelines and other quality-related issues.
- *Family Practice Management*, the Academy's new journal of practice management and socioeconomic issues, which frequently publishes articles on quality issues.
- The development and dissemination of explicit, evidence-based clinical guidelines and reviews of published guidelines.
- Courses designed to train family physicians in developing their own explicit, evidence-based guidelines and evaluating published guidelines.
- "Family Practice 2000," a series of monographs intended to help family physicians learn about issues ranging from capitation contracting to care management.

• "Vital Signs" is a monograph series that provides tools to help members measure and improve quality in several areas of their practice. The series currently includes five monographs:

1. Patient Satisfaction Surveys,
2. Assessing and Improving Your Cost-Effectiveness,
3. Medical Records Documentation,
4. Patient Tracking and Reminder Systems, and
5. Implementing and Measuring "Clinical Preventive Services."

Each monograph outlines the importance of measuring and improving quality in one area of practice and gives the reader tools to track and measure performance. The goal of this program is to help physicians improve and document the quality of care they provide. Together, the monographs are intended to help the practicing family physician lay the groundwork for a continuous quality improvement program, perform better in terms of the quality measurement instruments being developed in managed care, and, most of all, improve the quality of patient care. These monographs were developed with input from AAHP, NCQA, and WBGH; an attestation of support for the project signed by all three organizations appears in each of the monographs in the series (see sidebar previous page).

The "Fundamentals of Management" course, which enrolled its second and third classes in 1996, brings together family physicians who are beginning the

The following set of guidelines represents the Academy's policy framework for working with the managed care industry. It seeks to assure patient safety, appropriate physician impact on decisionmaking, and the sanctity of the physician-patient relationship. It is a "living" document, which is routinely modified and added to by the AAFP board of directors as the health care market evolves and creates new challenges and opportunities.

Requirements Related to Managed Care Plans, Utilization Review Programs, and Point of Service Plans:

1. Managed care plans should provide sufficient information about plan terms and conditions to allow prospective enrollees and patients to make informed enrollment decisions.
2. Physicians must be able to discuss any information, clinical or financial, necessary for their patients to make informed decisions regarding their medical care.
3. Managed care plans should demonstrate that they can provide sufficient access to physicians and other providers so that all covered medical services are provided in a timely fashion.
4. Managed care plans should develop contracting criteria for physicians. Such criteria should be available for review by physicians and should be utilized in determining physician selection, retention, and disenrollment.
5. Managed care plans should have sufficient financial reserves to ensure proper and timely payment for covered services.
6. Managed care plans should establish a mechanism by which physicians enrolled with the plan can provide input into the plan's medical policies.
7. Managed care plans should periodically provide to each physician data to evaluate his or her performance relative to stated plan performance criteria and in relation to a comparable group of plan physicians which are age, sex, and severity adjusted.

8. In regard to physician disenrollment, managed care plans must provide physicians with the reason for disenrollment, the right to appeal the disenrollment decision, and sufficient notice of disenrollment to allow the orderly transfer of patient care responsibilities.
9. Medical directors of utilization review programs should make coverage decisions based on clinically sound guidelines, however, physicians should have the right to appeal adverse coverage decisions and have such decisions reviewed by another physician with the same expertise and the same specialty.
10. Utilization review programs must respond to requests for prior authorization of a service within 2 business days.
11. Whenever practical, potential enrollees should have a choice of health plans, at least one of which should include a point-of-service option.
12. Managed Care plans may impose an additional, actuarially justified premium, and higher patient cost sharing requirement for "out of network" care.
13. Economic or capacity profiling of a physician must be adjusted to recognize case mix, severity of illness, age of patient, and other features of a physician's practice that may account for higher than, or lower than, expected costs.
14. Managed care plans should not discriminate against individuals with expensive long-term or chronic medical conditions by excluding such patients (i.e., pre-existing conditions).
15. Managed care plans should not discriminate against members of high risk, vulnerable, or other similar patient populations by excluding physicians with practices containing substantial numbers of such patients; and
16. Managed care plans should not utilize any criterion that excludes a physician based on sex, race, creed, national origin, or any other factor prohibited by law.

transition from full-time clinical practice of family medicine to roles that hold more management responsibilities. This is a longitudinal course that includes two didactic sessions that combine lectures, case studies, and small-group discussions to cover a range of topics that includes continuous quality improvement. These sessions are held approximately 10 months apart. Additionally, an individual management project, which addresses a problem or responsibility related to the participant's current or anticipated management position, must be completed. During the project, which is carried out in the months separating the didactic sessions, each student works with a family physician mentor who has extensive management experience. A number of the projects completed so far concern quality improvement.

Through the AAFP Commission on Health Care Services, the Academy continues to address policy issues that pertain to quality of care. Recent policies have included "Requirements Related to Managed Care Plans, Utilization Review Programs and Point of Service Plans" (see sidebar), a position paper on the family physician's role in disease state management programs, and one on the family physician's role in caring for patients with mental health problems.

FUTURE DIRECTIONS

As we look to the future, there are at least three quality themes that family physicians and their organizations must address.

First, family physicians and their organizations must maintain a focus on continuity of care and its relationship to overall quality. The current market demand for primary care physicians, and more specifically for family physicians, stems from the ability to provide value (defined as quality/cost). While many physicians believe that they can deliver this value in part because they tend to develop relationships with patients over long periods, physicians are only beginning to see data to support this. Family physicians must study the existing data and add to it in the process of finding ways to improve quality by emphasizing continuity. The AAFP Commission on Clinical Policies, Research and Scientific Affairs will address this issue.

Secondly, physicians must continue to be provided tools and incentives to measure and improve the quality of the care they provide. Although physicians may express initial reluctance to examine the quality of their own services, studies have shown repeatedly that when they are given data comparing their care to that of their peers or their outcomes to expected outcomes, they will adjust their behavior to move toward the desired outcome. As explicit clinical guidelines continue to be developed and evaluated, professionals also must focus on their dissemination and on their use by practicing physicians as tools to improve quality. Further, one must use the implementations of these guidelines to gather data that can be used in continuous quality improvement. In early 1997, the AAFP created an Ad Hoc Task Force on Quality Measurement and Improvement that will focus on the current and future state of the art in quality measurement and improvement with an emphasis on practicing primary care physicians. As part of this effort, physician education must move from increased knowledge only to a system that helps physicians achieve measurable improvements in patient care outcomes. Learning for its own sake will take a back seat to improved outcomes through learning in the managed care field.

Finally, AAFP must continue to work with patient groups, employers, and insurers to develop shared visions of quality. While each group will continue to view quality from a different perspective, AAFP must work toward developing a shared vision of quality and value in health care if health care is to be improved in the United States. The evolving field of quality measurement and improvement offers new opportunities to help ensure that the health care that patients receive is optimal, outcomes-based, provided in the appropriate setting by a quality provider, and meets the expectations of the patient. Unfortunately, at times, the cost pressures of managed care have focused efforts narrowly on how to reduce expenditures in the provision of health care services. AAFP believes that by placing more emphasis on quality improvement, quality care often will be the more affordable option.

Certainly as the knowledge base in medicine increases, opportunities to develop more outcomes-based performance measures will increase. However, while significant federal resources have been committed to biomedical research, little has been done to fund the primary care research agenda so essential to providing new tools to family physicians and other generalist physicians who provide comprehensive care for the millions of patients they see each year. Primary care research would assist physicians in streamlining the diagnostic process and increasing accuracy while simultaneously reducing the use of expensive, unnecessary, or potentially harmful medical tests. The Academy is deeply committed to AHCPR for its creation of a Center for Primary Care Research and will continue to work aggressively for significant increases in funding for the agency.

Chapter 8

Service Employees International Union

Managed Care Quality Assessment for Organized Labor

Directed by Peggy Connerton

The Service Employees International Union (SEIU) is an AFL/CIO affiliate that represents 1.1 million workers in a variety of service industries. SEIU and its locals across the country bargain for health care benefits on behalf of its members, nearly half of whom work in the health care sector. These factors make SEIU a major purchaser of health services and an informed leader in influencing health care issues within the AFL-CIO. SEIU therefore has considerable leverage in holding health plans accountable for both cost and quality of the services they provide.

This chapter is adapted from and includes materials originally published as a Service Employees International Union publication titled Demanding Quality.

Defining and evaluating quality are ongoing processes. SEIU actively participates in organizations like the National Committee for Quality Assurance (NCQA), working toward common understanding and goal-setting in this arena. As a tool for assisting their members in controlling health care costs while still preserving overall wages and benefits, the SEIU developed a systematic approach for evaluating quality in health care plans. This approach is organized in two parts:

- Part I: SEIU's Quality Principles, the basic features to expect from managed care plans; and
- Part 2: SEIU's Recommended Quality Measures, a blueprint for a good managed care report card.

The principles and measures described in this chapter offer a starting point for contract negotiators to feel comfortable in the role of demanding that certain questions be addressed by health plans. The result of several years' efforts, these principles and measures have influenced members and employers alike as they have provided a framework for negotiations regarding health benefits and cost-sharing arrangements.

This framework for quality evaluation benefits all levels of purchasers. Larger, more sophisticated purchasers of health care are most likely to use the volume of their purchasing power as leverage when demanding that specific criteria for quality are met. For these high-volume purchases, the criteria discussed in this chapter can be helpful in arriving at the best value—the nexus of cost and quality—within a health plan. Smaller purchasers tend to be concerned primarily with cost, making them less likely to insist on each of the principles and measures presented here in their entirety. Nevertheless, the framework can be helpful to these smaller purchasers by informing them about the most critical pieces for quality of service as they consider the cost versus quality tradeoff. In addition to facilitating contract negotiations with health plans, the SEIU principles and measures of quality in health care have been useful to other audiences, including union quality committees, policymakers, and direct consumers of health care services.

SEIU QUALITY PRINCIPLES

Principle One: Quality in All Settings

Consumers want confidence in the quality of their health care, particularly as anecdotal evidence increases that providers are favoring the bottom line over the interests of patients. Information about quality can be gleaned from two different, but related activities—accreditation and quality measurement. Both activities can help ensure that health care organizations are held accountable for the quality of care they deliver, and the information derived from them can begin to distinguish between good and poor performers.

Obtain Accreditation. All HMOs must be reviewed by the National Committee for Quality Assurance, all Preferred Provider Organizations (PPOs) by a national accrediting body, and all hospitals by the Joint Commission on the Accreditation of Health Care Organizations (JCAHO). Plans and hospitals must be accredited by a certain date, and those that fail to receive accreditation should be examined very closely to determine if they should be offered to SEIU members. Also, existing organization-specific accreditation summary reports should be forwarded to SEIU so that union leadership has a better understanding of a health plan's or hospital's strengths and weaknesses.

Collect and Report Quality Measures. Accreditation tells consumers that some agency approves of a managed care plan. Quality measures provide consumers with specific information they can use to reach their own conclusions about a plan's performance. A set of recommended measures is included in Part Two of this chapter. These indicators will be updated periodically as outcome and more consumer-relevant measures are made available.

Require an External Audit of Quality Measures. Plans obviously have strong incentives to portray themselves in the most favorable light. An audit improves credibility by ensuring that data is honestly and accurately reported.

Principle Two: Consumer Protection– Patients Before Profits

In a managed care environment, where providers face incentives to provide less care rather than more and where consumers are often "locked into" a plan, protections for consumers are vitally important.

Plans Must Not Have Formal or Informal Gag Rules. The type of gag rules prohibited include those that bar providers from disclosing their overall financial arrangement with the plan, those that bar discussions about treatment options, or anything that may be construed as "disparaging" the plan.

Plans Must Have a Responsive, Medically Informed Grievance System. All member grievances must be responded to in writing by the plan, and the following time lines must be observed. Plans must respond to urgent care grievances within five working days and to other grievances within 30 calendar days. Denial-of-care decisions must be made by physicians using established medical guidelines, and members have a right to appeal decisions made by the plan.

Plans Must Have Consumers on Their Board of Directors. Consumers must represent at least 20 percent of plan board of directors so that they can participate in plan governance decisions in a meaningful way. This standard has the potential to make plans more responsive to consumer concerns and requirements.

Principle Three: Accessible Medical Care

Managed care rewards physicians and health plans for withholding services. Physicians who receive a fixed sum of money for each person, regardless of services provided, will lose money on patients who require more intensive care. Health plans make a profit if their revenues from a company exceed the costs from treating the company's workers. Consumers need assurances that there are no barriers to getting the advanced or specialty care that they need, and that, if they so choose, they can gain access to out-of-plan or out-of-group physicians and hospitals.

Plans Must Offer a Point-of-Service Option. SEIU members and consumers overall place high value on being able to select a provider outside of a given network. A point of-service (POS) option addresses that need, giving members the option of picking an outside provider if they accept a copayment on those services.

Plans Must Contract With Network Hospitals That Have Specialty Units and Contract With Centers of Excellence Relevant to Their Enrolled Population. Health plans must contract with local or national hospitals that meet their members' current and potential needs for acute care and specialty services such as neonatal, trauma/burn, AIDS, coronary care, cancer, and other services.

Plans Must Provide a List of All Providers Included in the Network at Every Level of Care, including hospitals, physicians, long term care and residential facilities, ambulatory and outpatient treatment centers, and subacute care facilities, inclusive of both contractors and subcontractors. This list should be made available upon request to purchasers and consumers and should be updated at least annually.

Principle Four: Quality in the Workplace

As health care organizations seek to rein in costs—often by reducing the number of staff and changing their skill mix—consumers want assurances that their caregivers are adept, experienced, and able to give them necessary care and attention. Health care organizations that dedicate sufficient resources to ongoing education/training, that provide adequate numbers of staff, and that take the steps necessary to retain their staff are more likely to provide quality care.

Organizations Must Publicly Report Direct Care Staffing Levels. Staff is defined here to include physicians, nurses, and other licensed and certified caregivers.

Organizations Must Devote Resources to Education and Training. Specifically, they must channel more than 2 percent of their operating expense budget to nonmandatory staff level training and education activities.[1]

The Hospital Industry Must Adopt New Standards for Training and Certification. Many hospitals are redesigning their workplaces, leaving just three to four job titles, each with a broad span of duties. A recent study found that training for these new roles can range from two days to 12 weeks.[2] Industry norms are needed to assure adequate skill levels.

RECOMMENDED QUALITY MEASURES

The science of measuring quality is in its infancy and what we have today better reflects the interests of employers and health plans than of consumers. The best-known effort to create a managed care report card has been done by the NCQA. The NCQA has developed a report card with 50 quality indicators. The SEIU Recommended Quality Measures include many of the NCQA indicators, but also include new suggestions. To highlight the differences, NCQA measures will be marked ‡ in the tables that follow.

The 51 measures presented here begin to provide more information about issues that SEIU members and individual consumers care about, such as access to needed services, member satisfaction with their health care, the quality of providers that deliver care, and whether or not a plan has consumer protections in place.

The Recommended Measures fall into three broad categories—Quality of Care, Quality of Service, and Quality of Work. Although they do not correspond directly to the four Quality Principles listed in Part One, the underlying concepts are similar. These measures will evolve over time as negotiators meet with success in getting health care organizations to respond to their data requests, as plans' ability to report such information improves, and as the science of quality measurement improves.

While these measures have been developed with HMO plans in mind, many are relevant to nursing homes, hospitals, and other types of managed care plans. Plans deliver or contract for care and services across the entire health care continuum, including, for example, the delivery of behavioral health and nursing home services. However, they often do not provide adequate oversight of quality within these "delegated" arrangements. But, given that health plans are getting paid to manage the delivery of care and services across the continuum, they must be held accountable for quality across all settings.

The SEIU advocates that recommended measures be reported from the health plan to SEIU annually, using the previous calendar year's data. Given the complex web of plan contracting relations, the health plan should report recommended measures from a select number of network hospitals and nursing homes, namely two of the most often selected hospitals and nursing homes.

The local union leadership then can use this information in negotiations to monitor the plans and hospitals that their members use, and, in some cases, to inform consumers in the local community about the quality of plans, hospitals, and nursing homes in their area. The measurement results should be audited by an independent third party to ensure that they are honestly and accurately reported.

The Recommended Measures use NCQA measures, as well as key quality indicators, defined by other organizations.[3] NCQA's measures—known as the Health Plan Employer Data and Information Set (HEDIS)[4]—currently are being used by over 330 managed care plans for internal and external reporting. The decision to draw upon measures that are already in use is a practical one—it increases the validity of the results, the probability that there will be comparable data from like institutions, as well as the likelihood that an organization will comply with the data request. Wherever possible, information about related legislation also is included as a gauge of legislator and consumer support for a particular measure.

A description accompanies each grouping of measures to explain why they are relevant to consumers. At the end of each section, information is provided on which of the measures are already in widespread use, which are being field tested to ensure validity, and which measures are not in use on a large scale or have not yet been tested.

Finally, comparative data are provided as frequently as possible. The comparison numbers include industry averages, public health goals, and industry benchmarks ("best of class"), and help to answer the question: "In comparison to what?" The benchmarks come from the U.S. Public Health Service's *Healthy People 2000: National Health Promotion and Disease Prevention.* The industry averages come from various sources, including academic studies, NCQA, the Agency for Health Care Policy and Research, and the American Hospital Association. For many measures, however, there is no comparative information, primarily because the measures themselves have not been widely reported. Even when industry averages or nationals goals are unavailable, however, consumers can still benefit significantly from local data. In the short term, local data can be used to compare plans in an area. And over time, there will be a basis for tracking improvement or slippage in the performance of a particular plan.

Category I: Quality of Care

These 14 measures provide information about the quality of preventive and prenatal care delivered by a plan, about care related to chronic or mental health illnesses, as well as about hospital and nursing home quality. There are two long-term objectives for this category: to have a set that comprehensively spans the care continuum (health plan, hospital, nursing home, home health), and to collect information not only about how well a health care organization prevents illness or disease, but also how successful it is in restoring the health of those who become sick.

Quality of a Health Plan's Preventive Medicine. Preventive health screenings can help reduce death or illness related to breast and cervical cancer, as well as heart disease. In addition, childhood immunizations are a proven defense against serious illnesses such as measles, polio, tetanus, meningitis, and others. These measures assess how well a plan does on providing such preventive care to its members.

Quality of a Health Plan's Maternity Care. Timely and comprehensive prenatal care can help reduce the likelihood of delivering a low birthweight baby and also can identify any problems early in a pregnancy. Parents and providers seek to reduce the incidence of low birthweight babies because such infants are at risk for a range of illnesses, complications, handicaps, and congenital anomalies. These measures assess the quality of a plan's maternity care.

Table 1.

Quality of Preventive Care	HP 2000 Goal	NCQA Average
‡ 1) Mammograms (women: 52-64)	60%	About 70%
‡ 2) Pap Smears (women: 21-64)	85%	About 75%
‡ 3) Cholesterol Screening (adults: 40-64)	75%	About 65%
‡ 4) Childhood Immunizations (all vaccines)	90%	About 80%

Key:
Healthy People 2000 goals=The U.S. Public Health Service's Healthy People 2000 Goals; NCQA Average=Average of 21 plans that participated in the NCQA National Report Card Pilot Project.

Table 2.

Quality of Maternity Care	HP 2000 Goal	NCQA Average
‡ 5) Percentage of Low Birthweight Infants	5%	About 4%
‡ 6) Percentage of Women Who Receive Prenatal Care in the First Trimester	90%	About 90%

Quality of a Health Plan's Chronic Care Services. Complications related to chronic illnesses—such as diabetes and asthma—can be prevented if such illnesses are closely monitored and managed by providers and patients. Specifically, regular diabetic retinal examinations can reduce the likelihood of a diabetic person going blind. Conversely, if a plan is not doing a good job managing asthma, they are likely to have a higher asthma hospitalization rate than if they work closely with the patient and family to prevent such episodes. These measures give some indication of how well a plan manages chronic disease.

Table 3.

Quality of Plan Chronic Care Services	NCQA Average
‡ 7) Diabetic Retinal Screening	Approx. 45%
‡ 8) Asthma Hospital Admission Rate (2-19; 20-30)	About 0.2% and 0.05%

Quality of Mental Health Care. Regular follow-up after hospitalization for a mental illness is necessary to make sure that patients are successfully transitioning back to their home or work environment and that they have been prescribed the proper medication. This is one measure of how well a plan cares for those with mental illnesses.

Table 4.

Quality of Care for Mental Illness	HP 2000 Goal	NCQA Average
‡ 9) Plan Visit After Hospitalization for Major Affective Disorders	45%	Approx. 75%

Quality of Hospital and Nursing Home Care. Measures for hospitals and nursing homes have not been standardized to the same extent as they have been for health plans, nor have such measures been reported to the public to any significant degree. In fact, the Institute of Medicine (IOM) said in a recent report that they were "shocked by the lack of current data relating to the status of hospital quality of care."[5] The following are indicators of poor (as opposed to good) quality that hospitals and nursing homes have been tracking internally through their quality assurance (QA) programs.

These measures fall into three separate categories—measures related to complications, adverse incidents, and rework. The first two categories relate to both hospitals and nursing homes; the last category is relevant only for hospitals. Union leadership and consumers should raise questions if the rate of any of these measures is on the rise or if the particular institution had a significantly higher rate than others.

1. Measures related to complications:
   - Complications, defined here as those unrelated to the original diagnosis, can further increase a patient's discomfort, put him or her at greater risk, and drive up cost. Prevention of complications is tied to the adequacy of nursing care,[6] among other factors.

Table 5.

Measures Related to Complications	Comparative Information
10) Skin Breakdown Rate (Decubitus Ulcers; Stages I-IV)	Hospitals = 9.2% Nursing homes & Skilled Care Facilities = 23%[7]
11) Nosocomial Infection Rate (all types of infections that originate in the hospital including urinary tract, pneumonia, surgical wound)	No known comparative data exists.

2. Measures related to adverse incidents:
   - Generally, adverse incidents do not seriously affect a patient's health status, but on occasion they can result in significant problems or even death. Adverse incidents are tracked by hospitals and nursing homes because of their potential link to problematic policies and procedures and to staff issues. While nurses play a strong role in minimizing adverse incidents,[8] other disciplines and factors also play a part.

Table 6.

Hospital Adverse Incident Measures	Comparative Information
12) Patient Injury Rate (including medication errors)	Almost 4%[9]
13) Medication Errors	12 actual or potential drug injuries per 100 admissions[10]

3. A measure related to rework:
   - There is considerable interest in tracking hospital readmission rates because of the increased pressure physicians, nurses, and administrators face to reduce hospital lengths of stay. Patients that experience setbacks after being sent home and who have to be readmitted to the hospital are likely to suffer unnecessary duress and may be put at further risk. Readmissions are also costly.

Table 7.

A Measure Related to Rework	Comparative Information
14) Hospital Readmission	A literature search did not identify any comparative data.

4. How these measures relate to other initiatives:
   - All of the health plan-related measures are HEDIS measures. With respect to the hospital and nursing home measures, the JCAHO requires monitoring of nosocomial infections in hospitals, and both the JCAHO and the American Nurses Association are field-testing a nosocomial measure. ANA also is field testing measures related to skin integrity and patient injuries. Finally, both the JCAHO and ANA are testing a measure related to medication errors.

Category II: Quality of Service

These 24 measures indicate the accessibility of health services. For example, these measures assess plan members' ability to receive specialty care, to select a primary care physician, or to obtain care in an emergency. These measures also highlight what financial incentives are influencing doctors and plans and illuminate a plan's responsiveness to member complaints. Well-conducted satisfaction surveys can be an important additional tool to assess quality of service—they allow members and individual consumers to benefit from each other's experience with a particular plan or hospital.

Accessibility of Staff and Services. The following 10 measures provide information about the accessibility of medical and nursing staff, as well as needed services. Specifically, the measures look at how well the plan does in making sure that members visit a provider at least periodically; how easy it is to get an appointment; the availability of physicians, nurses, and other caregivers; whether or not members are readily able to get, or are covered for, necessary care beyond a routine office visit (e.g. specialty or emergency care); and the average number of days covered for vaginal and c-section deliveries. Also, there is a measure of how many plan providers speak a language other than English, given our country's diversity.

Although several of these measures lack comparative data, such data may soon be available.

Table 8.

		Accessibility of Staff and Services	Comparative Information
‡	1)	Percentage of plan enrollees (aged 23-39; 40-64) who visited a plan provider in the last three years	*NCQA Average:* Adults 23-39: 88% Adults 40-64: 91%
‡	2)	Ratio of primary care providers (PCPs) and specialists to plan members	Group/Staff Model HMOs = 808-824 members per PCP IPA/Network Model HMOs = 151-159 members per PCP No comparative data known to exist for specialists
‡	3)	Number/percent of primary care physicians accepting additional plan members to their panels, standards for appointment and telephone access for primary and urgent care, and standards for access to emergency care	No comparative data known to exist.
‡	4)	Health plan standards for geographic proximity of providers and hours of operation	No comparative data known to exist.
	5)	Ratio of nurses, LPNs/LVN, and aides to patients in hospitals[11]	RNs per patient = 1:4 LPNs/LVNs per patient = 1:25[12] No known data on aides exists.
	6)	Ratio of nurses, LVNs, and aides in nursing homes	RNs per patient = 1:65 LPNs/LVNs per patient = 1:37 Nurses aides per patient = 1:12[13]
	7)	Percentage of emergency room (ER) claims denied payment during the reporting year[14]‡	No comparative data know to exist.
	8)	Average days covered for a normal vaginal delivery	No comparative data know to exist.
	9)	Average days covered for an uncomplicated c-section delivery	No comparative data know to exist.
‡	10)	Percentage of plan providers able to speak a language other than English	No comparative data know to exist.

Measures 1, 2, 3, 4, and 10 are HEDIS measures. With regard to maternity stays, 10 states have passed related legislation. Seven of the 10 states require 48-hour minimum stays for vaginal delivery and 96-hour minimum stay for c-section deliveries.[15]

Financial Arrangements With Possible Links to Quality. With traditional (indemnity) insurance, physicians are paid more for providing more services.

Under managed care, however, financial incentives are structured to reward physicians for restricting services. Thus, many consumers worry that they won't be covered for the medical care they truly need. In addition, health care organizations increasingly are converting to for-profit status, with outside investors putting pressure on the organization to channel resources away from care and into profits. In isolation, the following measures do not give consumers a full picture of health plan quality. Instead, they should be looked at against other measures to see, for example, what the satisfaction level of members is in a plan that pays its doctors a bonus if they use fewer medical services.

Table 9.

Financial Arrangements With Possible Links to Quality		Comparative Information		
ǂ 11)	Percentage of Primary Care Physicians Compensated by: a salary; captivation; capitated withhold (%) or bonus; fee-for-service withhold (%) or bonus.	Primarily salary	=	8%
		Primarily capitation	=	37%
		Fee-for-service	=	31%
		Some arrangement that puts providers at risk	=	60%[16]
ǂ 12)	Medical Loss Ratio (% of total revenue dollars spent on medical/hospital services, as opposed to administration, marketing, and profits).	National medical loss ratio average	=	82%[17]
		Range of medical loss ratios is:	=	from 72.4%-98.3%[18]

These measures are both from HEDIS. In addition, Arizona and Wyoming now require plans to publish information related to physician compensation structures.[19] HCFA requires all plans with Medicaid and/or Medicare beneficiaries to publicly disclose the structure of provider financial incentive systems.

Member/Patient Perception of Care and Services. Well-conducted surveys of both health plan members and patients in network hospitals can provide an opportunity for consumers to learn from the experiences of others. In addition, both the percentage of enrollees who decide to leave a plan and those who join may be indicators of satisfaction. Finally, the last measure provides information on who is in the plan, which is useful to provide context for other measures.

The first is an NCQA instrument release in July 1995; the last three measures are HEDIS measures.

Table 10.

	Member/Patient Satisfaction	Comparative Data	
‡	13) For plans: NCQA's Annual Member Health Plan Survey	No known comparable data	
‡	14) For network hospitals: a survey fielded by a third party survey research organization with no stake in the outcome and that is conducted by mail[20*]	Comparable data is not relevant	
‡	15) Percentage of plan members who disenrolled over the last year	Median, all plans/1992= Median, non-profit/1992= Median, for-profit/1992 =	16.5% 16.5% 19.4%[21**]
‡	16) Number and percentage of new plan members over the last year	No known comparable data	
‡	17) Data on enrollment by age, gender, and payer (Medicare, Medicaid, and commercial)	No known comparable data	

*Research has shown that telephone and face to face surveys tend to be skewed with more positive responses. Ware JE. January 1995. "Data collection methods." *Medical Outcomes Trust Bulletin.* Vol. 2, No 6.

**GHAA (currently: American Association of Health Plans AAHP), 1994. "GHAA's annual HMO industry survey." Published in HMI Industry Profile. 1994 Edition.

Consumer Protection: Managed care enrollees have limited ability to influence a health plan's policies and procedures. If they are displeased with a plan's care and services, they can file a grievance, complain to the state agency responsible for HMO oversight, or, in some cases, vote with their feet by leaving. In light of the fact that most consumers are locked into a plan for at least some period of time, consumer protections are critical. Such protections are captured in Part One, including a prohibition against "gag rules" and standards for plan response to grievances. The following indicators attempt to measure plan grievance rates and assess plan responsiveness. Unfortunately, there is no known comparable data for these measures.

Table 11.

Consumer Protection	Comparable Information
18) Number of grievances filed per 1,000 members	No known comparable data
19) Number of grievances filed per 1,000 members related to denial of care	No known comparable data
20) Number of members who registered complaints with the state's department of insurance or similar regulatory body	No known comparable data
21) Average length of time in answering a denial of care grievance	No known comparable data
22) Average length of time in answering a grievance related to urgent care (an imminent and serious threat to the health of the patient)	No known comparable data

Twenty-one states have established time limits for grievance resolution that span from 15 to 180 days.

Plan Coverage and Financial Information. Members may not think about what a plan covers until they run up against some kind of limitation. Upfront disclosure of plan coverage limitations that is easy to read and understand can guide consumers when they are choosing among plans. In addition, most consumers do not consider a plan's financial health as pertinent; however, if an HMO goes out of business it can put a wrench into a member's ability to obtain needed care as well as to get paid for out-of-network services already rendered.

Table 12.

Plan Coverage and Financial Information		Comparable Data
23)	Disclosure of Benefit Coverage Limitations, including:	No known comparable data
	a) Policy on out-of-pocket costs for in and out of network care	
	b) Limitations on number of enrollee visits or dollar coverage	
	c) Limitations on dollar coverage or visits for specific illness or procedures	
	d) Limitations on types of procedures covered	
	e) Preexisting condition limitations	
‡ 24)	Select, relevant HEDIS financial measures:	No known comparable data
	a) Cost Per Member Per Month	
	b) Years in Business	
	c) Total Membership	
	d) Total Revenue(income generated from operations)	
	e) Net Income (excess revenue after expenses)	
	f) Net Worth (excess assets after liabilities)	
	g) Debt-to-Service Ratio (how well the plan is meeting debt obligations)	
	h) Overall Loss Ratio (% of premium revenue that goes to cover total expenses)	
	i) Administrative Loss Ratio (% of premium revenue that covers administrative expenses)	
	j) Operating Profit Margin (overall profitability)	

All the indicators in number 24 come from HEDIS.

Category III: Quality of the Work

These 13 measures indicate a health organization's commitment to attracting and retaining a qualified, effective staff of nurses, doctors, and other caregivers. Part of staff effectiveness relates to consistency, which is essential for continuity of care and for building strong, productive relationships with patients. These measures are particularly important in hospital settings where a growing number of managers are redesigning the jobs of direct caregivers, thereby increasing the demands on staff taking care of sicker patients who are leaving the hospital more quickly than ever before.

The majority of these measures are not found in existing, standardized measurement sets that focus predominantly on quality of care and services. The Institute of Medicine recommends, however, that standardized measures be developed that are "sensitive to nursing interventions and care."22

Education and Competency of Direct Care Staff. The first two of six measures use education as a proxy for the quality of physicians and ancillary staff. The third and fourth measures capture the mix of education levels among nursing staff, as research indicates that quality is enhanced with higher levels of RNs.[23] The fifth measure is a gauge of overall availability of the nursing staff. The final two measures provide an indication of how committed a hospital or nursing home is to ongoing staff-level education and training.

These six measures are increasingly important as hospitals experiment with different care delivery models that put more responsibility in the hands of ancillary staff, and as acuity levels rise in both hospitals and nursing homes. Consumers want to be certain that hospital and nursing home staff have the necessary qualifications to take care of them and are receiving ongoing education and training to be able to do so.

The federal government also has identified the issues of health care staff education/training as significant in today's rapidly changing environment. Specifically, the IOM described the issues of training and competency of hospital-based non-RN staff as "critical" and recommended that hospitals have "documented evidence that ancillary nursing personnel are competent and that such personnel are tested and certified by an appropriate entity for this competence."[24] Further, the IOM recommended that hospitals should be monitoring and evaluating changes in staff mix (broadly defined as work redesign) in relationship to clinical quality, patient satisfaction, and the satisfaction of nurses.[25] In addition, the IOM recommends that nursing homes enhance their overall nurse staffing levels in light of empirical evidence related to quality of care, and specifically that Congress require by the year 2000 24-hour RN coverage in nursing homes.[26]

The first measure is from HEDIS; the third measure is being field tested by ANA.

Consistency and Satisfaction of Staff Delivering Care. These measures assess staff turnover and provide information on hospital use of contingent workers. Research has shown that high turnover rates are linked to low levels of satisfaction, which may have a negative effect on quality. In addition, institutions that

Table 13.

Education/Competency of Direct Care Staff	Comparable Data
‡ 1) Percentage of Primary and Specialty Care Physicians that are Board Certified (have passed an examination in their area of expertise). Preexisting condition limitations	75% for Primary Care Physicians = NCQA average
2) Percentage of the Following Hospital Staff that are Certified: Nurses Aides/Assistants, Phlebotomists, Multi-Skilled Technicians.	No known comparable data
3) Ratio of Network Hospital RNs, LVNs/LPNs, and Unlicensed Direct Care Staff to overall direct care staff	No known comparable data
4) Ratio of Network Nursing Home RNs, LVNs/LPNs and Unlicensed Direct Care Staff to overall direct care staff	No known comparable data
5) Percentage of a Network Hospital's Operating Expense Budget Devoted to Education/Training	No known comparable data
6) Percentage of a Network Nursing Home's Budget Devoted to Education/Training	No known comparable data

employ a high percentage of contingent staff—part time, temporary, agency, or per diem—are less able to provide continuity of care, which also may have a negative impact on quality.

Individuals build relationships with their providers that they want to maintain, and research points to the positive effects that accrue from having consistent medical and nursing care.[27] Nursing homes have particularly high turnover rates as evidenced by a 1994 American Health Care Association survey that found a 100 percent turnover rate for aides, while rates for RNs and LPNs/LVNs were just above 50 percent. The IOM has identified high turnover as a contributor to poor quality and has called upon the nursing home industry to take steps to improve retention such as increasing wages and benefits.[28]

Staff turnover often is used as a proxy for satisfaction that is related to a range of factors, including everything from individual autonomy, to wages/benefits, to the degree of management support. Researchers have shown that settings where nurses are highly satisfied with their jobs provide a higher quality of care as demonstrated by better patient outcomes.[29]

The first measure is from HEDIS; the eighth and ninth measures are modified ANA measures.

Table 14.

Consistency/Satisfaction of Staff	Comparable Information
‡ 7) Rate of Annual Physician Turnover in the Health Plan	5% = NCQA Average
8) Rate of Annual Turnover for the Following Staff in Network Hospitals: RNs, LPNs/LVNs, nurses aides/assistants, and multi-skilled direct caregivers	Data exists but could not be located for publication
9) Rate of Annual Turnover for Nursing Staff (RN, LPN/LVN, nurses aide) in Network Nursing Homes	RNs = 56% LPNs/LVNs = 53% Nurses Aides = 100%[30]
10) Part-time, temporary, agency, and per diem RN and LPN/LVN direct care hours as a percentage of all RN and LPN/LVN direct care hours in network hospitals	No known comparable data
11) Part-time, temporary, agency, and per diem nursing aides or equivalent direct care hours as a percentage of all nursing aides or equivalent direct care hours in network hospitals	No known comparable data

Safety and Health Protections for Patients and Staff. These measures help to assess how committed network hospitals are to preventing patient/staff infections and exposure to chemical, biologic, environmental, and other hazards as defined by the Occupational Safety and Health Administration (OSHA). There is also evidence that staff fatigue related to overwork can contribute to injuries and cause omissions or mistakes (e.g., medication errors) that can have an unfortunate effect on patients.[31]

A survey conducted by the Bureau of Labor Statistics indicates dramatic increases among hospital and nursing home employees in injuries and illnesses, relative to the rest of private industry. Specifically, while such incidents per 100 full-time workers actually dropped among workers in private industry between 1980-1993, they rose 52 percent among hospital workers and 62 percent among nursing home workers.[32]

Table 15.

Safety and Health Protections	Comparable Information
12) A copy of the Network Hospitals' OSHA 200 Logs (captures all work-related deaths, illnesses, and injuries that meet certain conditions)	No known comparable data exists
13) Staff injury rate per 100 full-time employees per the Bureau of Labor Statistics definition	Hospitals = 11.8 per 100, 1993 Nursing homes = 17.3 per 100, 1993 Overall Rate for Private Industry = 8.5 per 100, 1993[33]

CONCLUSION

SEIU views the framework presented in this chapter as an important first step toward protecting its members as managed care sweeps the country. Issues related to quality are more urgent than ever before, and bargainers need tools that will help them get the best care for their constituents. SEIU's quality principles and measures assist contract negotiators in forcing health plans to focus not just on cost, but quality of care (clinical aspects), quality of service (consumer protection), and quality of work (the health care organization and its people).

Quality in health care continues to be an increasingly urgent priority for SEIU. The union has recently established a full-time Special Assistant to the President dedicated exclusively to quality in health care. Future efforts in this arena will include focusing on contract maintenance through the formation of labor management committees on quality.

A sequel to the document, *Demanding Quality*, from which this chapter is excerpted, is planned. Finally, former SEIU President John Sweeney, is current president of the AFL-CIO, which will facilitate the coordination of a broader effort on health care quality among union affiliates. Together with the quality measures and principles described in this chapter, these efforts will promote a new kind of competition in the health care industry: competition based on quality.

REFERENCES

1. A recent study of high-performance workplaces—those oriented toward creating high-skill, high-wage jobs—found that 5 percent of operating expenses typically went toward staff training and education. Appelbaum E and Batt R, *The New American Workplace*, ILR Press, Ithaca NY, 1994:85.
2. Greiner, Ann, "Cost and Quality Matters: Workplace Innovations in the Health Care Industry," Economic Policy Institute, Washington DC, 1995:24-55.
3. These other indicators include those of the JCAHO, which collects data for its own measurement set from more than 200 hospitals. JCAHO does not intend to make its hospitals' information publicly available. In addition, the American Nurses Association is in the process of field testing seven measures they have identified as possessing a strong theoretical link to quality.
4. National Committee for Quality Assurance, Health Plan Employer Data and Information Set 2.0/2.5, Washington DC, 1993, 1995.
5. Institute of Medicine. *Nursing Staff in Hospitals and Nursing Homes: Is It Adequate?* National Academy Press, Washington DC, 1996:116.
6. AHCPR. "Pressure Ulcers in Adults: Prediction and Prevention," Department of Health and Human Services, Rockville MD, 1992; Majesky SJ, Brester MH, Nishio, KT, "Development of a Research Tool: Patient Indicators of

Nursing Care," *Nursing Research*,1978:27(6):365-371; and McFarland GK, McFarlane EA, *Nursing Diagnosis and Intervention: A Model for Clinical Practice*, Mosby, St. Louis MOM, 1993:44-53, 160-169.

7. AHCPR, "Clinical Practice Guideline Number 33: Pressure Ulcers in Adults: Prediction and Prevention," Department of Health and Human Services, Public Health Service, May 1992.
8. Kramer M, Schmalenberg C, "Magnet Hospital: Part I, Institutes of Excellence," *Journal of Nursing Administration*, 1988:18(1):13-24, and "Magnet Hospital: Part II, Institutes of Excellence," *Journal of Nursing Administration*, 1988:18(2)11-19.
9. Brennan TA, Leape LL, Laire N, et al, "Incidence of Adverse Events and Negligence in Hospitalized Patients: Results from the Harvard Medical Practice Study," cited in *JAMA* Vol. 274, no. 1, pp. 29-34. July 5, 1995.
10. Bates D, Cullen D, et al, "Incidence of Adverse Drug Events and Potential Adverse Drug Events: Implications for Prevention," *JAMA* Vol. 274, no. 1, pp. 29-34. July 5, 1995.
11. Research has linked the inadequacy of nurse staffing to increased mortality, length of stay, and complications, including: Aiken L, "Charting the Future of Hospital Nursing," *Image*, 1990; 22(2):72-77; Flood SD, "Nurse Staffing, Patient Outcome and Cost," *Nursing Management*, 1988;19(5):34-41; and Prescott PA, "Nursing: An important component of hospital survival under a reformed health care system," *Nursing Economics*, 1993;11:192-199.
12. SEIU calculations based on AHA Hospital Statistics, 1994-1995.
13. SEIU calculations based on Harrington, Thollaug, Summers, 1995.
14. While the National Center for Health Statistics reports that a majority of visitors to an emergency room do not need immediate medical attention, a high ER payment denial rate may indicate that a plan doesn't make available appropriate alternatives (e.g., an urgent care center) or that a plan is deliberately seeking to hold down costs by routinely denying payment for ER services.
15. The American College of Obstetricians and Gynecologists, "State laws/regulations requiring insurance coverage for postpartum care: 1995-1996," March 1996.
16. Gold M, Hurley R, et al. December 21, 1995. "A national survey of the arrangements managed care plans make with physicians," *The New England Journal of Medicine*, vol. 333, no. 25, pp. 1678-1683. The survey was based on 108 managed care plans, was conducted in 1994, and asked the plan to list their predominant payment method.
17. Michigan State Medical Society. 1996.
18. Weiss Ratings. 1995. "Large HMOs skimp on spending premium dollars for members' care," *Medical Benefits*, January 30, 1996, p. 7.
19. Dallek G. 1995. "Consumer protections in state HMO laws," Center for

Health Care Rights, Los Angeles, p. 131.

20. Research has shown that telephone and face-to-face surveys tend to be skewed with more positive responses. Ware JE. January 1995. "Data collection methods," *Medical Outcomes Trust Bulletin*, Vol. 2, No. 6.

21. GHAA (currently American Association of Health Plans). 1994. "GHAA's annual HMO industry survey." Published in HMI Industry Profile, 1994 Edition.

22. Op. Cit., Institute of Medicine, pp. 122-124.

23. A number of studies have found a correlation between RN/nursing ratios and mortality/morbidity, length of stay, and complications. Among them: Hartz AJ, Krakauer H, Kuhn EM, Young M, et al. "Hospital Characteristics and Mortality Rate," *NEJM*, 1989; 321:1720-1725; and Prescott PA, "Nursing and Important Component of Hospital Survival Under a Reformed Health Care System," *Nursing Economics*, 1993;11-192-199.

24. Institute of Medicine. 1996. *Nursing Staff in Hospitals and Nursing Homes: Is It Adequate?* National Academy Press, Washington DC, pp. 102-103.

25. IOM, pp. 105-106.

26. IOM, p. 142.

27. Aiken LA, Smith HL, Lake ET, "Lower Mortality Among a Set of Hospitals Known for Good Nursing Care," *Med Care*, 1994;32:771-787. Kramer J, Schmalenberg C, "Magnet Hospital: Part I, Institutes of Excellence," *Journal of Nursing Administration*, 1988; 18(1):13-24, and "Magnet Hospital: Part II, Institutes of Excellence," *Journal of Nursing Administration*, 1988; 18(2):11-19.

28. IOM, pp. 160-161.

29. Aiken L, Smith H, Lake E. 1994. "Lower mortality among a set of hospitals known for good nursing care, " *Med Care*, Vol. 32, pp. 771-787; Kramer M, Scalenberg C. 1988. "Magnet Hospitals: Parts I and II, Institutions of Excellence," *Journal of Nursing Administration*, Vol. 18 (1&2), pp. 13-24 and 11-19, respectively; and Sandhu B, Kerouac S, Duquette A. 1992. "A case study of a nursing assignment pattern," *California Journal of Nursing Research*, Vol. 24(1), pp. 51-64.

30. ACHA. 1995. Survey conducted in January 1994.

31. Faqua R, Stevens K. 1988. "What we know about medication errors: a literature review," *Journal of Nursing Quality Assurance*, 3(1):1-17.

32. IOM, pp. 162-177.

33. *Ibid.*, p. 177.

Chapter 9

Washington Business Group on Health

Employer Purchasers Push for the Ideal Organized Health Care Delivery System

Robert F. Cole, PhD

American employers effectively have begun to bring the increase of health care costs under control by offering their employees emerging health delivery systems and encouraging these delivery systems to apply the arts and techniques of industrial organization. The power of the health care marketplace has driven these changes. As costs have leveled off, the question of quality and the value obtained for health care expenditures has come forward. The looming issue is to achieve a reasonable degree of price elasticity attributed to the performance outcomes of health care products.

Price elasticity based on the quality (as well as cost) of health care will begin when the behaviors of buyers in the marketplace—employer purchasers and the employees they represent—are affected by concerns for health care quality. Sorting out what quality will mean to the individual weighing the possibilities offered by the health professionals and their organizations to achieve and maintain the health of his/her household, or to the company making effective investments in the workforce as it represents human capital and productive capacity, is the key to affecting those critical buyer decisions. So quality-based price elasticity will need a set of broadly recognized terms that are applied and operational.

QUALITY TALK

We have no shortage of terms, languages, and dialects tumbling forward to fill this need. There currently are several levels of quality/performance measurement efforts—quality talk—active in the debates concerning the changing health care environment. It is important to distinguish them and the several emerging organizations proposing them. They might be characterized in an order that focuses on the particular to the more general, as follows:

- **Scientifically-based practice standards.** This refers to the state of the science and state of the art as represented in current journal literature. Provider professionals will refer to this literature as it provides the basis of peer review processes.
- **Plan-sponsored practice protocols.** Sophisticated health plans will adopt practice protocols based on the current literature as a guide for the plan's providers or provider networks. These protocols often are considered proprietary and used within the plan.
- **Condition- or disease-specific outcome measurement.** This refers to established uniform health care performance standards measuring treatment outcomes for specific diseases and conditions. The Foundation for Accountability (FACCT) establishes and promotes toolsets appropriate for this kind of measurement.
- **Quality assurance policies, procedures, and practice.** This refers to traditional quality assurance practices organized within the plan as appropriate for any health care facility. The purpose of these records, methods, and procedures is for the organization to be assured it is providing quality care to its members.
- **Continuous quality improvement.** Continuous quality improvement techniques as developed in industrial production have been introduced into advanced health care organizations. Their purpose is to control the production process through monitoring the details of specific operations. These techniques have little to do with what traditionally has been called health care quality, but they are very important in ensuring the effective operation of the health care organization.
- **Formal accreditation of health care organization.** Accreditation is undertaken at the plan's initiative in asking a recognized accreditation agency to provide an external review according to an accepted set of standards. Accreditation is used internally to set the agenda for orga-

nizational development and improvement and externally to represent the capability—but not the effectiveness—of the plan to its individual and corporate customers. NCQA, JCAHO (new standards for health care networks), and CARF (Commission on Accreditation of Rehabilitation Facilities) offer formal accreditation to plans.

- **Consumer satisfaction surveys.** Employer purchasers or the plans themselves regularly survey the plan's members to determine consumer satisfaction and to identify areas for improvement efforts. FACCT offers measurement tools for health risk and consumer survey measurement (satisfaction) with the purpose of setting a standard that will allow for comparability across plans and employers or purchasing sponsors (see Figure 1).

Figure 1. Quality Talk: Multiple Languages of Performance

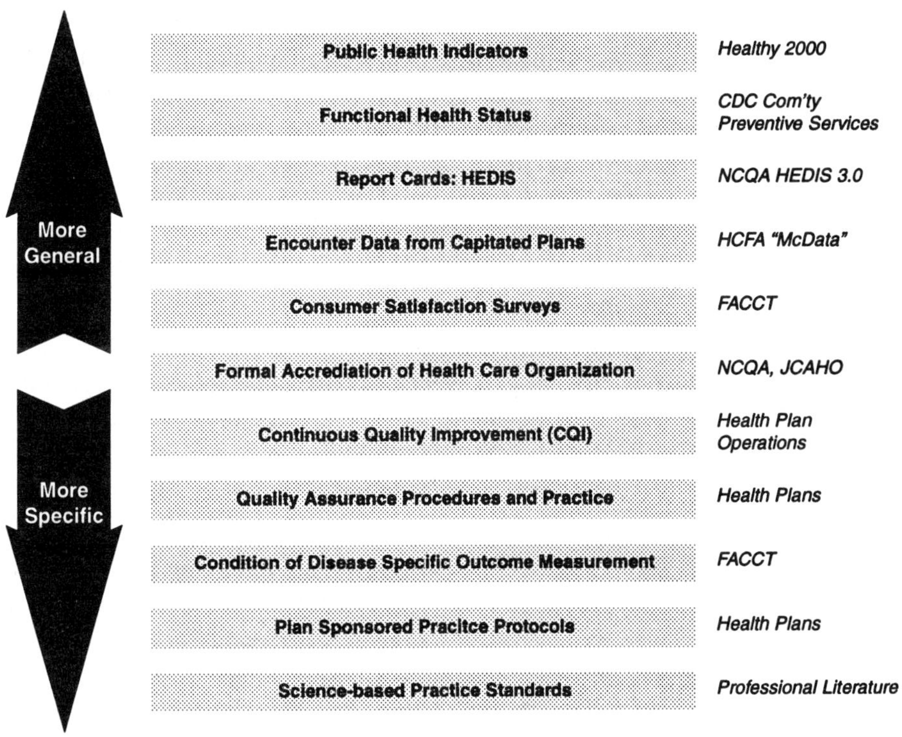

- **Encounter data from capitated plans.** Mainly public health care programs with a tradition of fee-for-service payment methods are tempted to develop data measures from encounter data comparable to FFS claims data. HCFA has promoted a "McData" dataset based on information collected through Medicaid and Medicare claims data.
- **Report cards: Health Plan Employer Data and Information Set (HEDIS).** NCQA has developed a limited dataset designed to make it possible for employers to compare the effectiveness of plans

offered to their employees in a given health care market. Over 350 plans are producing performance-based data using HEDIS measures. A Medicaid HEDIS has been developed that, of course, attends to persons with special health care needs and chronic conditions as reflective of that population. It tends, however, to be derived from encounter data from the state (claims payment) Medicaid management information systems as above. HEDIS 3.0, now in review, will bring together an integrated measurement set that is broad enough to respond to issues of acute and chronic care and to public as well as private purchasers and consumers. Among its "testing set" of new measures are measures that will seek to include in the report card format the results of systematic measurement of health care outcomes within the plans.

- **Functional health status.** This pertains to survey instruments that can measure the functional health status of individuals and populations and the health status of the community itself. The SF-12 and SF-36 are examples of this kind of measure. They can provide the basis of assessing population-based health care efforts or serve as a baseline to determine the effectiveness of a specific intervention or program. The Centers for Disease Control are developing a *Guide to Community Preventive Services*, which will work with effective services and service delivery methods to improve the health status of the community.
- **Public health indicators.** This refers to standard public health statistics reflecting the general health status of large populations. The federal Department of Health and Human Services and state health departments use these statistics, such as Healthy 2000, to frame public health policy and to set goals for public health efforts.

These different languages and all of this effort and activity speak to the urgency of need in the tense conditions of the emerging health care markets. The fact is, with the exception of accreditation practices and the use of HEDIS, very little of this activity and effort has been made operational on a widespread basis that could shape decisionmaking in the marketplace in favor of quality and performance. The cost of advancing any of these components of the quality spectrum to actual practice is not trivial. So it is essential to be strategic in identifying where emphasis should be placed to stimulate buyer behavior that is responsive to quality and performance issues. To understand the employer-purchaser's approach to this strategy, this chapter will review the employers' stake in health care performance measurement, the importance of the emerging role of the purchasing sponsor in health care financing, and the vision of the future health care system that has guided large health care purchasers—the organized system of care.

EMPLOYERS' STAKE IN HEALTH CARE PERFORMANCE MEASUREMENT

Employers need effective health care because they need productive workforces. Increasingly there is a realization that effective health care contributes to the value of the company's product. But it is critically important to be able to measure these relationships in ways that can justify business decisions. Correlations are being found between employee satisfaction (the healthy company) and workers' compensation claims and absenteeism. This opens the way to recast and integrate human resources functions within companies to further demonstrate the company's value.

For the health care portion of the human resource function, condition- or disease-specific outcomes measurement will provide the foundation for a "human resource metric" that will directly relate health care products with company productivity. When this is demonstrated it will provide the rationale for performance-based price elasticity in health care purchasing decisions by employers. So from the viewpoint of strategy, nothing is more urgent among all the efforts and activities on the quality spectrum as the systematic measurement of health outcomes if the objective is to shape purchasing decisions in the health care market. Performance-based price elasticity will be achieved when outcomes measurement becomes the currency of the health care marketplace.

STATE OF THE PURCHASING ART: THE HEALTH CARE PURCHASING SPONSOR

It is often pointed out that it is largely an accident that American employers during the decade of the 1940s assumed the responsibility for paying for health care. During the last decade and a half, as health care costs spiraled upward, a new role emerged for employers. They shifted from payer to purchaser. Through their benefits operations (or through outsourcing or coalition membership), they have assumed the role of health care purchasing sponsor, i.e. they have assumed the fiduciary responsibility to obtain, on behalf of their employees, value for the health care dollars spent for health benefits. This role of intermediary on behalf of the collective (of employees) makes it possible to achieve the advantages of a competitive market and to retain the insurance function—regularly collecting the resources for the entire risk pool.

Especially in progressive companies, sophisticated and aggressive purchasing techniques have developed. While each employer purchaser is unique and no one may employ all these techniques, cyclical purchasing and benefit management operations can include the following:

Plan qualification process. Progressive purchasing typically will require plans that wish to be offered to a company's employees to submit a detailed profile of the care system's capabilities, resources, reporting capacity, and cost structure.

Plan performance contracting. Plans and care systems that meet the company's standard will be offered a contract that often may have performance requirements to meet the needs and circumstances of the company's employees in a given market.

Member enrollment. The qualifying and contracted plans or care systems then are offered as an array of options to the company's employees in the annual enrollment process.

Performance monitoring. Each plan or care system will report on a periodic schedule on plan performance using agreed-upon formats such as HEDIS or other standard measures and also will report progress on specific performance benchmarks identified in the contract.

Member satisfaction surveys. Employer purchasers will survey, or commission a third party to survey, their employees as to their satisfaction with the services and care offered by the different plans and care systems.

Member communication and education. Results of satisfaction surveys and performance analysis systematically are made available to employees detailing the relative strengths of the plans and care systems offered, sometimes in relationship to the performance of health care organizations in the whole market or to national performance benchmarks.

Analysis and purchasing strategy formulation. Employer purchasers will undertake in the annual cycle strategic planning reviewing the performance of plans and setting targets for future performance. Long-term relationships with plans and health care systems are valued as are other kinds of suppliers with which a company works. Often, employee representatives or collective bargaining units will participate and help to set performance expectations for health care purchases.

The role of an effective purchasing sponsor is to create an environment of choice for the individual consumers it represents so that their decisions in choice of plan or provider within plans, use of flexible benefits, or participation in health risk prevention programs, etc., begin to shape the way health care products are delivered. The key information consumers need is clear—information on the strengths and weaknesses of plans and care systems in delivering effective health care (outcomes measurement).

Remarkable progress has been made to clarify and elaborate the terms and the information base upon which sophisticated purchasing can be undertaken. Major accreditation organizations have developed accreditation standards for comprehensive organized health delivery systems. Operational performance data have been standardized in the HEDIS measures and, as noted, over 350 plans are reporting uniformly on those measures. Purchasers and consumers have joined in sponsoring standardized toolsets to measure condition- or disease-specific outcomes and plans are being made to implement them in local health care markets.

The cumulative impact of these developments, especially the implementation of outcomes measurement, will be to tighten the "logic of value" in health care purchasing decisions. While standardized and increasingly refined operational performance measures will continue to benchmark health plans, condition- or disease-specific outcomes measurement will tie the knot for performance-based price elasticity in the health care market.

PERFORMANCE AND THE VISION OF THE ORGANIZED SYSTEM OF CARE

The implementation of outcomes measurement will create substantial demands upon plans—and plans are acutely aware of this burden. But these simply will not be added data collection demands. They will involve fundamental organizational development demands, similar to those experienced by American industrial organizations that have had to compete with quality products in global markets.

It is precisely this dynamic that employer purchasers find promising because, as health care organizations become competitive and achieve price elasticity based on performance measures, they will begin to achieve the ideals embodied in the vision of the organized system of care of the future (see Figure 2).

Figure 2. Organized System of Care

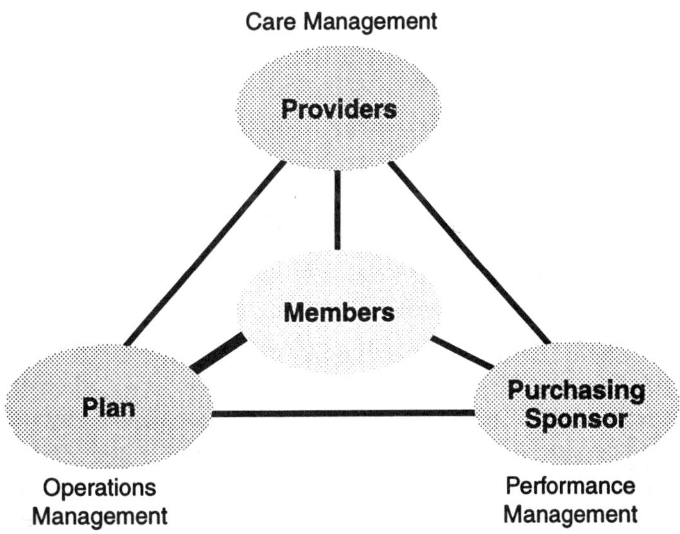

Organized System of Care

The OSC integrates the financing and delivery of a full continuum of care and is held clinically and fiscally accountable for the outcomes and health status of its enrolled population. The goal of the OSC is to provide quality, cost-effective care that improves the health status of the enrolled population.

For simplicity, characteristics have been grouped into the three broad organizational functions that must be carried out by all OSCs: care management, operations management, and performance management. Each is based on the mutual relationships between the members/consumers, the provider/clinicians, the organization/plan, and the purchasers representing the individual members in the collective (see Figure 3).

Figure 3. Language of Performance for the Organized System of Care

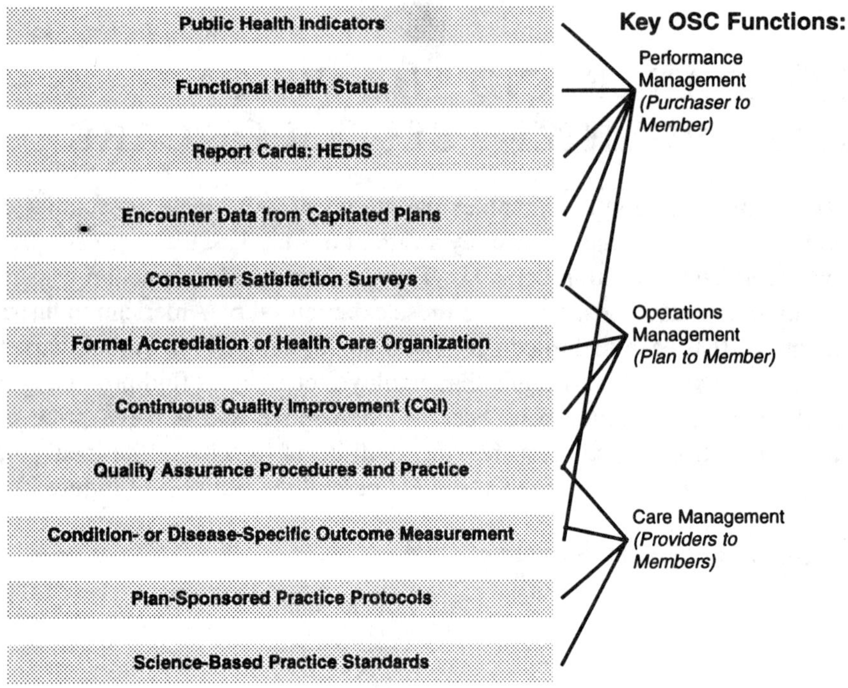

Key OSC Functions (and how they relate to the various formalities of quality and performance)

Care Management (Provider to Member). Care management refers to the processes used to influence the cost and quality of health care delivered to plan members. A distinguishing feature of an OSC is that care is patient centered. This involves all the mechanisms within the OSC that enhance the quality of care members receive: the peer review panels of clinicians and members, the process of design, and assessment of treatment procedures and policy. Of the quality formalities discussed above, science-based practice standards would be relevant because clinicians would be vigilant to bring the state of the medical art into the OSC's operations, especially shaping and constantly modifying the plan-sponsored practice protocols to reflect new developments in the field. The OSC also will incorporate condition- or disease-specific outcome measurement into its operations in order to enhance its care management function by systematically recording results of treatment. It also will constantly review results data in the context of its practice protocols as well as its clinicians' compliance with them. (The relationship of these reviews to the revision of the OSC's policies will affect its performance management functions.) Finally, traditional quality assurance procedures and practice will bring external reviewers into the plan through accreditation agencies to assess and confirm how well the OSC is doing in performing its care management functions. (Accreditation review also serves as an important part of the OSC's operations management function.)

Operations Management: (Plan to Member). The efficient management of OSC operations requires an integrated approach to functions such as provider credentialing, alignment and contract management, purchasing sponsor contract management, enrollment and patient satisfaction, clinical management and quality improvement, and cost accounting and other financial monitoring. Specifically, the OSC uses medical records, cost and financial data, and enrollment and eligibility data to drive and coordinate care, set goals, measure outcomes, and monitor performance. Again, in terms of the quality formalities discussed above, the OSC's operation management function includes condition- or disease-specific outcomes measurement and science-based practice protocols; but it will use its continuous quality improvement (CQI) processes to account for the results and outcomes of treatment and to feed back to its clinicians how well they comply with the endorsed protocols. As noted, the operations management function will oversee the implementation of quality assurance procedures and practice and organize the formal accreditation of health care organization by independent accrediting agencies. Member services will be performed under the operations management function, and consumer satisfaction surveys will be undertaken in this context. (The importance of consumer satisfaction information on OSC policy also will figure in the OSC's performance management function.) Finally, operations management will use these quality improvement activities as part of its negotiations and operating relationships with purchasers and network or affiliated provider clinicians.

Performance Management: (Purchaser to Member). Performance management refers to the processes by which OSCs demonstrate accountability for improving health plan operations and the health status of enrolled populations. Continuous improvement is a key concept guiding the OSC's performance management activities. Performance management is the seat of organizational policy for the OSC, directing its internal operations but also establishing its position with its customers and the community as a whole. The importance of consumer satisfaction surveys and condition- or disease-specific outcomes measurement for external relationships with purchasers has been noted. In cases in which comparisons with fee-for-service data are still relevant to purchasers, encounter data from capitated plans may be useful, and, increasingly, report cards such as HEDIS are relevant to health care purchasers. Finally, purchasers of health care are holding OSCs accountable for the functional health status of the covered population of its members and in the context of broader community responsibilities for their performance measured by public health indicators.

ACCOUNTABILITY PROCESSES

The test of achieving performance-based price elasticity for health care will require that the systematic and routine measurement of health outcomes become operational on a widespread basis. The strategy of starting with outcomes measurement will, in the context of the delivery system, bring along all of the elements of the quality spectrum, and implementation will entail more than just measurement and data collection. Implementation will require the development of effective accountability processes within the community/market and within the health care delivery system through which consumers, purchasers, and providers participate in the exercise of choices based on health outcomes and delivery system effectiveness that influences policy and practice. The employer-purchaser's vision of the organized system of care projects a model of an advanced health care organization that is an organic whole including members, their purchasing sponsors, and the provider community—interconnected with the plan administration and fully and appropriately participating to establish and maintain the health of the community. The accountability processes that will bond this organic whole together will involve all the participants and activate every element of the spectrum of quality and performance measurement.

Chapter 10

The Consumer Coalition for Quality Health Care

A Consumer Agenda

Andrew Webber

The organization of health care delivery and financing through managed care plans is revolutionizing the American health care system. This revolution is not fueled by consumer interests in ensuring access to high-quality health services, but by purchaser interests in containing escalating health care costs. In response to competitive pressures and rising budget deficits, employers and large public purchasers, including the Medicare and Medicaid programs, turned to managed care plans to help control health care expenditures.

The health care consumer was sadly relegated to the sidelines in this transition to managed care. Consumers, while not generally understanding the financing arrangements and the economic incentives of managed care, are acutely aware that their own health care delivery system is changing. Like much of health care, consumer reaction to managed care is highly personal and experience based. The following examples are typical of the range of consumer encounters with managed care:

- the disgruntled employee who finds that the company's new and only health care plan does not include his or her longstanding physician in the preferred network of physicians;
- the grateful welfare mother who, after years of trips to the emergency room, finally has a designated family physician for the care of her child;

- the frustrated individual attempting to cope with the endless approval process to see a specialist, particularly the disabled or chronically ill patient with special care needs;
- the relieved parents who are no longer saddled with arcane and unreadable insurance forms and exorbitant out-of-pocket expenses; and
- the angry mother opposed to being discharged from the hospital within 24 hours of childbirth.

As these consumer experiences illustrate, managed care represents both great risks and great opportunities for the health care consumer. The Institute of Medicine analyzed the impact of managed care on quality in this way: ". . . the paradigm shift call for health plans to provide needed services to a population in the face of stringent resource constraints, and the incentive will likely be to underserve people. These changes make monitoring the quality of care imperative, especially for the sickest individuals and other at-risk populations." The potential for managed care plans to impede access to needed services and health care professionals is the leading consumer concern under managed care.

Managed care also shows promise. By moving away from the fragmented and unmanaged fee-for-service system and emphasizing an integrated and multidisciplinary approach to disease management and preventive care, managed care plans have the potential to produce high-quality care at lower costs. Moreover, this new paradigm holds a single delivery system accountable for maintaining and improving the health status of a defined population.

This chapter, drawing on the work of the Consumer Coalition for Quality Health Care and the perspectives of consumer advocates from around the country, attempts to outline a policy framework for protecting, assuring, and improving quality under managed care. This recommended policy framework for managed care is reliant on the science of quality measurement, a subject well chronicled in previous chapters of this book. As previous authors have noted, the challenge of developing valid and reliable quality measures is in itself a complex task requiring ongoing investment and research. But the ultimate challenge, and one that can not be deferred in the search for the perfect measurement tool, is to efficiently and effectively apply quality measures in the establishment of a comprehensive system of quality accountability. That is the aim of this chapter.

QUALITY ACCOUNTABILITY SYSTEM

There is a natural chronology to the policy principles and recommendations that follow in designing a system of quality accountability. To enter the market, managed care plans must meet certain internal quality and structural standards in order to be licensed. This chapter recommends minimum plan standards that all plans must meet to participate in public programs and private markets for managed care.

Plans entering a highly competitive market succeed or fail on the basis of plan selection. To choose plans that match their needs and expectations, consumers must have access to quality-based information comparing the performance of plans across multiple indices. This chapter recommends a health care information system for the purpose of producing annual comparative reports on plan performance.

Consumers enrolled in managed care plans are entitled to certain rights, none more important than the right to file complaints and appeal plan treatment determinations. This is particularly important in the managed care setting because of capitation incentives and the potential for underservice. This chapter recommends a comprehensive complaint and appeals system that ensures an enrollee's right to an independent review of plan determinations.

Consumers enrolled in managed care plans do not have the clinical expertise to evaluate the technical quality of care provided by health plans, particularly on a systemic basis. Health care plans and practicing health care professionals within plans need to keep abreast of the ever-changing medical knowledge base and need help in identifying best practices. This chapter recommends an independent quality monitoring and improvement program that monitors quality and access to care, holds plans accountable for achieving ever-improving patient care results, and assists plans in quality improvement initiatives.

Consumer empowerment and the need for individual self-determination over one's own health care are essential characteristics of a patient-centered and accountable health care system. Consumers unfamiliar with managed care need help in navigating this new world of health care delivery and financing. This chapter recommends an independent managed care assistance program to serve as the consumer's advocate and to assist consumers in selecting plans and understanding their rights and responsibilities as plan members.

The recommended system for quality accountability in managed care is driven by an important policy principle—shared responsibility. Managed care plans and the health professionals and workers delivering care at the bedside must do their part to deliver compassionate and ever-improving quality care to the populations they serve. Government must provide common sense and efficient regulation of the managed care market. Purchasers—small and large employers and the Medicare and Medicaid programs—must be committed to expanding informed choice for consumers and monitoring the quality of care provided by all participating plans. The health care consumer must take responsibility for full participation in the health care decisionmaking process, including choice of plan, provider, treatment, and lifestyle.

Pieced together, the following policy principles and recommendations shape both a regulatory environment that demands quality and a competitive environment that rewards quality. Without both carrot and stick incentives for holding plans accountable for quality, the current managed care market will continue to be driven by competition to produce the lowest premium price—not by competition to achieve desired outcomes for the health care consumer.

HEALTH PLAN QUALITY STANDARDS

Policy Principle

The establishment of quality-oriented health plan standards—through state licensing, private accreditation, and Medicaid and Medicare conditions of participation—is an important first step in assuring quality health care in the managed care setting. The scope is limited, however, because the process attempts to measure a plan's internal capacity to deliver quality health care services. It cannot measure the actual provision of care, including timely access to care, effective treatment, and achievement of expected outcomes.

Discussion

Health plan market entry is an appropriate starting point for discussion of quality accountability in managed care. The McCarran-Ferguson Act gives states the primary responsibility to regulate the insurance industry. A managed care plan must be licensed by a state in order to conduct business in the private commercial marketplace.

The licensing process typically is conducted by a state insurance commissioner and is based on the establishment of health plan standards that must be met as a condition of market entry. Plan standards typically cover a wide spectrum of plan activities from fiscal solvency, to provider network adequacy, to marketing practices. The National Association of Insurance Commissioners (NAIC) is influential in this process by recommending model plan licensing standards that individual states routinely adopt.

The Health Care Financing Administration also certifies HMO plans for participation in the Medicare and Medicaid programs by using "conditions of participation" that look very similar to licensing standards established by states.

In recent years, large employers have moved beyond the state licensing process by demanding that any HMOs under contract for the provision of health services to their employees be privately accredited by independent entities, typically the National Committee for Quality Assurance (NCQA). Accreditation standards are similar and may exceed the licensing standards established by states.

The procedure for state licensing, private accreditation, and federal certification usually entails review of a plan's written application and typically an onsite evaluation of a plan's operation. States renew plan licenses on a periodic basis and major changes in a plan's operations must be approved. State licensing is self-supporting through the assessment of licensing fees on health plans. State and federal enforcement mechanisms typically include the ability to curtail or stop plan enrollment, assess financial penalties, and suspend or revoke a plan license. The gravity of enforcement mechanisms vary by state.

Concerns with the quality of care provided by managed care plans have led many states to enact legislation establishing plan standards. Prohibitions on gag rules and permitting mothers the choice of 48-hour maternity stays in hospitals are two well-publicized examples of legislative activity at the state and federal level.

Recommendations

1. State insurance commissioners, the Medicare and Medicaid programs, the Labor Department (with regulatory authority over self-funded ERISA plans), and private accrediting bodies should work together to develop a comprehensive and national set of plan standards that apply to all managed care plans. Over time, this could lead to a uniform procedure for licensing plans and approving participation in Medicare, Medicaid, and ERISA programs.
2. At minimum, plan standards should be developed for fiscal solvency, provider network adequacy, quality assurance and improvement, utilization review, member rights, provider credentialing, and marketing practices.
3. Mergers and acquisitions leading to the downsizing of the health care workforce merit vigilant oversight in today's managed care environment. Adequate staffing requirements should be established for all managed care plans and for any institutional provider in a plan's network.
4. Regulators should discourage the current plan practice of shifting financial risk to network providers because it increases the potential for underservice, perpetuates an already fragmented delivery system, and reduces incentives for plans to create an integrated system of quality improvement and accountability. All plans should be required to make contracts with providers publicly available upon request, and limitations should be placed on capitation incentives at the individual physician level.

INFORMED CONSUMER CHOICE

Policy Principle

Choosing a health plan should be the responsibility of individual employees and beneficiaries, not employers and public purchasers. Employers and purchasers should be responsible for ensuring that all plans offered to employees and beneficiaries meet minimum quality standards and for providing comparative performance information to guide individual plan selection. Such an informed-choice strategy will lead to quality-based competition in the marketplace. It also will send a strong signal to managed care plans that quality is a distinguishing factor in plan selection and future market success, thus encouraging plan investments in quality improvement. But despite recent advances in quality measurement and information disclosure, it will be many years before informed consumer choice drives a quality-based competitive marketplace for managed care plans. Quality measurement science is still in infancy and consumers will need an expanded choice of plans and intensive education and training to understand and use sophisticated comparative information. Regulatory oversight is needed to supplement informed-choice strategies and to assure the quality of health care in managed care plans.

Background

Managed care plans that become successfully licensed in states enter a highly competitive marketplace. Plan selection, by purchasers and those individual consumers with the luxury of choosing plans, determines market success or failure.

In an ideal world, plan selection would be based on a consumer's determination of plan value, as measured by price, covered benefits, quality, and customer satisfaction. Managed care plans that produce better value for their customers would reap the rewards through increased enrollment and revenue. All consumers would benefit from plans competing to generate ever-improving quality and service at lower prices.

Experts agree that the textbook model of value-based plan competition does not exist in today's market. Many consumers either do not have health insurance, their employer selects a plan for them, or their choice of plan is limited. Moreover, consumers with choices typically select a health plan based on cost, benefits, and the provider network within a plan. Information on quality-based plan performance and customer satisfaction is not available, leaving the current marketplace dominated by price competition. This has negative consequences for quality health care as plans squeeze important investments in internal quality assurance and improvement programs, reduce staffing levels, and shift financial risk to network providers to stay price competitive.

Recently, however, there has been a renaissance in the field of quality measurement that shows promise for producing consumer reports (often called report cards) on quality-based plan performance. The Agency for Health Care Policy and Research (AHCPR), NCQA, the Foundation for Accountability (FACCT), Medicare peer review organizations (PROs), academic groups, research corporations, and specialty societies are just some of the groups involved in practice guideline development, performance and outcome measurement, consumer surveys, and other significant quality measurement activities.

AHCPR currently is sponsoring a five-year Consumer Assessments of Health Plans Study. CAHPS is a major effort to: (1) develop and test questionnaires to assess health plans and services from the point of view of consumers; (2) produce easily understandable reports for communicating survey information to consumers; and (3) evaluate the usefulness of these reports for consumers selecting health care plans and services.

HCFA recently announced its commitment to develop comparative reports on plan performance to help guide beneficiary selection of Medicare HMOs. Information from HEDIS 3.0 (NCQA's performance measurement system for managed care plans) and the CAHPS enrollee satisfaction survey will be included in the reports to beneficiaries. Large employers, like GTE and Federal Express, have led the way in informed-choice strategies by expanding plan choices and preparing comparative guidebooks for employees during open enrollment periods. Medicaid state agencies also are committed to report cards as increasing numbers of Medicaid clients move into managed care plans.

NCQA recently released "Quality Compass"—its first report card on the comparative performance of 226 health plans providing services to 26 million individuals. "Quality Compass" combines the results of NCQA accreditation and HEDIS information (HEDIS is NCQA's performance measurement system for health care plans). Major employers have indicated that they will integrate "Quality Compass" information into plan descriptions and comparisons provided to employees.

State government is becoming more active in the informed-choice arena through the establishment of managed care information advisory committees, boards, and councils responsible for the collection and public release of information on provider performance. For several years New York state's health department has published a risk-adjusted report card on hospital and individual physician performance on heart bypass surgery. Minnesota, Florida, and Utah are all engaged in comparative reports card development for managed care plans licensed in the state.

Recommendations

1. The federal government should be responsible for developing a consumer information agency responsible for the development and dissemination of comparative public reports on health plan performance. This agency should be supported by an information council that is responsible for selecting plan performance measures. To the degree possible, selected quality measures should be consistent with quality measures being mandated in the private sector, particularly NCQA's HEDIS measures. All self-reported plan performance data should be independently audited to ensure the data accuracy and integrity.
2. Valid and reliable plan performance measures should be established in the following areas: price/copayment, benefits, provider network, clinical quality, service quality, and consumer satisfaction. Clinical quality information should include access, process, and risk-adjusted outcome measures. Service quality should include comparative waiting and appointment times, disenrollment rates, and complaint and appeals statistics.

3. Federal and state legislation should require a minimum patient encounter database for managed care plans as a condition of state licensure or participation in Medicare or Medicaid. A patient encounter database would support report card development and external monitoring of plan performance.
4. The ability to service and treat sick and vulnerable populations enrolled in managed care plans should be the litmus test for managed care plans. Quality measurement efforts should focus special attention and additional resources on evaluating the care received by such populations—particularly the disabled, the chronically ill, and individuals with rare diseases. Enrollee satisfaction surveys should be conducted of valid samples of vulnerable populations. Individuals leaving plans also should be independently surveyed to make certain that plans do not encourage disenrollment by frustrating access to needed services for vulnerable populations.
5. Plan competition on avoiding risk rather than managing risk will continue as a major obstacle to quality-based competition until plan premium payments reflect the health risks of enrolled populations. Risk-adjusted premium and provider payment methodologies must be implemented to encourage enrollment and appropriate treatment of vulnerable populations.
6. Consumer choice of plans should be expanded. The development of purchasing alliances among small businesses and the mandating of multiple-choice options through federal and state legislation should be encouraged.

COMPLAINT AND APPEALS SYSTEM

Policy Principle

Every managed care plan licensed in a state should have a fair and rapid system for resolving enrollee complaints and appeals. The need for such a system is particularly compelling in managed care arrangements where the plan actually provides services and greatly influences the decisions about what medical care a covered person will receive. The financial incentives of capitation encourages plans to limit the use of services and, as a result, many covered persons are at risk of a wrongful denial of care. An effective complaint and appeals system is a critical consumer protection and right under managed care.

Discussion

Once consumers enroll in a managed care plan, protecting an individual's right to all covered benefits and the provision of high-quality service and treatment becomes a paramount concern.

Consumers that enroll in managed care plans enter a new and unfamiliar world of health care delivery and financing. Under the fee-for-service system, there was a reasonable expectation that the interests of consumers in receiving health services were aligned with the financial interests of providers. The incentives of capitation changed this dynamic to the point where consumers now question whether physicians have greater allegiance to their contracted plan or to their patient.

Access to a complaint and appeals system is an important consumer right under any delivery system but particularly under managed care. To counterbalance managed care incentives to underserve, all enrollees must have the right to challenge the health care plan if they believe that medically necessary services are being denied, reduced, or terminated. Consumers also must have the opportunity to air complaints if they feel mistreated or believe that have received poor quality service or treatment.

Current complaint and appeals mechanisms for individuals enrolled in managed care plans are not well established. In the private commercial marketplace, most states require that managed care organizations have an internal complaint system but do not mandate specific procedures, like second-level reviews by independent peer panels. In the absence of regulatory standards, managed care organizations are left as judge and jury for the care they provide.

The NAIC has developed model complaint and appeals standards for states to adopt. NAIC recommendations include: uniform standards for initiating complaints, first- and second-level review requirements with timeframes, expedited reviews in the case of service denials that may jeopardize the life or health of an enrollee, appeals to the designated state agency, and rights to judicial review.

The current NAIC model authorizes establishment of a second-level review within the health plan and stipulates that a majority of the panel shall be comprised of persons who were not previously involved in the complaint. Consumer advocates argue for an independent review outside the plan and for the continuation of benefits at no cost to the enrollee during dispute resolution.

The structure and design of the managed care complaint and appeals system is a contentious political issue at the state level. The managed care industry is well organized to fight comprehensive and independent complaint/appeals procedures, and consumer advocacy groups are beginning to organize around the issue. In New York state, the industry was successful in blocking legislation pushed by consumer groups that would have granted independent appeal rights to managed care enrollees.

The Medicare and Medicaid programs represent the best currently operating model for a meaningful appeal systems. Both programs require review by an entity outside the plan and, where necessary, independent outside medical review. However, certain safeguards are lacking. For example, the Medicare program, which has an independent outside contractor review all medical issues arising between a beneficiary and an HMO, still does not have enough time limits for resolving cases where treatment has been denied, reduced, or terminated and the beneficiary is not receiving care.

In addition, the Heath Care Financing Administration has been lax in communicating to beneficiaries what their rights are, and in requiring that managed care plans fully implement the procedures required under current law. A Medicare beneficiary class-action suit—*Grijalva v. Shalala*—against the Secretary of the U.S. Department of Health and Human Services was won by beneficiaries and will lead to an improved appeals process in the Medicare program through regulatory rulemaking.

Recommendations

1. A complaint and appeals system should apply to every type of enrollee grievance or dispute within a managed care plan.
2. Written notices should be given to enrollees for any decision to deny, reduce, or terminate services requested by the enrollee or by the provider. The notice should state the specific reason for the decision and describe the appeals process available to the enrollee.
3. A model appeals process should include: (a) a first-level review by the health plan; (b) a second-level review by individuals who have not participated in the first level and, in instances of medical necessity or appropriateness, a second-level review by an independent peer panel or entity having no connection to the plan or financial interest in the review outcome; (c) an appeal to an administrative law judge; and (d) judicial review.
4. Expedited review mandates and timeframes should be established for any care denied, reduced, or terminated by a health plan that is appealed by the enrollee. In an expedited review, the appeals procedure should be completed as rapidly as the situation requires, with a maximum allowable time of five working days from the day expedited review was requested to the time the second-level review is completed.
5. Independent review by a peer panel or independent entity for all appeals involving medical necessity and appropriateness should be required. Health plans should be required to pay for this independent review, thus giving plans the incentive to resolve complaints internally.
6. Enrollees in managed care plans should have access to second opinions with minimal cost-sharing requirements. Second opinions should be free for Medicaid beneficiaries.
7. Information on the complaint and appeals process should be required in all marketing materials developed by plans and should be posted

prominently in managed care facilities and physician offices. The number of individual complaints, the number of appeals at all levels, and the results of appeals should be provided as comparative data in consumer reports on plan performance.

QUALITY MONITORING AND IMPROVEMENT

Policy Principle

Consumers enrolled in managed care plans do not have the clinical expertise to evaluate the technical quality of care provided by plans, particularly on a systemic basis. Health care plans and participating providers find it difficult to keep abreast of the ever-changing medical knowledge base and need help in identifying best practices. An independent quality monitoring and improvement program is needed to track patient access to appropriate care, facilitate internal and cross-plan quality improvement initiatives, and hold managed care plans accountable for achieving ever-improving patient care results.

Discussion

Competition among managed care plans is most likely to improve the visible, service quality aspects of health care delivery, such as waiting times, geographic proximity and convenience, and interpersonal communication with patients. It is far less likely, until consumers are educated to understand sophisticated quality measures, to affect complex technical issues in quality of care.

Most consumers recognize that they do not possess the clinical knowledge and expertise to evaluate the quality of health care services. An effective complaint and appeals system will provide some protection against egregious cases of denied access or poor quality, but it cannot begin to uncover the potential universe of systemic quality concerns. Particularly under managed care, the average consumer will not know when medically necessary services are being withheld or that treatments received did not meet accepted practice guidelines. This concern is exacerbated for those who most need good health care—the disabled, chronically ill, and the disadvantaged.

Managed care plans, and their participating network of providers, face uncertainty of their own in understanding the complexity of clinical medicine. It is difficult for plans and providers to keep abreast of an ever-changing medical knowledge base as medical research produces new understandings about health and illness along with new tests and treatments. Widespread variation in medical service use, treatment, and outcome is the predictable result but one that is little understood by the public. Plans and their participating providers and facilities need help in integrating new medical knowledge into active practice and in identifying quality benchmarks.

Independent quality monitoring and professional oversight is a well-accepted principle in most industries. In the context of managed care, with the incentives to underserve, the monitoring of access to care becomes imperative, particularly for vulnerable populations. Efficient and effective population-based methodologies, such as the small area variations technique pioneered by John Wennberg, MD, are well established to monitor utilization rates within managed care plans, although they are dependent upon the availability of patient encounter databases. Population-based monitoring of plan adherence to accepted practice guidelines is also needed to ensure the quality of care enrollees receive.

Independent professional oversight also can hold plans accountable for their stated commitment to continuous quality improvement and facilitating improvement activity. The application of quality improvement science to the health care industry shows the promise of accelerating patient care results for the largest number of health care consumers. Independent monitoring entities, with expertise in quality improvement, could help facilitate plan improvement initiatives by disseminating new medical knowledge and best practices and organizing community-based quality improvement initiatives across all plans licensed in the state. The sharing of best practices among plans often is frustrated by competitive and proprietary factors that can be overcome with the active involvement of independent entities that have the backing and endorsement of public and private purchasers.

Independent quality monitoring and oversight is well established in the public-sector health insurance programs. Since the early 1970s the Medicare program has contracted with independent, state-based, peer review organizations for quality monitoring and review of Medicare's fee-for-service system.

Since the late 1980s, PROs also have reviewed the quality of care provided by Medicare HMOs. Current PRO review of Medicare HMOs is focused on monitoring and facilitating plan improvement activities through local improvement projects. National projects are under way to improve breast cancer screening and the management of heart disease and diabetes. PRO efforts, particularly population-based monitoring of patient access to needed care, have been hampered by HCFA's unwillingness to mandate HMO reporting of patient encounter data.

By federal mandate, state Medicaid agencies also must contract with external quality review organizations (EQROs) for the evaluation of managed care services provided to Medicaid beneficiaries. External quality monitoring for managed care in both the Medicaid and Medicare programs are relatively new initiatives with few published results to date.

In the private sector, independent oversight of the quality of care is not a well-established principle, although organized quality improvement activities working with health plans are well established. The Breakthrough Series of the Institute for Healthcare Improvement, directed by Donald Berwick, MD, is a leading private-sector model of collaborative plan and provider initiatives to lower costs and improve outcomes. Employers and employer coalitions also have organized state and local outcome initiatives to facilitate and promote improvement activities among plans at the community level, but initiatives are isolated and results are not published.

Recommendations

1. Congress should enact a nationally designed but locally implemented quality monitoring and improvement program to assure and improve the quality of care in managed care plans.
2. The core functions of an independent quality monitoring and improvement program should be: (a) monitoring access and quality in managed care plans using population-based methods; (b) holding plans accountable for systemic improvements in the quality of care through documenting plan progress in achieving quality improvement results; and (c) facilitating plan quality improvement activity through the identification and feedback of best practices and the organization of community-wide improvement projects.
3. An independent quality monitoring and improvement program should be required to share information with regulatory bodies when systemic patterns of poor quality or undertreatment are uncovered. Independent monitoring entities should not possess regulatory authority but should be empowered to recommend enforcement action by federal and state entities.
4. Quality monitoring and improvement functions should be performed by state-based, private-sector, nonprofit organizations governed by a board of all parties in the health care system, including consumers, purchasers, and health care professionals. The staff expertise of independent entities should include individuals with credentials in: quality improvement, epidemiology, medical statistics, performance measurement, practice guidelines, and provider and consumer education.

CONSUMER ASSISTANCE

Policy Principle

The managed care system is an inherently unbalanced playing field in terms of knowledge, access to information, and power. A consumer-based continuum of education, support, and representation at the individual, plan, and system level is needed to empower consumers to take responsibility for their own health and health care choices.

Discussion

Consumers need help navigating the new world of managed care—particularly vulnerable populations who have the greatest health care needs and the most to lose under managed care arrangements.

Consumers have very basic questions about managed care: What is managed care? How is the delivery of health care services different in a managed care plan? Will I have a choice of my own physician? Can I receive care outside the network of plan providers? How do I select a plan? What are my rights as a member of a health plan? What do I do if I have a complaint about the plan or believe that services are being denied me? How do I file a complaint or appeal a treatment decision? Can I leave a plan at any time if I am dissatisfied? What is the process of enrollment in a new plan?

The concept of an ombudsman has a long history in health care. In the context of managed care, an independent assistance and ombudsman program could play a valuable role in empowering health care consumers. First, a consumer assistance program could educate, train, and assist consumers in selecting managed care plans. Individuals on staff to an assistance program could lead consumers through a structured needs assessment tool for the purpose of matching individual and family health care needs with plans that perform well in identified health service arenas. Trained staff could help consumers understand sophisticated quality-based performance information and use such information in making plan, provider, and treatment decisions.

Second, a consumer assistance program could play a valuable role in assisting individuals as enrollees of a plan. Trained staff could help enrollees resolve complaints and understand their rights as members of a plan. An ombudsman could act as an important consumer liaison with managed care plans—advising plans on systemic concerns that enrollees are encountering with the provision of health services, while running interference with plans for consumers with individual grievances.

Finally, an independent managed care ombudsman program could help consumers organize around managed care issues. Such assistance could take the form of helping enrollees petition, at the plan level, for improvements in the delivery system and, at the systemwide level, for needed consumer rights and regulatory protections. Plan enrollees need assistance in organizing their interests and encouraging plans to fully include enrollees in all plan policymaking activities, including shared decisionmaking at the individual treatment level. Ombudsman could advocate for the inclusion of enrollees on the governing boards of managed care plans and the creation of enrollee advisory committees.

Enrollees that suffer from the same disease or illness also could use assistance in organizing support groups that would provide continual feedback to plans on patient experience and suggested improvements in treatment processes. At a systemwide level, an assistance program could help organize consumers to petition legislative and regulatory bodies for public policies that advance consumer protections and quality oversight systems in managed care.

The State Long Term Care Ombudsman Program created by the Older Americans Act represents a useful model that could help inform the design of an ombudsman initiative under managed care. The current program is more narrowly focused on patient advocacy in long term care facilities, but its functions and responsibilities can be easily translated to managed care settings.

Another relevant program created by the Older Americans Act and funded by the Health Care Financing Administration is the Health Insurance Counseling Assistance Program. HICAPs assist the elderly in understanding Medicare's insurance and payment policies, Medigap insurance policies, and the Medicare HMO option available to seniors. As Medicare HMOs become more broadly available to beneficiaries, HICAPs have experienced a marked increase in inquiries and requests for assistance. HICAPs, particularly those that are linked to legal assistance programs, also are involved in identifying systemic problems that the elderly consumers encounter with managed care plans and have become effective advocates for consumer rights in these settings.

With the dominance of employer-based insurance in the private sector, employers typically assume the role of an ombudsman for their employees. This is particularly true for large employers, where personnel and benefit administration offices organize information for employees on plan selection, provide education on health plan member rights, and often play interference for employees that have concerns and complaints with their plan. Small employers have a more difficult time providing needed assistance to employees because of limited resources and therefore might be convinced of the advantage of a publicly sponsored ombudsman program. Employees working for large or small employers would benefit from an independent consumer assistance program.

Recommendations

1. Federal, state, and local governments should support the establishment of a national network of local consumer assistance programs for enrollees of managed care plans. Such programs should be financed by a small assessment on plan premiums.
2. A managed care consumer assistance program should have three critical functions: insurance and plan selection counseling, the traditional ombudsman function of complaint investigation, and the organization of advocacy efforts at the individual plan and systemwide level.
3. A national center should be established for the purpose of training the staff of local managed care assistance programs. A major focus of the training center should be to educate the staff of assistance programs to: use managed care plan report cards, understand enrollee rights and responsibilities, investigate enrollee complaints, and organize consumer advocacy efforts.
4. Managed care plans should be required to include enrollees on their governing boards. At minimum, all plans should be required to establish consumer advisory committees for the purpose of actively soliciting input and recommendations on plan policies, utilization review procedures, treatment and disease management protocols, and plan operations.

CONCLUSION

Purchaser interests and a cost containment imperative have driven the first generation of managed care. It is the hope of this author that a new era in managed care is approaching, driven by consumer interests and a quality-of-care imperative. No longer should managed care's success be measured by meeting the bottom-line demands of business and government; it should be measured by its ability to ensure access to high-quality and ever-improving health care services—particularly to vulnerable populations.

To accomplish this aim, a system of quality accountability is needed for managed care. Such a system would, by creatively applying the emerging science of quality measurement, produce a market environment that rewards quality and a regulatory environment that demands quality. Quality-of-care measurement and management science also would be used by managed care organizations to accelerate health care professional learning and quality improvement activities within integrated systems of care. The ultimate beneficiary would be the health care consumer.

Chapter 11

Allina Health Systems

Measuring and Improving Organizational Performance

Bryan Bushick, MD, MBA

Health care organizations are becoming more complex through growth and consolidation. It is increasingly difficult to balance cost, quality, and access in the face of an aging population, technology advances, and cost-shifting tensions between the public and private sectors. Given this reality, it is more difficult, yet more important, to understand organizational performance and the factors that drive it. This insight is challenging enough to achieve within a single operating business, such as a hospital or health plan, where structure and mindset commonly reinforce departmental distinction and suboptimization often occurs. The resulting toll on overall organizational effectiveness is characterized by inefficiency, rework, unfocused efforts, and a wealth of missed opportunities for innovation. As operating units are combined during integration, the challenge of understanding and managing organizational performance dramatically increases.

This chapter describes the implementation of a key performance indicator initiative in an integrating health care system. This effort's fundamental principles are associated with sustainable performance excellence and include a focus on customers, the use of evaluation cycles to promote learning, an emphasis on data-based management, and an orientation toward results. The core values and concepts outlined in the 1995 Malcolm Baldrige Health Care Pilot Criteria provide an excellent overview of these fundamental principles.[1] The key performance indicator initiative is based on the premise that the leading health care entities for the next century will be those that can instill such fundamental principles within the very fabric of their organizations. Performance measurement at Allina supports this quest.

To clarify, performance measurement is not about assuring or controlling health care quality. It is not about quality as a feature or attribute of a service or product. It does not pertain to the traditional view of quality in health care—and many other industries—as the work of a department or dedicated group of staff. To the contrary, it is about improving the functioning of an entire system. In the context of what is trying to be accomplished, the insight gained from the analysis of performance can be used to achieve sustainable performance excellence. Clarity of organizational intent—as outlined in the vision, mission, and strategic plan—and a deep commitment to the ongoing evaluation of performance and the systematic reconsideration of strategy are required.

Key indicators are intended to reflect performance across multiple dimensions. As a set, they should help leaders and staff understand performance and better predict future performance and subsequent results. While some aspects of this work previously have been described,[2] this chapter will highlight the development and use of key performance indicators in an emerging integrated health care system and one of its major components, the managed care operating unit. In this case, the performance measurement agenda was principally intended to foster integration throughout an organization as it was forming. Without the luxury of a stable culture, structure, and strategic priorities, this initiative is intended to help manage change, maintain performance during the transition, and lay the foundation for ongoing high performance.

BACKGROUND

To fully appreciate the approach and challenges, one must understand the context. In a market known for its experience and innovation in managed care, Allina Health System was created in 1994 through the merger of a multihospital system, HealthSpan Health System, with Medica, a local HMO serving the state of Minnesota. (HealthSpan itself was the product of a merger of two hospital organizations in 1993.) A combination of external and internal factors were conducive to Allina's formation. External factors included a state health policy environment that supported managed care and the creation of integrated care systems, an active and informed purchasing community, and continued provider-side reconfiguration to meet market demands for access, accountability, and overall value. Internally, both HealthSpan's and Medica's management teams reached independent but simultaneous decisions to pursue the next level of performance in care management and health improvement.[3] This was sought in an environment characterized by extensive managed care penetration, where consumers enjoyed a high general standard of care at costs below many major metropolitan markets throughout the United States.

Allina currently is comprised of hospitals, physician practices, ancillary health care businesses, and a health plan that offers a range of products throughout the region. Details regarding the system and the populations served are included in Figure 1. Since Allina is a not-for-profit organization, the board of directors and senior management team maintain shared responsibility for stewardship of Allina's resources and more than $2 billion in revenue. Allina's vision to become "the recognized innovator in community health improvement"[4] will occur through collaboration with stakeholders. The vision's reference to "community" encompasses members and employer groups served by the health plan as well as geographic areas and selected special-need groups of individuals throughout the region.

Figure 1. Allina Health System Characteristics

- *19 owned and managed hospitals (30,000 admissions)*
- *56 owned clinics (over 425 physicians and 1.4 million visits)*
- *7 nursing homes*
- *Ambulance, home health care, and other ancillary companies*
- *Network-model HMO (over 6,000 contracted physicians)*
  - *840,000 commercial members*
  - *100,000 Medicare members*
  - *60,000 Medicaid members*
- *$2.1 billion net revenue (1995)*
- *20,000 employees*

As Allina emerged, support grew for the creation of a new function, one without precedent in either HealthSpan or Medica. This area, Performance Measurement and Improvement (PM&I), provided system-level coordination to support Allina's desire to be accountable—internally and externally—for its performance. This accountability was needed to provide ongoing management and execution of strategic priorities and to demonstrate Allina's value to community stakeholders. As defined at its creation, the PM&I agenda does not concentrate on traditional quality assurance. Although attentive to the expectations of state regulators and accrediting bodies such as the Joint Commission on Accreditation of Healthcare Organizations (JCAHO) and the National Committee for Quality

Assurance (NCQA), external reporting is not the objective. The focus intentionally reaches beyond the boundaries of traditional quality improvement or quality assurance functions to promote a fundamental set of principles for achieving true performance excellence. PM&I's goal is to understand past and present performance from multiple dimensions as a basis for identifying the true drivers of organizational success.

A rich and varied set of experiences pertaining to "quality" resided within HealthSpan and Medica at the time of the merger. Some business units were more evolved than others. Consequently, leaders, quality professionals, and employees from throughout Allina were engaged in 1995 in an effort to reconcile differences in terminology, clarify philosophy, and ultimately create a unifying foundation for proceeding with Allina's commitment to being "quality-driven." The result was the Blueprint for Quality. Beyond articulating principles, the Blueprint included specific tactics in support of six strategic planks (Figure 2). Not surprisingly, given the commitment from Allina's executive office, the roles of leadership, measurement, and customer feedback were reinforced.

Figure 2. Long-Range Strategic Planks

1. *Cultivate shared leadership throughout Allina to steward its commitment to quality principles and establish accountability for improvement (e.g., boards, senior management, employees, unions, affiliated providers).*
2. *Engage physicians, actively and meaningfully, in Allina's commitment to excellence based on quality principles.*
3. *Transform strategic planning processes to reflect and reinforce quality principles.*
4. *Enhance Allina's capacity to gather, refine, and disseminate "customer knowledge" as the basis for decisionmaking and action.*
5. *Establish the organizational infrastructure, including technical and facilitative resources, educational vehicles, and communication channels, to support Allina's evolution.*
6. *Advance the systematic rigorous measurement of Allina's internal and external environments, its efforts, and their results.*

Significant change has continued to take place in Allina's environment. This has only added to the challenges of managing this complex undertaking. Provider-side consolidation has continued and realignment of physician groups has accelerated. A local employer coalition, the Buyers Health Care Action Group, has shifted from its initial encouragement of integrated systems to the pursuit of more direct relationships with providers, a move that could alter the roles of health plans and providers. In addition, there is continued call for increased accountability by purchasers and consumers concerning the performance of providers and managed care organizations. This activity principally is focused within the Minnesota Health Data Institute. The Institute is a public-private partnership to collect, analyze, and report health care performance data and support health care industry electronic commerce. Finally, cost pressures have escalated, with significant current and future implications for providers and health plans. This challenging environment clearly reinforces the need for effective mechanisms to understand and improve performance.

KEY PERFORMANCE INDICATORS

Key performance indicators are a set of measures that provide a view of organizational performance—past, present, and future. Taken together, they should relate directly to an organization's strategy and priorities. The indicators balance short- and long-term horizons on performance and include a mix of lagging and leading measures. As summarized by Kaplan and Norton, lagging indicators typically reflect outcome measures that are consistent with strategy. Such measures often convey goals that are common to many organizations and tend to reflect past performance such as market share and profitability.[5] Leading indicators are measures that are thought to have some association—ideally, predictive power—with the desired outcomes. When linked to true performance drivers, such leading indicators can provide early feedback on an organization's progress in achieving strategic priorities.

In translating strategy into actionable terms, the key performance indicators serve as a bridge from strategy to tactics.[6] Once implemented, the key performance indicators are intended to become the core of an organization's management system. [7] The primary customers for system-level key indicators are senior leaders and governing boards. Ideally, analysis will reveal associations among key indicators, and this insight can be used to enhance performance and refine the key indicators over time. Additionally, as implementation continues, one should expect more explicit linkage of system-level key indicators with tactics and frontline efforts through operating unit key indicator sets and departmental plans.

The Allina key performance indicator initiative was influenced significantly by three sources. First, Kaplan and Norton's seminal work regarding the balanced scorecard provided critical foundational material and highlighted experiences from other industries.[8, 9, 10] Second, the perspective of Heskett and his associates on the "service-profit chain" provided important direction.[11] Third, a unifying framework for Allina's quest to be quality-driven was provided by the Malcolm Baldrige National Quality Award criteria.[12] Reaffirming parallels were noted between Allina's six strategic planks (Figure 2) and the seven Baldrige categories. In particular, Baldrige Category: Information and Analysis, was reinforcing for this initiative. It confirmed the importance of integrating diverse information that pertains to all strategies and key operations for use in establishing targets, demonstrating success relative to customer requirements, and identifying business drivers. The vital role of comparative data also is highlighted, as is the critical leadership practice of routinely assessing performance. Finally, the importance of relating customer data, improvements in service, and process enhancements with relevant indicators of overall performance—that include financial as well as other market indicators—is emphasized.

For any organization, the initial benefit of developing key performance indicators is the communication that it sparks. Efforts to identify a limited set of key indicators provoke internal dialogue regarding strategy and the overarching direction of an organization. As demonstrated in Figure 3, it is vital that insights into customer requirements provide the foundation for strategy and that effective feedback loops exist to ensure the strategy is refined as needed. Once confirmed, strategy provides the basis for key performance indicators. At Allina, this stage was particularly challenging given the organizational and environmental complexities that existed. The resulting clarity, as reflected in the specific key indicators, then can be used to help align the efforts of numerous operating units and focus the organization on a discrete number of priorities.

Figure 3. Context for Key Performance Indicators

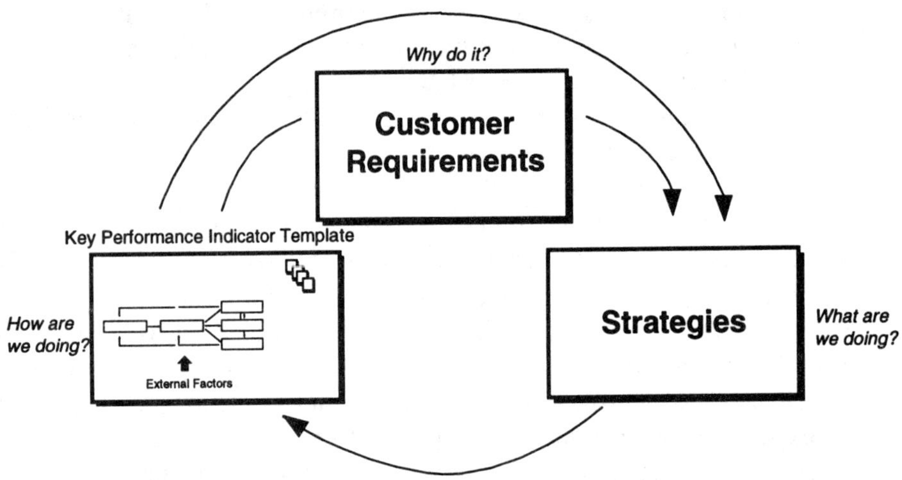

Through the experience in applying key indicators at many levels throughout the organization, Allina expects to be able to:

1. identify potential problems earlier in their course,
2. promote transfer of innovations more efficiently across the system,
3. identify drivers of performance as well as high-leverage processes and uses of resources,
4. demonstrate success across many dimensions of performance, and
5. challenge hypotheses upon which strategy is based, thereby routinely refreshing the critical thinking and assumptions that drive Allina.

With this foundation, Allina has proceeded with the simultaneous creation of multiple sets of key performance indicators within Allina's major operating components (Figure 4).

Figure 4. Parallel Development Efforts Throughout Allina

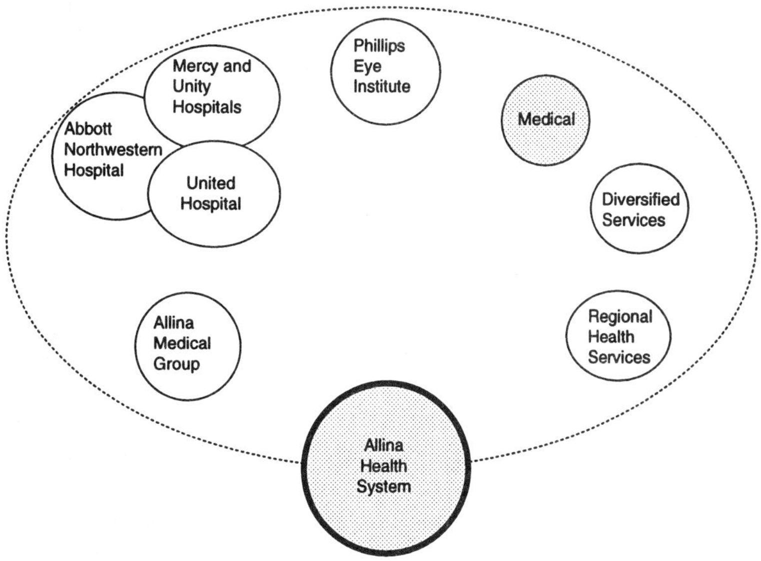

NOTE: Shaded components represent the subjects of this chapter.

Although complex, this parallel process was used to:

- build on the varied experiences that exist throughout the organization,
- foster alignment around categories from the template and specific indicators, and
- expedite full implementation in response to a rapidly changing environment.

A participative process was used to support development of the unifying Allina template and the design and implementation of key performance indicators throughout the organization. The template, which is explained in detail in the following section, consists of five major categories and provides a mechanism for organizing this work. Representatives were involved from all major operating areas as well as key staff functions including information services, finance, and human resources. The experiences of other organizations inside and outside of health care were reviewed.[13–24] Additionally, reporting sets and criteria such as those from the Health Plan Employer Data and Information Set (HEDIS), JCAHO, Foundation for Accountability, Minnesota Health Data Institute, and other external parties also were considered.[25–29]

Not surprisingly, early design efforts confirmed a major gap between available data and what was desired. In acknowledging this gap, considerations spanned from data definitions and completeness to the efficiency of retrieval and time lag in collection. Throughout the development process, a balance was sought between using currently available information to begin testing this model and learning from the use of key indicators and waiting until data gaps were filled for key indicators that were desired, but not available. In light of the complexity of Allina and challenges facing the organization, the decision was made to proceed using data that were easily retrievable. This tact enabled Allina to gain experience, fully expecting that additional data would be added and refinements made over time.

The ongoing challenge will be to manage this tradeoff, recognizing the complexity and costs associated with generating meaningful key indicator data. As feasibility testing proceeds for indicators that are desired, a "placeholder" is maintained in the key indicator report. Beyond signifying a future intent to measure an area, this placeholder reinforces the importance of the topic and supports internal communication of this message.

KEY PERFORMANCE INDICATOR TEMPLATE

The primary vehicle for stimulating alignment of key indicators throughout Allina is the key performance indicator template (Figure 5). The template consists of five categories and was used to help identify and organize system-level key indicators. In the template, categories of "Internal Competencies and Capabilities" and "Core and Support Processes" include leading indicators, providing a more upstream reflection of performance. Ideally, if leading indicators accurately reflect the drivers of business, information from these categories will help predict important outcomes (signified by lagging indicators) in the "Clinical and Community Health Improvement," "Customer Satisfaction and Loyalty," and "Financial Health" categories. One also would expect interrelationships to be documented between indi-

Figure 5. Allina Template for Key Performance Indicators

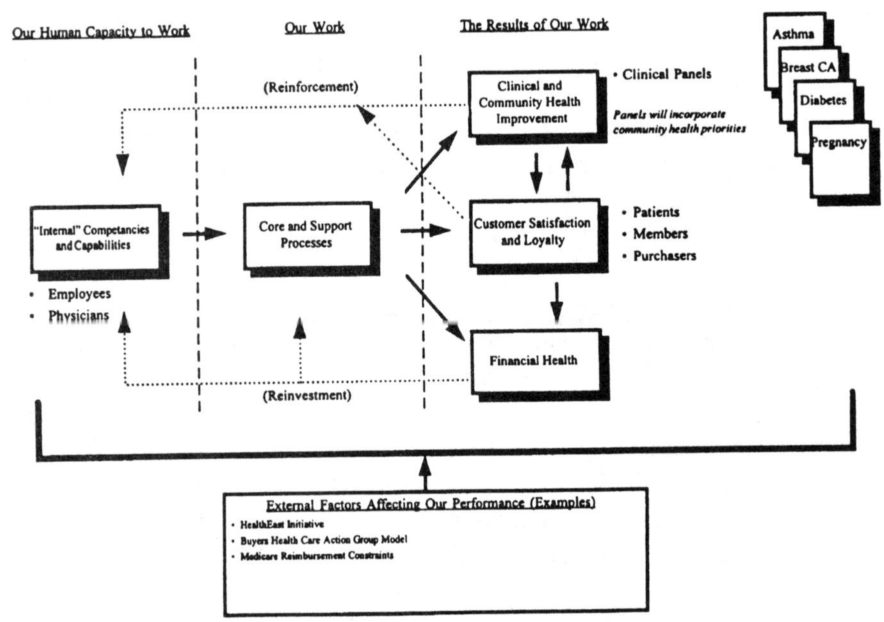

cators in the three downstream results categories. For example, enhanced customer loyalty will increase the potential for improving health through risk reduction due to the prolonged customer relationship. This, in turn, would increase the financial return of such investments in health improvement. An additional benefit of the template is the reinforcement for considering work processes and their inputs as the basis for improving results. The template also highlights the critical consideration of employee perspectives and the voice of the customer in understanding performance.

The themes represented by the Allina key performance indicator template are consistent with the long-range strategies that served as a guide during Allina's organizing stage (Figure 6). Additionally, the key indicator themes are consistent with—and serve to reinforce—the three core competencies currently being examined within Allina:

1. Acquiring, analyzing, and disseminating comprehensive information to enable informed decisionmaking by employers, consumers, and providers;
2. Implementing Allina's clinical care approach consistently throughout the committed system; and
3. Creating customer loyalty through demonstrable service excellence.

Figure 5. Allina 1996-1999 Goals—General Themes

- *Market-driven products/services*
- *Provider relationships*
- *Community health improvement*
- *Medical cost management*
- *Long-term financial viability*
- *Workforce flexibility, diversity, motivation and training*
- *Information systems support (of above)*

ALLINA HEALTH SYSTEM KEY PERFORMANCE INDICATORS

Based on the template, Figure 7 outlines the indicators assembled for the initial report. Recalling the intention to represent the entire system, one will note inclusion of indicators pertaining to delivery and managed care operations. In those instances in which desired data are not yet available, developmental efforts are under way and a placeholder is maintained in the report.

One major component of the system-level key indicator set merits further discussion. In Allina's efforts, the design of clinical performance indicator sets warranted special attention. Building on the existing physician engagement strategy, an approach was created for identifying a set of indicators for each Allina-wide clinical priority. Consequently, implementation is under way for indicators per-

Figure 7. Allina Health System Key Performance Indicators (Version 1.0)

Topic	*Indicator*
Internal Competencies and Capabilities	
Employee Health	➲ Work injuries/100 FTEs
	➲ Risk factor status for employees [consider in '97]
Employee Perspectives	➲ Topic: information needed to do job
	➲ Topic: Allina values
Physician Commitment	➲ % admissions in Allina facilities
	➲ % network with Partner or Affiliate contracts
Physician Perspectives	➲ Topic: Information needed for patient care
	➲ Topic: Commitment to Allina delivering sites and Medica
Core and Support Process	
Process Management	➲ Days revenue in receivable (unadjusted for payer mix)
	➲ Medica products: Days/1,000; Admissions/1,000
	➲ % of events not meeting target for one priority process in each business unit
	➲ % liabilty claims/exposure units
Clinical and Community Health Improvement	
Health Improvement	➲ Clinical performance indicator for Allina priorities
	➲ Risk factor status for members [consider in '97]
Customer Satisfaction and Loyalty	
Customer Satisfaction	➲ Patients: overall and by dimension
	➲ Members: overal and focus on access
Customer Loyalty	➲ % of commercial accounts renewing
	➲ % of Medicare members voluntarily disenrolling
	➲ Pull-through: among those obtaining care, % members obtaining services from Allina hospitals/clinics in last 12 months
	➲ Inpatient market share (metro)
	➲ Health plan market share (by product)
Financial Health	
Costs	➲ Clinic expense per visit
	➲ Costs per adjusted admission
	➲ Medical trend by product
	➲ Administrative expense (corporate and operating unit)
Revenue	➲ Pre-financing earnings as % of revenue
	➲ Cash flow (year-to-date); by obligated group and remainder of Allina
	➲ Return on average invested capital

taining to pregnancy, childhood asthma, diabetes, acute myocardial infarction, breast cancer, and colon cancer. As with the organizational key indicators, sets of measures pertaining to clinical populations and spanning the continuum of care will provide a more meaningful reflection of performance than any single clinical indicator. As an example, simply tracking cesarean section rates tells little about a true management of pregnancy and actually can be somewhat misleading without greater context.

Examples of clinical indicator sets for breast cancer and childhood asthma are included in Figure 8. Detailed specifications regarding definitions, exclusion criteria, relevant time periods, etc., are in development and being tested for each indicator. The key feature of this work is the engagement of health care providers actually caring for patients with the targeted conditions in indicator selection and prioritization. Involvement by providers during the design phase should increase interest in these data on an ongoing basis. It also confirmed the anticipated value of such data to those best able to use them and sensitized providers to the complexities and costs of gathering meaningful clinical indicators.

Figure 8. Clinical Performance Indicators: Recommended Sets For Feasibility Investigation

Breast Cancer

1. Rate of eligible patients who receive a mammogram:
   - In calendar year
   - During prior two-year period
2. Rate of eligible women who received a breast exam in the calendar year.
3. Rate of eligible patients with cancer at Stage 0, I or II (stage at which breast cancer was detected) at presentation.
4. Rate of eligible surgical patients who receive consult by an oncologist within two weeks pre- and post-surgery
5. Rate of eligible patients:
   –Satisfied to specified degree with overall care
   –Able to make informed decisions regarding treatment options
   –Reporting adequate communication
   –Satisfied with timeliness of results reporting
   –Satisfied with access to specialists
   –Satisfied with access to support services
   –Reporting desired role/involvement of family

Pediatric Asthma Care

1. Rate of inpatient asthma admissions (age 2-19).
2. Rate of eligible children with to-be-specified number of ER visits annually.
3. Rate of eligible children with moderate to severe asthma on anti-inflammatory prescriptions.
4. Rate of eligible children with to-be-specified compliance with their asthma care.
5. Cost/member/month (stratified by asthma severity).
6. Rate of eligible children whose parents self-report:
   –having a written asthma plan for their child
   –satisfaction to a to-be-specified degree with received asthma care - having a peak-flow meter for their child

Formatting considerations concerning key indicators were considered early in the process, with the resulting desires outlined in Figure 9. As with the issue of data availability, the format for key indicators will evolve as Allina gains experience and assembles additional internal and external data.

Figure 9. Desired Characteristics of Key Performance Indicator Reporting

- *common definitions*
- *causative linkages with desired outcomes*
- *trended data*
- *targets*
- *drill-down detail (when meaningful)*
- *comparative data*
- *tests of significance (e.g., control limits when appropriate)*
- *interpretative commentary*

FUTURE FOCUS FOR THE ALLINA SYSTEM-LEVEL SET

Now that the transition has been made from design to implementation, the Allina senior management team will review and discuss the Allina system-level key indicator report, which is scheduled to be produced quarterly. As experience is gained and refinements are made, more frequent consideration of these data is likely to evolve. Even with quarterly review of the key indicator set, the senior management team may have more frequent discussions concerning various indicators, drill-down analyses, and improvement interventions.

Three areas of focus exist for 1997:

1. Ensure that goals or targets are established for all key performance indicators at the Allina system-level and within the major operating areas. Where possible, assemble comparative information as a context for interpretation.
2. Clarify the accountability for managing those aspects of Allina's operations that affect the key indicators. Identify a spokesperson from the Allina senior management team for each system-level indicator.
3. Establish more explicit linkages between the indicator sets for Allina and those from its operating units, as well as between the operating unit indicator sets and departments functioning within those areas. This will ensure greater alignment throughout the organization, reinforcing the unifying role of Allina's strategy.

A network of leaders sponsoring key indicator work from each operating unit will be maintained as a foundation for the continued refinement of this work and as a way to accelerate learning regarding the use of key indicators.

Details regarding the purpose and composition of the Allina key indicators will be communicated throughout the organization. This is required if the benefits of alignment and focus are to be realized. The cascading relationships that link system-level and operating unit key indicators should continue so that departmental and, eventually, personal objectives incorporate aspects of the key performance indicators that are applicable to the work being done. This will enable employees to identify how their work contributes to the overall direction of Allina. This linkage is also important since another potential development is the association of key performance indicators with compensation.

As Allina gains experience with key performance indicators, various types of analyses will be necessary. The objective will be to test relationships between the key indicators themselves, while another will be to identify drivers of individual indicators ("drill-down") within the operations or staff functions of Allina. These analyses, combined with continued reconsideration of the indicator template, will enable leadership to test the integrity of current strategy and modify indicators to reflect future strategic direction. Consequently, consideration of Allina's key indicators in the planning process becomes a logical extension of this work.

While it is hoped that the key indicator template will remain relatively stable, the template and specific key indicators are subject to change. The key indicators will evolve based on four primary factors:

1. modification of Allina's strategy,
2. clarification regarding a unifying business model for Allina,
3. analysis of data that suggests more meaningful leading and lagging indicators of overall performance or identifies more specific "drivers" of performance from within the organization, or
4. enhanced capacity to efficiently collect and report desired data.

In managing ongoing refinement, it will be necessary to balance a major tradeoff of using an indicator long enough to get meaningful trends and insight into its benefits and limitations through analysis, with introducing or investing in new indicators that are thought to be important due to shifting priorities.

MEDICA'S KEY PERFORMANCE INDICATOR EFFORTS

A microcosm for the key indicator initiative is provided by Medica, Allina's managed care organization. The size and diversity of Medica's operations—spanning seven product lines and covering more than one million members—presents fertile ground for implementing key indicators. Beyond the need to align organizational efforts across departmental boundaries, Medica faces the additional challenge of effectively engaging thousands of contracted health providers and scores of facilities and other network components. The approach used within Medica exemplifies the relationship between system-level and operating unit key indicator structure and identity. It also demonstrates the potential power of drilling indicator categories and specific measures from the system-level to the front line.

Medica's key performance indicator initiative was largely influenced by the Service-Profit Chain concepts.[30] This influence is reflected in Medica's Excellence Pathway, the organizing vehicle for its key indicator work (Figure 10). The Pathway was introduced and explained at all employee meetings, an example of the communication required to achieve alignment. While some terminology varies, there is considerable consistency between the Allina template and the Medica pathway. As the key indicator work evolves, one will see greater overlap in terminology, organization, and content between the Allina system-level and Medica key indicators.

Figure 10. Medica Excellence Pathway

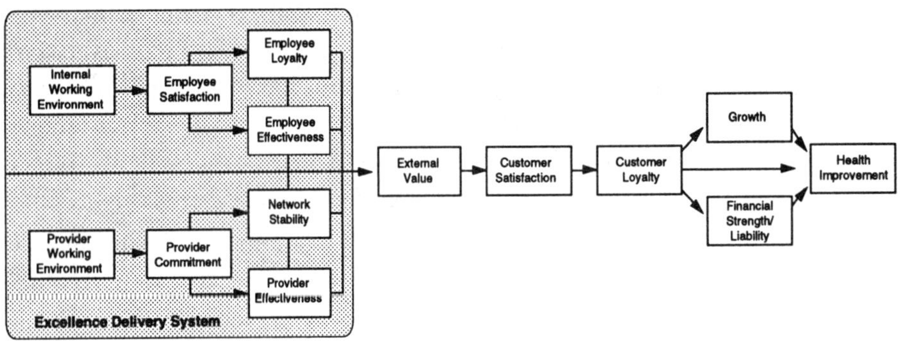

Medica has more than one year's experience with the monthly production of its report. The specific indicators are listed in Figure 11 and are directly associated with categories from the Excellence Pathway. The data are shared with the 40-member general management team and have been regularly discussed at meetings of Medica's president and other senior leaders. While general support existed from the start, issues concerning the rationale for pursuing this initiative were revisited during many initial discussions. Early discussion also focused on indicator formatting rather than data interpretation. Nonetheless, the effort advanced with refinements based on collegial input, and dialogue eventually moved to the substance of the report.

Figure 11. Medical 1996 Key Performance Indicators

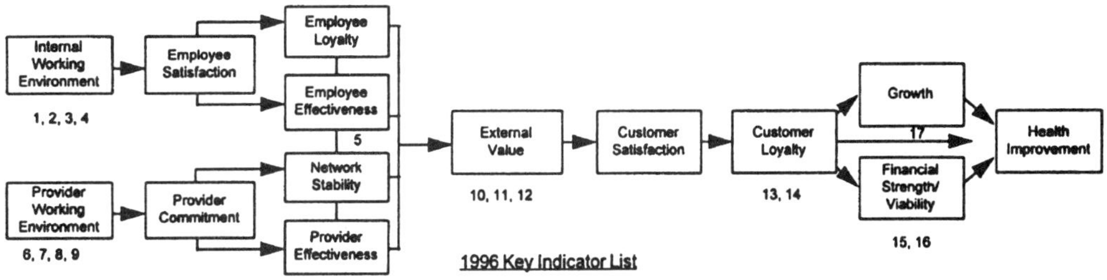

1996 Key Indicator List

1. Employee satisfaction
2. Employee loyalty (survey-based)
3. Employee effectiveness (survey-based)
4. LAN availability
5. Administrative expense
6. Provider service average wait time
7. Provider service call abandonment rate
8. Claims adjustments
9. Pended claims
10. Customer service average wait time (by product segment)
11. Mammography rate
12. Health care cost trend
13. Commercial members leaving Medica
14. Medicare members leaving Medica
15. Operating income percentage
16. Medical loss ratio by product
17. Membership

The Medica Key Indicator Report also has been shared with Medica's board of directors. Although there was significant interest among board members, the decision was made to forgo routine discussion with the board until the management team gained additional experience with the use of key indicators and management of their underlying processes. Much of the key indicator report content still is shared with the board in other contexts such as HEDIS reports, financial statements, and marketing summaries. It is anticipated that the report will be regularly shared with the board in 1997.

As a pilot, electronic distribution of Medica's Key Indicator Report to selected senior and general managers was implemented using the Local Area Network. The objectives of the pilot included:

1. Promoting alternative mechanisms for distribution of key indicators,
2. Encouraging electronic means of information dissemination, and
3. Identifying future needs and desired capabilities of information system-based tools for applying key indicators.

Acrobat was the software application used, providing a display and distribution mechanism but not supporting on-line analysis or queries. Features of this approach included hypertext linkages to indicator definitions, interpretive commentary, and help screens.

An evaluation of the pilot revealed that although there was general support for Medica's key indicators, a number of issues required further consideration:

- **Key indicators should be "verified."** Irrespective of the distribution mode, confidence was building in the belief that the initial report included the key indicators of Medica's overall performance. The pilot's timing—early in the evolution of key indicator implementation—appeared to undermine broad interest in testing this distribution mechanism.

- **Indicator data must be current.** At most, Medica indicators were updated monthly. In some cases, the information was refreshed less often. Consequently, little impetus existed for accessing the data more often than monthly. A resulting enhancement involved identifying the date of last update for each indicator so that recipients were prompted to focus their attention.
- **The electronic version must be available before—or in place of—hard copy.** Although the pilot was intended to test an additional means for distributing information, the hard copy version continued to be available. As a result, little reason existed for accessing the data on-line, since the report was circulated in the more traditional manner at the same time it was available electronically. This was particularly true for individuals who were not inclined to use a PC frequently.
- **Every senior manager should commit to trying the electronic version.** Continued use of the paper report by some leaders diluted the energy necessary to test electronic distribution. In fact, at the time of the pilot, only a few of the senior managers routinely used information technology such as e-mail. Solidarity would increase the likelihood that "late adopters" would overcome their dependence on the paper-based report. The role and value of a paper-based report should be clarified as a basis for planning enhancements of paper and/or electronic versions.
- **Additional information technology resources are needed.** Some individuals typically used evenings to review information such as the key indicator report. Those lacking appropriate computer resources faced an obvious barrier. Since the report was periodically discussed in meetings, some leaders were accustomed to making notes on the report and/or referring to previous notations made when reviewing the information in advance. Since notebook or laptop computers were not widely used, an added disincentive existed. Finally, drill-down and query capabilities were requested to increase the value of this resource and effectively support leadership decisionmaking. While cumbersome, this is often possible with paper-based reports.

As with the work at the Allina system level, the initial design of Medica's report was based on currently available data. This provided experience in using key indicators without requiring significant investment. Given the intent to provide feedback about performance that was closer to "real-time" than many traditional means, the initial requirement was that data be available at least quarterly and, preferably, monthly. Other key indicators were identified during the initial design process for inclusion over time, as resources were invested to produce information not currently available.

Future direction for Medica includes the increased use of control charts where warranted to assist with interpretation of variation seen in the data. With each planning and budgeting cycle, consideration will be given to indicator refinement and the resource investments necessary to provide data thought to be valuable but not currently available.

In retrospect, the Excellence Pathway, Medica's initial structure for organizing key indicators and reinforcing the focus on service, has been useful. Although the practice of systematically discussing key indicators is evolving, the underlying concepts and initial design have stimulated more "systems thinking" regarding Medica's functioning as a whole (versus the traditional departmental orientation). Furthermore, appreciation has grown for potential cause-and-effect relationships and the importance of process management as a basis for improving performance. A dose of reality—the cost of additional indicator data—has been sobering and has limited the evolution of Medica's report. Despite progress, the reliance on traditional financial indicators has been difficult to break. This has been particularly true as Medica faces financial challenges.

OVERALL INSIGHTS

Although progress has occurred within Allina, a number of major insights have surfaced or been reinforced. When possible, consideration of these factors should precede initiatives involving key performance indicators.

- **Merger challenges:** The significant cultural and organizational change associated with mergers provides a multitude of distractions. Even though the initiative at Allina was intentionally pursued as a means to support integration and improve performance, the upheaval was significant and the uncertainty accompanying Allina's creation impeded progress.
- **Strategic ambiguity:** A well-defined strategy is an essential foundation for development of key performance indicators. In the case of an emerging health system such as Allina, it is critical that at least meaningful organizing principles and strategies are in place. While this was the case, the rapidly changing environment, combined with unanswered questions concerning Allina's overall business model, raised questions regarding the meaningful key indicators. This experience punctuated the vulnerability caused when organizational direction and focus are not clear or are interpreted differently by senior leaders. This is certain to be uncovered when defining indicators of organizational performance. It should be noted that the dialogue associated with developing meaningful key indicators can help surface important issues and clarify critical questions as an aid to strategy formulation. With this in mind, expectations regarding implementation of true key indicators must be held in check.

- **Data gaps:** Paradoxically, many health care organizations do not lack data. They do lack information that is linked to their overall strategic direction and priorities and is available in a format and time that supports effective decisionmaking for planning, target setting, performance assessment, etc. Data must be more efficiently collected, analyzed, and disseminated with clear definitions and a useful context for interpretation. Unfortunately, within emerging organizations the expected barriers associated with information systems are heightened by the increased complexity and numerous competing demands. The resources required to fill gaps can be significant. Leaders must carefully weigh options when identifying meaningful indicators, but cannot be constrained by using only data that are already available. This would severely limit the value of key indicators in most cases since many important issues are not currently quantified.
- **Health care nuances:** Other industries have significant experience using key indicators and leadership systems that rely on such information. Application of this approach is relatively new in health care and is complicated by the nature of the services provided by health care organizations. Even with improvements in some measurement instruments and techniques such as risk adjustment, efforts to quantify outcomes and the health status of individuals and populations are still in their infancy. Even with improved metrics and a consensus regarding the definition of the "product" and its "customers," attribution of the responsibility for clinical results remains a challenge. Given the great range of factors that influence organizational results, some of which are directly controlled by the customer, assignment of causality in the search for performance drivers must proceed cautiously. Finally, the not-for-profit status of many organizations, with the resulting obligation to the community, might diffuse focus and clarity of organizational aim.
- **Leadership involvement:** The adoption of key performance indicators requires a shift in the individual roles and financially-dominated mindset of many leaders. Direct involvement of senior leaders in the design and use of key indicators is the single greatest catalyst. In light of the complexity and cycles of analysis required, leaders are looked to for long-term commitment to such an initiative. They must refine the skills necessary to effectively use such information and stimulate dialogue with their colleagues.
- **The natural catch-22:** A significant barrier exists that can limit the viability of key performance indicator development. A "chicken and egg" argument can ensue in which some key stakeholders want assurance that indicators included in the initial design are, in fact, the critical ones needed for the organization. The utility of the key indicators can be challenged before the first report is even produced, with lead-

ers wanting assurance of value before buying into the overall approach. Obviously, given Allina's decision to restrict early versions to data that were easily retrievable, it was extremely unlikely that the initial indicators would be the "right" ones. Further, it is the personal engagement of senior leaders and dialogue with other colleagues and critical external stakeholders that is needed for optimal design. Lack of leadership investment can almost ensure the effort will fall short of its potential.

- **Critical mass of investment needed:** Use of key performance indicators should never become an end in itself. It is simply a means to promote sustainable performance excellence. Consideration should be given to the time needed for effectively engaging leaders in the design process and for reviewing, discussing, and refining key indicators on an ongoing basis. Mechanisms are needed to enhance leaders' skills for processing the information. Resources also are required for data collection and analysis, as well as for ongoing communication as a basis for alignment. With the need for efficiency and increasing demand for customized analysis, information system support is vital. Development efforts should be given high priority so that some important data gaps are filled early to support desired indicators. If key performance indicators are to assume a central position in an organization's management processes, one would think the investment is justified. Nonetheless, there are often considerable constraints caused by resource limitations as early development occurs outside the mainstream of many organizations' leadership practices. Below a certain point, inadequate investment to support this effort will threaten survival of the initiative.
- **Dissemination complexities:** Key performance indicator sets typically contain sensitive information. Opinions vary regarding the appropriate audiences for such work. Dependence on nonemployee relationships, such as those with physicians contracting with a health plan or admitting patients to a facility, further complicate the issue of dissemination. Because alignment requires some degree of communication, thought should be given in advance as to how such information will be shared and how recipients will be prepared to act on such information.

SUMMARY

Since 1995, efforts have been under way at Allina Health System to implement related sets of key performance indicators for the system and its major components. The premises at the root of this work contend that:

1. Current performance must be understood if future performance is to be improved
2. Although traditional financial metrics are useful, they are not sufficient for assessing overall performance, and
3. The process of establishing key indicators in an emerging organization can help clarify overall direction by provoking dialogue and assuring a common view of strategy among those sharing responsibility for performance, the board and senior managers.

Key performance indicators, as a core component of the management system, help align an organization. They link operations to strategy using a tangible, cause-and-effect model. The KPI template is applicable at multiple levels of an organization: system, business unit, and department. It conveys important themes and reinforces the need to enhance processes and their inputs to affect desired organizational outcomes.

Leaders of increasingly complex health care organizations need more effective mechanisms for aligning efforts of staff throughout the organizations. They also require information to support effective and timely decisionmaking. Key performance indicators are intended to respond to these needs, while themselves being responsive to changing organizational direction. With the foundation in place at Allina and its operating units including Medica, the challenge now turns to maintaining constancy of purpose. In an environment filled with distractions, unyielding senior management support will be necessary for thorough implementation, credible analysis, investment to fill data gaps, and ongoing cycles of indicator refinement so that the potential can be fulfilled and sustainable performance excellence can be achieved. The true test remains, with the benefits accruing to the customers and communities that are served.

REFERENCES

1. Health Care Pilot Criteria. Malcolm Baldrige National Quality Award, American Society for Quality Control, Milwaukee WI, 1995.
2. Bushick B. "Performance Indicators for Achieving Goals at Allina." *The Quality Letter.* Capitol Publications, Volume 8, Number 5, June 1996.
3. Bushick B. "Creating an Integrated Health Care System as a Basis for Managed Care Breakthroughs: The Health Plan's Perspective." *Managed Care Quarterly*, Volume 3, Number 1, Winter, 1995, pp. 1-10.
4. Allina Health System Vision Statement, 1996.
5. Kaplan R. and Norton D. *The Balanced Scorecard.* Harvard Business School Press, Boston MA, 1996.
6. *Ibid.*

7. Kaplan R. and Norton D. "Using the Balanced Scorecard as a Strategic Management System." *Harvard Business Review*, January-February, 1996, pp. 75-85.

8. *Ibid.*

9. Kaplan R. and Norton D. "The Balanced Scorecard—Measures that Drive Performance." *Harvard Business Review*, January-February 1992, pp. 71-79.

10. Kaplan R. and Norton D. "Putting the Balanced Scorecard to Work." *Harvard Business Review*, September-October 1993, pp. 134-147.

11. Heskett J; Jones T; Loveman G; Sasser, E; and Schlesinger, Leonard. "Putting the Service-Profit Chain to Work." *Harvard Business Review*, March-April 1994, pp. 164-174.

12. Health Care Pilot Criteria. Malcolm Baldrige National Quality Award, American Society for Quality Control, Milwaukee WI, 1995.

13. Kaplan R. and Norton D. "Using the Balanced Scorecard as a Strategic Management System." *Harvard Business Review*, January-February, 1996, pp. 75-85.

14. Kaplan R. and Norton D. "The Balanced Scorecard—Measures that Drive Performance." *Harvard Business Review*, January-February 1992, pp. 71-79.

15. Kaplan R. and Norton D. "Putting the Balanced Scorecard to Work." *Harvard Business Review*, September-October 1993, pp. 134-147.

16. Heskett et al. Ibid.

17. Eccles R. "The Performance Measurement Manifesto." *Harvard Business Review*, January-February 1991, pp. 131-137.

18. Luttman R; Siren P; and Laffel G. *Assessing Organizational Performance. Quality Management in Health Care*, Aspen Publishers, Inc., 1994, pp. 44-53.

19. Nelson E; Batalden P; Plume S; Mihevc N; and Swartz W. "Report Cards or Instrument Panels: Who Needs What?" *Journal on Quality Improvement*, Volume 21, Number 4, April 1994, pp. 155-166.

20. Provost L. and Leddick S. "How to Take Multiple Measurse to Get a Complete Picture of Organizational Performance." *National Productivity Review*, Autumn 1993, pp. 477-490.

21. Rose K. "A Performance Measurement Model." *Quality Progress*, February 1995, pp. 63-66.

22. O'Rourke L. and Bader B. "Principles for Developing Governance Reports on Quality and Performance." *The Quality Letter*, Capitol Publications, Volume 5, Number 2, March 1993.

23. O'Rourke L. and Bader B. "A Process for Developing a Board Quality and Performance Report." *The Quality Letter*, Capitol Publications, Volume 5, Number 2, March 1993.

24. Brown M. "Is Your Measurement System Well Balanced?" *Journal for Quality and Participation*, October/November 1994, pp. 6-10.

25. Health Plan Employer Data and Information Set Version 2.0, National Committee for Quality Assurance, Washington DC, 1993.
26. "1995 Comprehensive Accreditation Manual for Hospitals," Joint Commission on Accreditation of Healthcare Organizations, Oakbrook Terrace IL, 1994.
27. Foundation for Accountability, Portland OR, 1995.
28. Minnesota Health Data Institute, St. Paul MN, 1995.
29. Buyers Health Care Action Group, Bloomington MN, 1996.
30. Heskett et al. *Ibid.*

ACKNOWLEDGMENTS

The author wishes to acknowledge the Allina Key Performance Indicator Learning and Advisory Group members for their insights, contributions, and resilient support; other speakers and participants at the September 1996 Balanced Scorecard Conference (Boston MA) for providing additional perspectives into current application of these concepts and an opportunity to confirm the direction of the Allina initiative; VHA System-Wide Measurement Working Group convened by Jim Roberts, MD, for the sharing of experiences and ideas; and the assistance of Michelle Fredrickson in preparing this manuscript.

Chapter 12

Aetna U.S. Healthcare

Patient-Centered Models for Providing Quality

Carol C. Diamond, MD, and Nicholas A. Hanchak, MD

There is growing interest in information concerning the quality of care provided by managed care organizations. This is hardly surprising—quality health care is important to those who receive it, those who provide it, and those who pay for it. There are, however, a number of issues raised by the measurement of quality, including such basic concerns as how to do it, who should do it, and who should have access to the results. In 1990, U.S. Healthcare, Inc. (now Aetna U.S. Healthcare) formed a subsidiary, U.S. Quality Algorithms, Inc. (USQA), to assist in the development and application of health care performance measures. Several examples of USQA's research efforts in the areas of quality measurement and physician performance assessment that have been implemented as programs within Aetna U. S. Healthcare's medical delivery system are featured in the following pages.

Founded seven years ago as the quality measurement subsidiary of U.S. Healthcare, USQA is recognized as a leading performance and outcomes measurement company. The pairing of U.S. Healthcare and Aetna has opened the door to a world of tremendous opportunities for USQA. Almost overnight, USQA has grown from a small 30-person research and development unit to an organization of more than 280 devoted to developing performance measurement tools and information products and services.

Measuring performance to improve the quality of care, measuring medical costs to improve the value of care, and delivering sophisticated information products and services are the linchpins of USQA's mission. Accomplishing these tasks will ensure Aetna U.S. Healthcare success in its goal to deliver high-quality, affordable health care services. Above all, improving the health outcomes for Aetna U.S. Healthcare members is USQA's ultimate goal.

USQA's roots are in researching, analyzing, and identifying opportunities to provide increased value, either by improving physician performance, studying medical costs, or improving outcomes. USQA's work will continue to include refining established performance-based compensation models that reward providers for improving their performance on the basis of specific quality measures. In addition, through the development of risk-stratification methodologies, Aetna U.S. Healthcare will get a better sense of who's at risk for costly hospitalizations or emergency room visits. Knowing which members need to be more closely case managed for acute exacerbations allows Aetna U.S. Healthcare to use its resources more efficiently and better manage patients' conditions through case management programs. This chapter reviews the evolution of performance measurement research at USQA and previews what's in store for the future as USQA continues setting the standard in quality measurement efforts in managed care.

UNDERSTANDING THE PREVALENCE OF CHRONIC DISEASES IN AETNA U.S. HEALTHCARE

There are a number of widely recognized quality measurement systems, such as HEDIS and the Foundation for Accountability measures, that serve as important public yardsticks by which health plans may be compared. USQA believes that in addition to these measures Aetna U.S. Healthcare's own internal resources should be applied in order to improve the health of members. This chapter, therefore, initially will concentrate on methodology and examples of using the company's database to determine and manage the health status of Aetna U.S. Healthcare members. First, the authors introduce USQA's Health Profile Database and how it can be used to determine and manage the health status of Aetna U.S. Healthcare members. Second, the authors discuss USQA's approach to performance measurement of its health care professionals and institutions.

As a managed care organization, Aetna U.S. Healthcare assumes responsibility for both the financing and delivery of health care. In addition to maintaining financial solvency, MCOs have accepted an explicit commitment to monitor and attempt to actively improve the quality of care their members have access to. Because MCOs have been active in controlling resource utilization, they have come under sharp scrutiny from patients, employers, and accrediting organizations for the quality of care delivered to their members.[1] The assessment of care is challenging because the organizational arrangements between providers and

MCOs vary. MCOs must be innovative in measuring physician performance and quality of care and in implementing quality improvement programs.[2] A key requirement of managing the financing and delivery of health care services and assessing the quality of care is a sophisticated information system.[3]

In contrast to traditional quality assurance programs, which rely on retrospective review and abstraction of medical charts, quality-of-care activities can be enhanced with data collected by an MCO.[4] Although these approaches still have benefit, the approach to quality measurement in the era of managed care is rapidly changing.[5] Data collected by MCOs can be quite extensive, with different data obtained from multiple sources. Financial and administrative data systems, such as those containing billing and membership information, hold important clinical data that can help contribute to measuring the quality of care delivered to patients. The challenge for MCOs is to link the multiple sources of data to obtain relevant clinical information and apply it to their quality assessment and improvement efforts.[6,7,8,9]

A key aspect of improving quality and controlling costs is the ability to identify and manage patients with specific needs due to certain clinical conditions.[10] Efficiently managing patients with chronic illnesses, in particular, has considerable impact on both quality and cost for MCOs. Aetna U.S. Healthcare's information systems—databases filled with potentially important clinical information—serve as the starting point for determining at-risk patients. The various information sources and their strengths are listed below:

- An encounters database provides information about the diagnoses and procedures of patients who seek care from providers, both primary care physicians (PCPs) and capitated specialty providers.
- Claim databases gather diagnostic information about patients who utilize noncapitated resources and also provide insight into the number and types of procedures that providers use to treat certain conditions. Both outpatient claims, generally submitted on a HCFA 1500 standard claim form, and inpatient claims, which utilize the standard UB82/UB92 formats, contain diagnostic and procedural information. They also furnish information about the episodes of care, including the dates of service and the responsible providers.[11]
- MCOs maintain a membership database that allows for the identification of certain demographic and benefits variables that may influence access to care and the utilization patterns of specific health care resources, as well as help identify patients at increased risk for certain conditions or adverse outcomes.
- Pharmacy data are an important source of clinical information, in some cases allowing for the identification of specific disease states, and they provide information about the prescribing patterns of physicians in treating specific diseases.
- Laboratory data also can be used in identifying patients with specific diseases and understanding the outcomes of certain processes of care.

Most approaches to using administrative databases to evaluate the quality of medical care take a provider-centric approach and solely rely on claims data. Services received by a patient are aggregated to the provider level, and utilization patterns for individual providers are compared with other providers. The availability of data on multiple providers yields a reference distribution for the establishment of expected or normative behavior. Deviations from the norm are flagged as potential problems.[12]

Using providers as the unit of analysis is a necessary part of a quality assessment program, but it is not sufficient. A comprehensive approach requires integration with other analyses that focus on the patient as the unit of analysis and incorporates all available data. Without this integration of provider and patient-centered analyses, and without the inclusion of information from multiple data sources, there are limitations to the conclusions that can be drawn about the delivery of quality medical care.

USQA has chosen to implement a patient-centric approach to performance measurement and quality improvement through its data warehouse. The data warehouse is at the hub of USQA and Aetna U.S. Healthcare (see Figure 1). When fully constructed, Aetna U.S. Healthcare's data warehouse will be the largest health care database in the world and one of only approximately 10 terabyte-range warehouses. The data in the warehouse provide both a clinical and financial view of all services provided to Aetna U.S. Healthcare's members. Membership information is contained here, along with provider, quality-of-care, service-level information, revenue, and expense data.

Figure 1. The USQA Data Warehouse

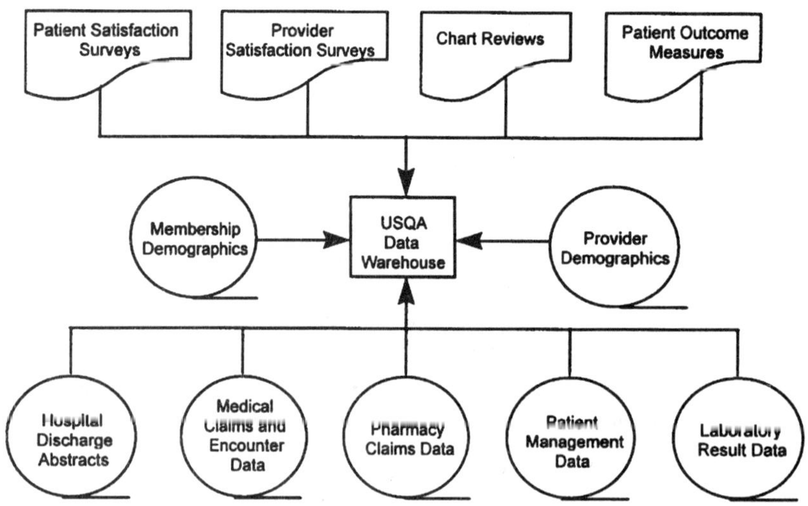

Identifying Chronic Diseases in the Population

There are many strengths in a patient-centric approach to profiling clinical administrative data. The USQA Health Profile Database is a tool that was developed taking these strengths into account. A patient-centric approach tends to be more inclusive, with a more complete capture of members with important conditions. Moreover, the ability to use data from five or more years and providing the common link (i.e., the member identification number) improves the sensitivity of identifying and risk stratifying members with certain diseases.[13]

The intent of USQA's Health Profile Database is to profile members within the Aetna U.S. Healthcare health plan who have chronic diseases. Members who suffer from chronic diseases likely will need ongoing medical care. Ongoing care means higher costs, and the costs of caring for members who suffer from chronic illnesses represent significant expense to a health plan. Nevertheless, the quality of care that providers within a health plan are able to deliver is perhaps best demonstrated by their ability to take care of members with chronic diseases.

Although acute illnesses represent a significant burden to the members within a health plan, they do not allow for assessing and improving the quality of care of specific patients because they are of limited duration and, therefore, difficult to identify from retrospective claims data with sufficient timeliness. Acute illnesses are critical for provider-centric analyses, however. USQA currently is developing methods to incorporate multiple sources of data for the identification of episodes of acute illnesses, and ultimately a comprehensive view of the burden of illness in a primary care provider's patient panel.

There were no prior assumptions made about the inclusion or exclusion of certain conditions into the Health Profile Database. The selection of illnesses is, in fact, an iterative, ongoing process. The selection process began with an analysis of individual claims and identified illnesses that were prevalent in terms of number of members with that disease or health care encounters for that disease. The prevalence criterion was secondary to the cost requirement so that the need for high prevalence was relaxed for diseases in which there were high costs per patient.

A second consideration for inclusion in the Health Profile Database was that selected diseases be candidates for improvement in the processes of care that would ultimately lead to better outcomes.[14] In other words, preference was given to diseases in which practice guidelines had been developed and proven to be both efficacious and effective in improving the health of a population with a given disease. Through better compliance with these performance standards, the health of a specific at-risk patient population potentially can be improved.

High-cost chronic conditions were identified and their potential for improved processes and outcomes were evaluated. The results of a literature search were incorporated with the clinical judgments to identify and quantify those diseases with potential for improved outcomes. In addition to medical conditions that are chronic in nature, certain other conditions were included in the Health Profile Database because of the interest in the care obtained by patients with those conditions (e.g., lung cancer, breast cancer). A total of 64 different chronic diseases have been identified to be of sufficient importance to track within the Aetna U.S. Healthcare membership. The list of chronic conditions currently included is shown in Figure 2. Other conditions that present opportunities for improvement in quality, cost, or both will be added to this list.

Figure 2. The Health Profile Database List of Chronic Diseases

1. Diabetes Mellitus
2. Asthma
3. Congestive Heart Failure
4. Chronic Obstructive Pulmonary Disease
5. Ischemic Heart Disease
6. Otitis Media
7. Peptic Ulcer Disease
8. Atrial Fibrillation
9. Hypertension
10. Benign Prostatic Hypertrophy
11. Epilepsy
12. Hypothyroidism/Hyperthyroidism
13. Down's Syndrome
14. Alcoholism
15. Depression
16. Cholelithiasis
17. Iron Deficiency Anemia
18. Breast Cancer
19. Osteoarthritis
20. Rheumatoid Arthritis
21. AIDS
22. Colon Cancer
23. Lung Cancer
24. Hypercholesterolemia
25. Cerebrovascular Disease
26. Migraine and Other Headaches
27. Chronic Renal Failure
28. Kidney Stones
29. Diverticular Disease
30. Back Pain
31. Nonspecific Gastritis/Dyspepsia
32. Sickle Cell Anemia
33. Multiple Sclerosis
34. Crohn's Disease
35. Hemophilia
36. Systemic Lupus
37. Prostate Cancer
38. Ovarian Cancer
39. Endometrial Cancer
40. Cervical Cancer
41. Hodgkin's Disease/Lymphoma
42. Leukemia
43. Brain Cancer
44. Malignant Melanoma
45. Head/Neck Cancer
46. Esophageal Cancer
47. Stomach Cancer
48. Pancreatic Cancer
49. Pancreatitis
50. Hepatitis
51. Peripheral Vascular Disease
52. Endometriosis
53. Ventricular Arrhythmia
54. Lyme Disease
55. Female Infertility
56. Menopause
57. Bladder Cancer
58. Glaucoma
59. Low Vision and Blindness
60. Cataract
61. Any Cancer
62. Dementia
63. Allergy
64. Osteoporosis

Using the disease selection specifications, the identification program used to populate the USQA Health Profile Database queried the encounters, claims, pharmacy, and laboratory databases. A member record is generated for any member who meets the necessary specifications for one or more diseases. The Health Profile Database is updated on a monthly basis by running the clinical algorithms against the entire membership with a retrospective sweep dating back to 1990.

Enrollment updates also occur on a monthly basis, and all the demographic data are fully replaced each month to keep the database consistent with the enrollment data. Information on members no longer enrolled in the health plan is also maintained in the database, and the members' inactive status so indicated. The Health Profile Database is a starting point to define the burden of illness in the member population of the health plan.[15,16]

As with any system of quality measurement that relies solely on administrative data, it is necessary to determine the accuracy of the data and the methodologies employed in analyzing the data as they are converted into meaningful information.[17, 18] The process of validating the Health Profile Database will be illustrated using diabetes mellitus. To begin to validate the selection criteria used in the identification of diabetic patients (see Figure 3) primary care physicians who participated in the previous U.S. Healthcare health plan were sent a list of the members in their practice identified as having diabetes by the administrative selection criteria. Physicians were asked to identify false positives (i.e., those on the list who did not have diabetes) and false negatives (i.e., those who were not on the list but who had diabetes).

Figure 3. Diabetes Mellitus Selection Criteria

Diagnosis Criteria (ICD-9 Codes)

- 250-250.93 (diabetes mellitus with various manifestations)
- 357.2 (polyneuropathy in diabetes)
- 362.0 362.02 (diabetic retinopathy)
- 366.41 (diabetic cataract)

Procedure Criteria (CPT-4 Codes)

- C82985 (glycated protein) and/or C83036 (glycated hemoglobin)
- occurring twice in any 12 consecutive months, at least 90 days apart
- CJ1820 (diabetic injectable medications)
- CW0070 (oral hypoglycemic medications)
- CW0071 (antidiabetic products (miscellaneous)
- C5190D (registered nurse diabetic visit)
- C5205D (certified diabetes educator)
- C9890A (diabetes education program)
- CE0607 (home blood glucose monitor)

Pharmacy Criteria (NDC Codes)

- Insulin
- Sulfonylurea
- Biguanides

A total of 292 physician offices responded to the questionnaire, for a response rate of 8 percent. The response rate was low because only offices with significant errors on their lists were asked to respond. The number of diabetic patients identified by the initial selection criteria in the panels of these responding physicians was 4,172. The total number of capitated patients cared for by these physicians was 220,298. The positive predictive value (i.e., percentage of positive tests that accurately reflected the disease state) for the selection criteria was 84.2 percent, and the sensitivity (i.e., the percentage of the time that the presence of a disease state was accurately reflected by a positive result) was 97.3 percent, based on a total of 115 diabetic patients who were added because of the physician response.[19]

Although the sensitivity and specificity of the individual criteria can be calculated, the results must be interpreted with caution because of certain biases in physician responses. Error rates were probably magnified due to selection bias, whereby physicians with more errors on their lists might have had greater reason to respond. The ratio of false positives to false negatives was likely inflated as well. This is due to the fact that it is easier to recognize a patient as not having a disease when presented with the patient name, as opposed to identifying patients with a disease from a panel who were left off the list.

There are differences in the ability to identify diseases from administrative data. Some diseases such as diabetes can be readily identified by any of several database sources (i.e., claims, encounters, pharmacy, lab). Others, such as osteoarthitis or sickle cell anemia, are only diagnosed by ICD-9 diagnosis codes from claims or encounters. Generally, however, each additional database available improves the sensitivity of profiling members. Using information from all four databases—claims, pharmacy, encounters, and laboratory—greatly improved the accuracy of identifying members with diabetes (Figure 4).

Figure 4. Incremental Detection of Various Databases

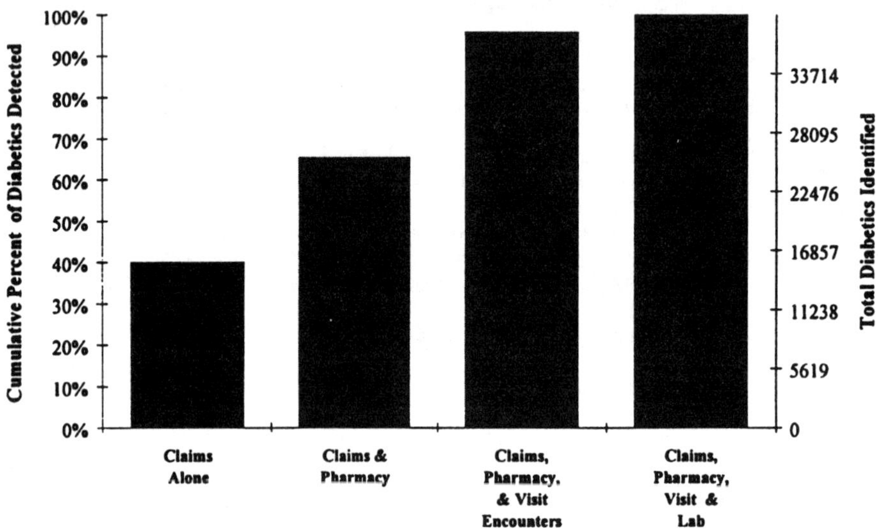

Applying the USQA Health Profile Database

The applications of the Health Profile Database for assessing physician performance and quality also will be illustrated using diabetes. Within the group of chronic diseases, diabetes mellitus provides one of the most significant opportunities for effective patient management. The Diabetes Control and Complication Trial provides firm evidence that good glycemic control, especially for Type 1 diabetics, leads to better outcomes.[20] Individuals with diabetes are at risk not only for complications resulting from hyperglycemia and hypoglycemia, but also for cardiac and peripheral vascular disease, end-stage renal disease, retinopathy, and peripheral neuropathy.

The USQA Health Profile Database was used to conduct a study to assess the prevalence and costs of diabetes in the Aetna U.S. Healthcare member population.

Assessing the quality of care provided to diabetic patients by Aetna U.S. Healthcare's contracted providers was also an important goal of the study. The results of this study have important implications for management decisions aimed at providing improved care to diabetic members.

The calculation of the prevalence of diabetes is complicated by the time lag between when a member joins the health plan and when data that identify the disease reach the administrative databases. This time lag can lead to an underestimate of the true prevalence.

USQA determined the prevalence estimate of diabetes in the Aetna U.S. Healthcare membership to be 3.1 percent. This was calculated by limiting the denominator and numerator to those members belonging to Aetna U.S. Healthcare for at least 12 months. To improve the sensitivity, this calculation was further limited to those members on the pharmacy plan. Aetna U.S. Healthcare's 3.1 percent estimate is consistent with other figures appearing in the medical literature of the estimated prevalence of diabetes.[21, 22]

The prevalence rate of diabetes in our population was calculated based on members who currently are enrolled for each of the specified minimum time periods. Limiting the prevalence calculation to those members who were health plan members for at least one year begins to address the decreased sensitivity of administrative data associated with a shorter period of active time in the health plan (see Figure 5). Note that the prevalence curve continually increases and never appears to "flatten." The suspected reason for this phenomenon is that the increase in the prevalence curve is caused by the increase in the incidence rate of diabetes among the Aetna U.S. Healthcare population.

Figure 5. Prevalence Based on Varying Membership Time Periods

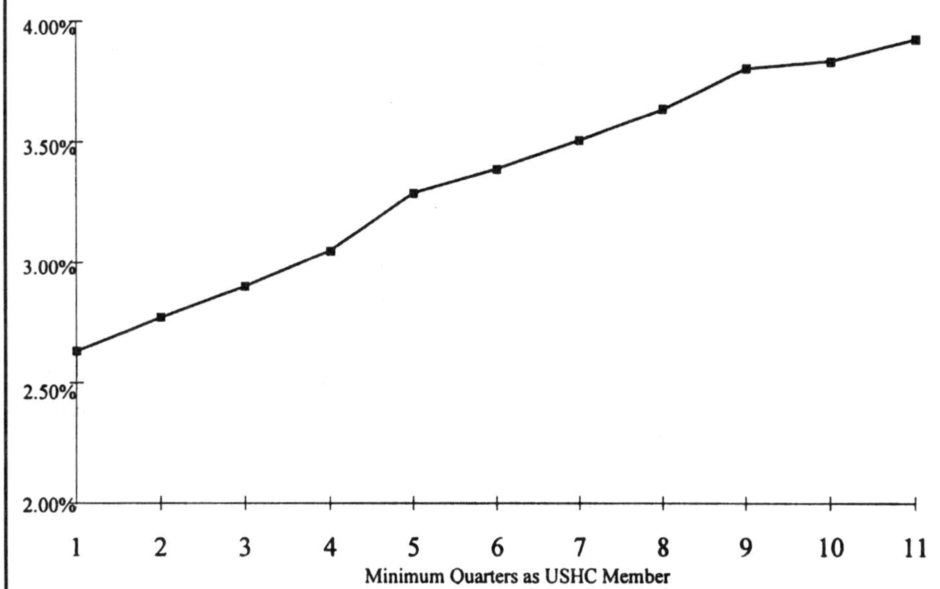

Costs related to diabetes constitute an important proxy for the burden of illness experienced by diabetic patients. These costs also can help to estimate the proportion of health care resources used by diabetic patients. The total noncapitated costs for these patients can be calculated using the Health Profile Database. The direct facility and professional costs for inpatient care, emergency room care, short procedure unit care, and outpatient care for diabetic patients versus the average member are shown in Figure 6. In this figure, indirect and unrelated costs are combined. Indirect costs are for conditions related to diabetes, such as kidney disease and heart disease. Unrelated costs are all costs other than direct (for diabetes) and indirect costs. In addition, the following costs were excluded (both medical and societal): capitation paid to PCPs, radiologists, laboratories, podiatrists, and mental health providers; pharmacy costs; nursing home costs; costs for undiagnosed diabetics; and loss of income due to illness, disability, and premature death.

Figure 6. Comparison of Total Fee-For-Service Costs

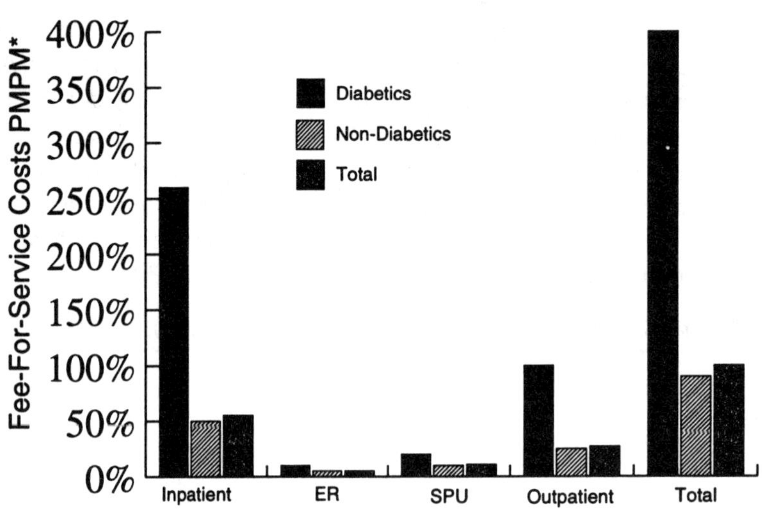

*Adjusted scale equates total fee-for-service costs for average U.S. Healthcare member at 100%

The cost estimates reflected in Figure 6 represent one advantage of using a patient-centric approach rather than a claims-centric approach to evaluate the quality of care. When using a claims-centric approach, only direct disease-related costs can be calculated since members with a disease are not first identified.

Figure 7 presents the cumulative diabetes-specific costs associated with the 2,000 presumably sickest diabetics during the 12-month reporting period. Although these 2,000 diabetics represent only 4.9 percent of the U.S. Healthcare diabetic population, they account for 91.9 percent of the yearly direct diabetes-specific expenditures. The top 400 sickest diabetic patients (one percent of diabetics) account for 58.7 percent of the yearly noncapitated diabetes-specific expenditures. This highly disproportionate utilization of medical resources suggests the potential return to be gained by concentrating aggressive case management efforts on the sickest diabetic patients.

Figure 7. Incremental Costs of Diabetic Patients

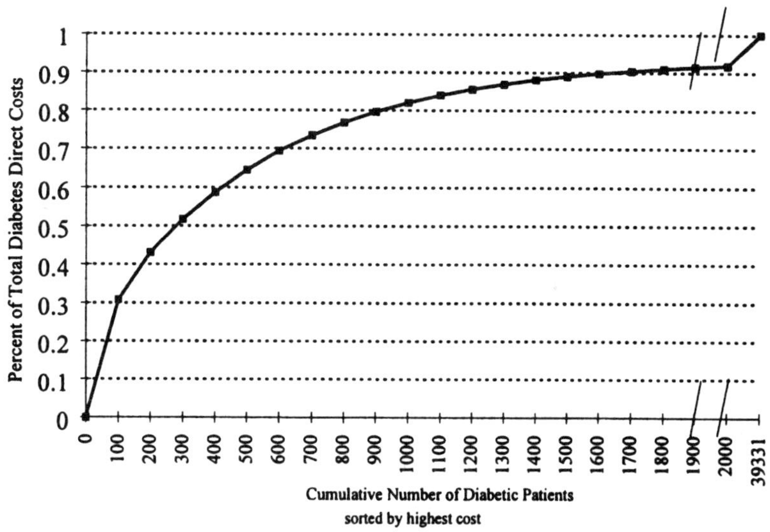

USQA's Approach to Risk Stratification

Identifying chronically ill members is foremost to delivering high-quality health care. Once identified, high-risk members can be enrolled in patient management programs designed to help maintain or improve their health status. Health insurance companies, in general, have used a number of methods to identify members for participation in case management and educational programs. Usually, however, methods are largely subjective or limited to information available to a primary provider.

Using administrative data that are likely to be available to managed care organizations, USQA developed a statistical model that objectively, quantitatively, and accurately identifies those with asthma who are at the highest risk of hospitalization.[23] Such members have the most to gain from case management and increased education.

Building on methodologies designed to identify members with chronic diseases in the Health Profile Database, USQA risk-stratified Aetna U.S. Healthcare members who have one or more chronic diseases. Separating members with chronic diseases into severity levels identifies even more precisely those who can gain the most from disease management programs. For instance, individuals who are at lowest risk for an acute exacerbation can be aggressively supported and educated via these programs. Case management and rigorous education of high-risk members result in better health outcomes and more efficient use of health care resources.[24,25,26]

This risk-stratification methodology builds on previous research by USQA. It is among the first disease-specific stratification study to use a database rich with disease-specific prior utilization information, including pharmaceutical and health system encounters, as well as demographic information that does not depend on respondent recall and is thereby free of recall error. Prior utilization is an acknowledged predictor of future health services utilization.[27,28,29] Databases containing an individual's prior utilization of services are generally available to MCOs. When used in a methodologically valid manner, these data can help identify individuals who are at highest risk for hospital admission. In turn, these individuals can be enrolled in a case management and education program designed to help keep patients out of the hospital and help them lead healthy lives. Additionally, the methodology provides information that can be applied with relative ease and low cost in terms of data acquisition.

Asthma will be used here as an example chronic disease to which the MCO applied a regression-based approach for risk stratification. Once asthmatics were identified in the USQA Health Profile Database, statistical models were created to determine the relationship between certain patient characteristics and the risk of an acute exacerbation requiring hospital admission. Extensive literature, clinical, and statistical reviews were conducted to identify the variables that would help distinguish patients who were most at risk for an acute exacerbation.[30, 31, 32, 33, 34] The presence of certain comorbidities, along with patient demographic information, prior utilization, and prior pharmaceutical use, were common predictors for an exacerbation in most chronic diseases. The list of variables that were determined empirically to predict the probability of an acute exacerbation among asthmatics is included in Table 1 (see following page).

The logistic regression dependent variable was whether the asthmatic was admitted to the hospital in 1994 specifically for an asthma-related condition. The initial sample included 1,000 Aetna U.S. Healthcare asthmatics who met the criteria. Thirty-four independent variables, largely indicated by the data, were included in the model. Variables with significant statistics at the .05 level were included in the model based on a stepwise logistic regression. Variables considered but not reaching the .05 threshold included 60 additional comorbidities defined by the Health Profile Database, primary care provider visits in 1992, and each of the geographic regions other than New York.

This model-building strategy was appropriate since the company was not interested in interpreting individual parameter estimates. Rather, Aetna U.S. Healthcare is interested in the predictive capabilities of the model as a whole. Again, variables were selected for the model based on their level of significance in a stepwise regression. Also contributing to these particularly low levels of significance is the large sample size. The overall model fit the data with a $P < .0001$. The study included selected variables that did not meet this criteria if they were part of a statistically significant group of variables or were considered to be clinically important regardless of statistical significance.

Five risk strata or levels were defined by the model. Individuals with asthma in the first risk category have the lowest risk for hospital admission, while those

Table 1. Variable Definitions and Means

Variable	Mean
DEPENDENT VARIABLE	
Admitted $_t$	.018
Not Admitted $_t$ ✔	.982
INDEPENDENT VARIABLES	
Demographic	
Gender	
Male	.47
Female ✔	.53
Age $_{t-1}$	22.12
Medicaid Status	
Medicaid subscriber $_{t-1}$	.01
Non-Medicaid subscriber $_{t-1}$ ✔	.99
Service Area	
New York Service Area $_t$	.21
Other Service Area $_t$ ✔	.79
Comorbidities	
COPD $_{t-1}$	.02
Ischemic Heart Disease $_{t-1}$	.02
Severity of Illness	
No pharmacy plan $_{t-1}$	.14
Level 1 $_{t-1}$ ✔	.56
Level 2 $_{t-1}$	.04
Level 3 $_{t-1}$	.15
Level 4 $_{t-1}$	.10
Level 5 $_{t-1}$	.01
No pharmacy plan $_{t-2}$	.28
Level 1 $_{t-2}$ ✔	.52
Level 2 or Level 3 $_{t-2}$	.12
Level 4 or Level 5 $_{t-2}$	.07
Prior Utilization	
Admissions	
Zero asthma-specific admissions on record $_{t-1}$ ✔	.97
One asthma-specific admission $_{t-1}$	.02
Two or more asthma-specific admissions $_{t-1}$	.003
Zero asthma-specific admissions on Record $_{t-2}$ ✔	.93
One asthma-specific admission $_{t-2}$	.05
Two or more asthma-specific admissions $_{t-2}$	.01
ER Visits	
Zero asthma-specific ER visits on record $_{t-1}$ ✔	.95
One asthma-specific ER visit $_{t-1}$	.04
Two asthma-specific ER visits $_{t-1}$	
Three asthma-specific ER visits $_{t-1}$	
Four or more asthma-specific ER visits $_{t-1}$	.001
Zero asthma-specific ER visits on record $_{t-2}$ ✔	.97
One asthma-specific ER visit $_{t-2}$	.03
Two or more asthma-specific ER visits $_{t-2}$	.01
Primary Care Visits	
Zero primary care provider visits on record $_{t-1}$ ✔	.76
One primary care provider visit $_{t-1}$	.15
Two primary care provider visits $_{t-1}$	.05
Three primary care provider visits $_{t-1}$	.02
Four or more primary care provider visits $_{t-1}$	.02
Outpatient Visits	
Fewer than four specialist outpatient visits on record $_{t-1}$ ✔	.90
Four or more specialist outpatient visits $_{t-1}$	.10
Administrative Information	
Length of Enrollment	
< One half year $_a$ ✔	.03
At least one half year and < one year $_a$	.13
At least one year and < three years $_a$	.32
At least three years and < five years $_a$	.27
Five or more years $_a$	.25
Primary Care Provider Type	
Pediatric patient $_t$	.36
Nonpediatric patient $_t$ ✔	.64

✔ Indicates reference category in the logistic regression analysis.
$_t$ Indicates during 1994 (e.g., admission during 1994)
$_{t-1}$ Indicates during 1993 (e.g., utilization during the year prior to risk year)
$_{t-2}$ Indicates during 1992 (e.g., utilization during the year two years prior to risk year)
(a) Length of enrollment is measured from December 31, 1993.

in the fifth risk category face the greatest odds of being hospitalized. Asthmatics with at least a one in five chance of being hospitalized (20 percent or above) are in the fifth risk stratum. Asthma sufferers with a probability of hospitalization of between 10 and 19 percent are included in the fourth level. Those with a probability of between 5 and 9 percent are included in the third category. The second risk level includes asthmatics with a probability of hospitalization between 2 and 4 percent. All others are included in the first stratum. Figure 8 displays the distribution of asthmatics in each of the five risk strata. As shown, the majority of asthmatics are in the least severe category and have the lowest chance of hospitalization.

Figure 8. Risk Stratification for Asthmatics

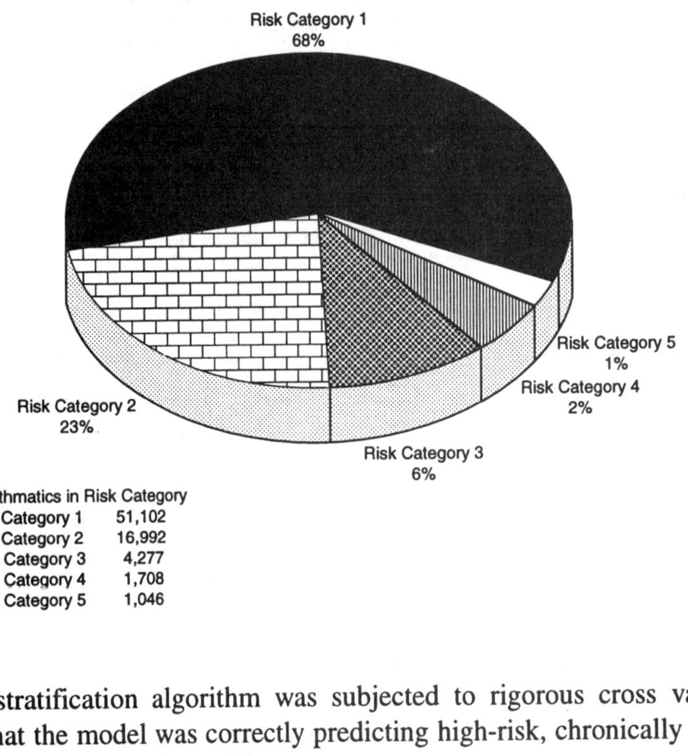

Asthmatics in Risk Category

Category 1	51,102
Category 2	16,992
Category 3	4,277
Category 4	1,708
Category 5	1,046

The stratification algorithm was subjected to rigorous cross validation to ensure that the model was correctly predicting high-risk, chronically ill asthmatics. Validation was performed by:

- Reevaluating the statistical relationships with data from other years not used in developing the models. This ensured that these relationships were not specifically related to the data used for modeling, but rather generalizable to the entire population.
- Evaluating the literature and clinical results to ensure that statistical relationships were not random.
- Comparing the predicted probabilities of an acute exacerbation with actual experience in the same datasets to measure the model's accuracy.

Figure 9 displays the actual probability of admissions in each of the five risk categories. The actual experience values were obtained for each stratum at the end of the year. As evidenced by the graph, the proportion of those who were hospitalized increases with each successive stratum. In fact, those in risk stratum five are about 30 times more likely to be admitted when compared with those in risk stratum one. Chi square goodness of fit tests were calculated and statistically reflect the accuracy of the stratification algorithm to appropriately predict the chances of an acute exacerbation.[35]

Figure 9. Validation of Risk Strata—
Actual Probability of Hospital Admission

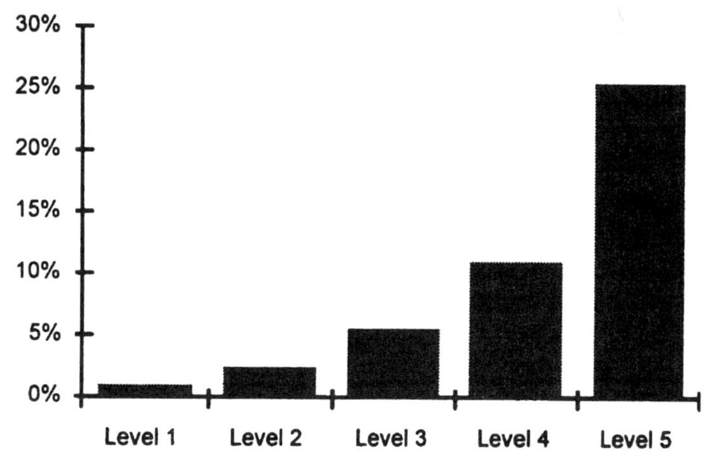

To more efficiently and effectively utilize health care resources, it is important that managed care organizations be able to maximize the return on investment by way of improved health outcomes for members.[36] Identifying the highest-risk members who stand to benefit the most from case management and increased educational efforts is one way Aetna U.S. Healthcare can help to improve the health of their members and realize cost savings. While several other hospitalization risk-stratification models exist in the literature, the USQA models are the first validated disease-specific ones that use only administrative data.

The USQA risk stratification methodology accurately identifies chronically ill members who are at the highest risk for an acute exacerbation. The application of this model can be used to better match disease management resources with patient needs and help managed care organizations better allocate their case management and educational resources. For example, asthmatics with a high probability of an acute exacerbation could be proactively enrolled in an intense disease management program that makes full use of the most intense interventions, including case management and home-based patient education and treatment. Those at low risk for an acute exacerbation could be enrolled in a less intense program—but one appropriate for their specific needs and level of severity—such as a general health education program, a member mailing, or a population-based outreach program. This ability to stratify members by severity and then target the appropriate interventions is clearly a significant milestone in managing the chronic diseases of a population.

USQA'S APPROACH TO PERFORMANCE MEASUREMENT

USQA has devoted resources to developing population-based measures for evaluating the performance of all key providers within the medical delivery system: PCPs, specialists, and hospitals. Aetna U.S. Healthcare uses the availability of performance information to provide peer comparison, to set benchmarks for attainable performance, and to stimulate providers to continuously improve their performance. USQA's tools for measurement include report cards, profiling systems, and performance-based contracting.

Overview of the Measurement of Quality

The issue within the new managed medical delivery system is accountability, and the Health Plan Employer Data and Information Set (HEDIS) is widely recognized as a driver in this new era. But HEDIS addresses just one level of the medical delivery system—the health plan. Provider organizations and physicians also must be accountable for the quality and costs of care they provide. The following overview briefly describes some of the terms and concepts that are currently in use.

Avedis Donabedian's taxonomy of structure, process, and outcome provides a good starting point for discussing the dimensions in which quality is measured.[37, 38] Structure can be thought of as how well the system or provider of interest is arranged so that the highest quality care can be provided and the best outcomes can be achieved. An example would be the difference in outcome that might be expected for a patient requiring emergent angioplasty if there is an interventional cardiologist on call within a hospital with a catheterization laboratory, as opposed to a hospital where the cardiologist has to travel from home. Process measures of quality can be described as how well providers are following certain proven performance standards, such as immunization rates for eligible children within a pediatrician's practice. Outcomes of care can be described simply as whether or not the most desirable results are achieved by the care provided. Outcomes can relate to clinical issues, such as the ability to effectively control a patient's asthma, thereby avoiding visits to the emergency room or hospital admissions. In addition, outcomes can relate to nonclinical issues surrounding the quality of a patient's life and functional status, such as the ability of a patient with severe asthma to work full time or have better attendance in school or the ability of a patient undergoing hip replacement to ambulate fully in the postoperative period.[39]

Within the medical delivery system, hospitals have been most subject to measurement and accountability. Accreditation by the Joint Commission on

Accreditation of Hospital Organizations traditionally has concentrated on the structures in place within the hospital; however, JCAHO and MCOs have begun to measure the quality of hospital care along other dimensions. Hospital care is important both in terms of its role in taking care of patients at their sickest and in the enormity of dollars spent on that care.

Figure 10 shows an example of a report card used by Aetna U.S. Healthcare to measure the quality of care of hospitals. In addition to describing some of the structural aspects of hospital care, the report card measures three important dimensions of quality: efficiency, effectiveness, and satisfaction. The costs of care are partly measured by the length of stay—a measure of the efficiency of the care process. Effectiveness of care is measured by the complication rate and the mortality rate. Service levels of quality are measured by the satisfaction rates of the patients admitted to the hospital as well as those of the attending physicians.

Figure 10.

Memorial Hospital of XYZ County

Hospital Report Card Ratings

Administrator: John Doe, President **Hospital Type:** Non-Government, Not for Profit

Address: 75 Avenue **City:** Anytown **State:** NJ **Zip:** 08060

Telephone: 555-1212

Admissions: 18,033 **Beds:** 365 **Births:** 2,216 **Employees:** 1,969 **Occupancy Rate:** 76%

PRODUCT LINE	Length of Stay	Adverse Event Rate*	Mortality*	Satisfaction**	Combined Rating
MEDICINE					
Cardiology	l	l	n		l
Gastroenterology	n	r	m		r
General Medicine	l	r	n		n
Hematology/Oncology	l	l	n		l
Medical Oncology	l	r	n		n
Neurology	l	n	l		l
Pediatrics	l				l
Pulmonary	l	r	r		n
Total Medicine Rating	l	n	n	n	n
OB/GYN					
Gynecology	r	n			n
Obstetrics	l	n			n
Total OB/Gyn Rating	n	n		l	n
SURGERY					
CT Surgery	l	r	r		n
General Surgery	l	r	n		n
Neurosurgery	n	r	n		n
Orthopedics	n	n	n		n
Otolaryngology	l	r			n
Urology	l	m	n		n
Vascular Surgery	n	r	n		n
Total Surgery Rating	l	r	n	n	n
OVERALL RATING	l	n	n	n	n

* Blank cells appear in product lines where USQA does not model performance.

** Too few surveys were collected for individual product lines to allow accurate rating.

m	r	n	l
Lowest Rating			Highest Rating

The report card measures overall hospital performance along with individual specialty performance. Hospitals are measured in comparison with their peers and receive a score of 1 to 4 for each of the individual measures, which are casemix and severity-adjusted for important characteristics of the patients admitted to the hospital. Additionally, each major physician specialty within the hospital is measured. More and more hospitals are turning to this type of information in an effort to improve the quality and cost-effectiveness of care provided within their institutions. Because an administrative dataset containing clinical information is generated for every patient discharged from the hospital, this information is readily available to examine the overall quality of care provided by the hospitals and the practice patterns of individual physicians. As a result, physicians have become more accountable for the care provided to their hospitalized patients.[40]

With health plans being accountable to employer groups and provider organizations being accountable to health plans, it stands to reason that under the new managed care system individual physicians also will be held accountable. Physicians must understand the changes that are taking place at the health plan and provider organization level and the implications for their own individual practices. MCOs and provider organizations that seek to optimize the quality of care while maintaining or decreasing costs must scrutinize the physicians with whom they do business, either through contractual or ownership relationships. The development of methods to measure the physician-specific costs and quality of care allows an enhanced level of accountability, which the individual practicing physicians will be asked to maintain.[41,42,43,44]

In order for the individual physician to be accountable for the care that is provided, the goals and expectations of the MCOs and provider organizations must be understood. Most, if not all, of these expectations make sense because they represent the common goal of high-quality, cost-effective care.[45] There has been a lack of consensus about what defines and how to measure high-quality care. However, the focus remains on process and outcome measures of care that are quantifiable. Many of the processes of care have been proven to lead to better outcomes: immunizations, cancer screening, early prenatal care, anti-inflammatory control of asthma, and tight glycemic control of the diabetic.[46, 47] These areas of care must be followed closely, and measurement must take place to determine which physicians are the best practices for certain types of care and how others can learn from them. In addition, outcomes of care have included measures of utilization and member-based health status and quality of life.

At USQA, measuring physician performance evolved from the ability to understand the membership with chronic diseases using the Health Profile Database, described earlier in this chapter. In addition to providing prevalence and utilization statistics outlined previously, the Health Profile Database forms the basis of measuring and reporting the quality of care provided to members with chronic diseases. That process is explained below.

In Aetna U.S. Healthcare's managed care system, each member chooses a PCP who coordinates the member's care. The PCP is expected to focus on health maintenance and early identification of disease and to make medically appropriate decisions that facilitate the management of patients by the most suitable provider and place of service. Moreover, since each PCP is responsible for a defined patient population, USQA can measure, with a fairly large degree of accuracy, the performance of each individual physician when it comes to caring for these patients.

An example of USQA's work in evaluating physician performance can be illustrated using diabetes. USQA developed a physician performance report for PCPs, which evaluated the degree to which care they delivered to diabetic patients followed the accepted standards as promoted by the American Diabetes Association. The report measured physicians' use of various preventive tests, the percentage of diabetics who visited their PCP, and the average number of visits per diabetic member, as well as outcome and satisfaction measures.

Other measures easily calculated using the Health Profile Database included the prevalence of beta blocker use in ischemic heart disease and end-stage renal disease in diabetic patients. In essence, the Health Profile Database provides a denominator and broadens ability to choose a variety of numerators to calculate important rates that add to the range of process and outcome measures of quality. The annual occurrence of lower extremity amputation, diabetic nephropathy, and blindness/impaired vision also have been calculated.

Using this approach, all diabetic patients within a PCP office are identified. The physicians within that office are evaluated on their performance in providing high-quality care to their diabetic patients. Finally, the performance of physicians is compared with the practice-based norms of their peers.[48, 49]

Figure 11 shows an example of the two-year Diabetes Performance Report. This version of the report provides results for a U.S. Healthcare region for 1994 and 1995, based on continuously enrolled members identified with diabetes from the Health Profile Database. This report is unique in the sense that it represents USQA's initial effort to run performance measures two years in a row. For the first time the company was able to observe important trends that support the claim that feeding back performance measurement to physicians is an important step in quality improvement. Over the two-year period, there was significant improvement in several of the indicators across many regions and providers in the network.

By using clinical data stored in administrative databases, Aetna U.S. Healthcare and USQA have demonstrated that physician performance can be measured and quality improvement can be tracked. USQA recognizes that performance measures can assist purchasers and consumers in evaluating health care and provide physicians with an ability to identify and prioritize areas for improvement. The purpose of the Diabetes Performance Report was not to single out physician outliers but to provide educational feedback so that physicians could improve their performance. Providing physicians with performance information on key quality measures for chronic diseases can positively affect practice patterns. Feeding back data to physicians can be effective in altering their practice patterns when it is part of a comprehensive program of quality improvement. Equally important, performance measurement can be quantified and tracked over time, as demonstrated by this two-year Diabetes Performance Report.

Figure 11. Diabetes Performance Report—U.S. Healthcare

Report time period: 1/1/94-12/31/95
Number of Current USHC members identified with diabetes: 29,384

PREVALENCE MEASURES	1994	1995
1. Estimated overall prevalence of diabetes	3.0%	3.1%
2. Diabetics on insulin with pharmacy plan	36.2%	29.2%
3. Estimated overall prevalence of diabetes, age 0-19	0.2%	0.2%
4. Estimated overall prevalence of diabetes, age 20-39	1.0%	1.0%
5. Estimated overall prevalence of diabetes, age 40+	7.0%	7.1%
ACCESS MEASURES		
6. Members with any diabetic disease seeing the PCP at least once	91.2%	93.5%
7. Average Number of annual PCP visits per diabetic	4.79	6.73
8. Members with any diabetic disease seeing the endocrinologist at least once	11.2%	11.9%
PROCESS MEASURES		
9. Average number of annual glycated hemoglobin tests per diabetic	1.82	2.34*
10. Diabetics with at least two glycated hemoglobin tests	40.8%	49.6%*
11. Diabetics receiving a retinal eye exam	40.3%	39.9%
12. Diabetics receiving cholesterol screening	43.9%	46.9%*
13. Diabetics receiving microalbuminuria screening	11.3%	13.7%*
OUTCOME MEASURES		
14. Emergency room visits specifically for diabetes/1000 diabetics/year	10	10
15. Admissions specifically for diabetes/1000 diabetics/year	26	25
16. Admissions for ketoacidosis, hyperosmolar coma, or other coma/1000 diabetics/year	3.50	3.22
17. Admissions for hypoglycemia/1000 diabetics/year	1.45	1.26
18. Admissions for cellulitis/1000 diabetics/year	17	16
19. Inpatient days (acute) specifically for diabetes/1000 diabetics/year	130	101
SATISFACTION MEASURES*		
20. Overall satisfaction with medical care a the PCP office of diabetic members	97.7%	97.9%
21. Satisfaction with the ability to make appointments for illnesses	97.1%	97.2%
22. Satisfaction with the response to an emergency call within 30 minutes	94.2%	94.4%

*Percent responded with good, very good, or excellent — *p<.01

It is apparent from the results of this Diabetes Performance Report that information on quality indicators, provided directly to PCPs, can be a factor in improving the care delivered to diabetic members. Aetna U.S. Healthcare has demonstrated marked and significant improvements in many of the performance measures evaluated over time. One of the most encouraging findings of this study, however, is that in addition to an improvement in many of the process measures, access to ambulatory care for diabetic members increased while inpatient days decreased. It is hoped that clinically significant improvements in care will continue to evolve as a result of sharing performance information with providers.

The ability to evaluate the epidemiology of chronic diseases and measure the performance of network physicians on important process and outcome measures is crucial to the success of managed care plans. Such analyses can help MCO leaders make informed decisions on whether and how to apply resources to physician education and patient management programs. These analyses also can help determine the potential impact from proposed interventions and justify anticipated costs of these interventions.

Studies of the epidemiology of the other diseases in the USQA Health Profile Database, along with performance reports to evaluate the care provided by PCPs to patients with asthma, hypertension, atrial fibrillation, congestive heart failure, and ischemic heart disease, have been done. Performance measures for the majority of the major specialties also have been developed by USQA and shared with providers.

Other Measurement Tools

The quality of care that individual physicians provide can be measured by other methods. Graphs similar to the one in Figure 12 are used to identify variations in practice patterns. This graphical display of performance plots individual physician offices against their case volume for measures such as c-section rates, average length of stay, and readmissions. Each point represents an individual office. The expected benchmark level of performance is shown with a horizontal line, and the broken lines surrounding it are the 95 percent confidence intervals. Using this graphical display, both MCOs and physicians can evaluate the performance of individual physicians and, with some statistical certainty, can identify practice patterns that are truly different. This type of performance measurement will become increasingly important as MCOs feed back information in the quest for continuous quality improvement.[50]

Figure 12. Cesarean Section Rate vs. Vaginal Deliveries

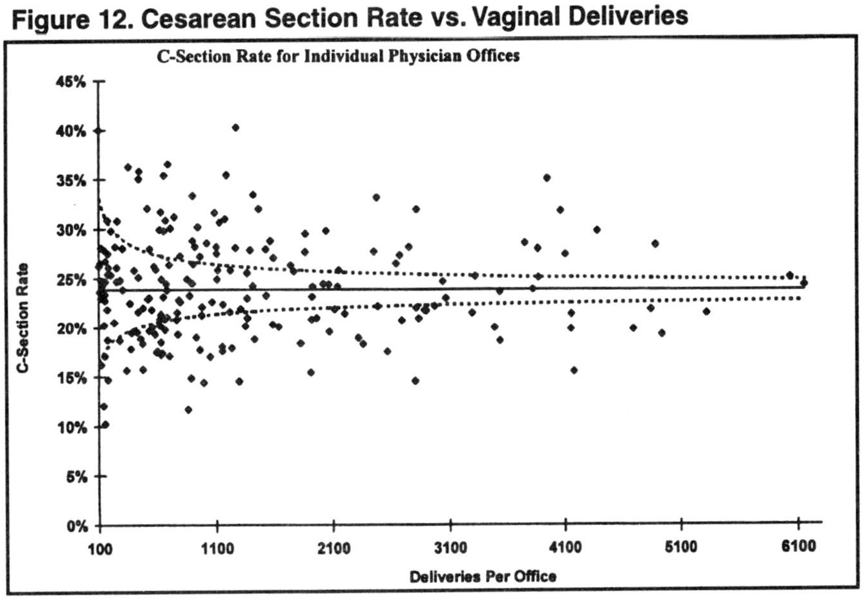

Figure 13 displays an example of a performance report of obstetrician/gynecologists within Aetna U.S. Healthcare. In this report, an individual office's performance is compared with the 90 percent level within its peer offices for six measures that Aetna U.S. Healthcare's Ob/Gyn Specialty Quality Assessment Committee has deemed important in representing quality care.

Figure 13. The US Healthcare Obstetrics/Gynecology Performance Report

Performance Measure	Your Office's Performance	90th Percentile Performance	Range of Performance
C-section Rate	32%	16%	10% - 59%
Office-based Work-up for Abnormal Uterine Bleeding	91%	92%	20%-100%
Average Length of Stay	2.3	1.9	1.8-4.2
Readmission Rate	14%	1%	0% - 20%
Physician Vists per Members Seen	1.3	1.2	1.1 - 1.6
Precertification Rate	74%	90%	72% - 100%
Member Satisfaction	87%	94%	80% - 97%

One of the biggest concerns voiced by physicians who are faced with having their own performance and practice patterns measured is that their patients may be sicker than average and, therefore, their performance might appear below average because of the patient population they serve. In addition, they may have a special expertise or core competency that makes their patient population different from providers who otherwise might be considered their peers. The casemix and severity of illness of patients being cared for by a specific physician do need to be taken into account in order to draw valid inferences about differential performance.[51, 52]

Performance-Based Compensation

Increasing physician accountability also means MCOs are beginning to incorporate measures of how well their expectations are met into their compensation arrangements with providers. Performance-based contracting aligns financial incentives with the quality goals of the health plan and leads to improved performance.[53,54] Aetna U.S. Healthcare generally pays all PCPs by capitation. Capitation refers to a payment methodology in which the PCP receives a prepaid, set amount to cover the cost of caring for each Aetna U.S. Healthcare member in his or her practice. The payment amount is adjusted for the age and sex of that member and is paid irrespective of the number of services the member utilizes.

Aetna U.S. Healthcare introduced the measurement of performance of PCPs into its compensation model in 1987. Since the introduction of this PCP Quality

Care Compensation model (QCCS), Aetna U.S. Healthcare participating PCPs have the opportunity to receive additional distributions above their capitation amount based on their measured performance in providing quality care to Aetna U.S. Healthcare members. This PCP QCCS has undergone further refinement since its initial introduction and is currently in its third generation. Most recently, the MCO has incorporated burden of illness casemix adjustment methodology into the PCP QCCS model.

Additional distributions are dependent on a PCP office's overall Quality Factor. The Quality Factor for the office is derived from three components: Quality Review, Comprehensive Care, and Utilization (see Figure 14). The Quality Review component includes measures related to member satisfaction and derived from member surveys, member transfer rates, focused medical chart reviews, and the PCP office's philosophy of managed care. When conducting chart reviews, USQA looks for compliance with health maintenance standards, such as providing recommended immunizations and cholesterol screening tests in the appropriate age groups.

Figure 14. The Primary Care Physician Quality Care Compensation Model

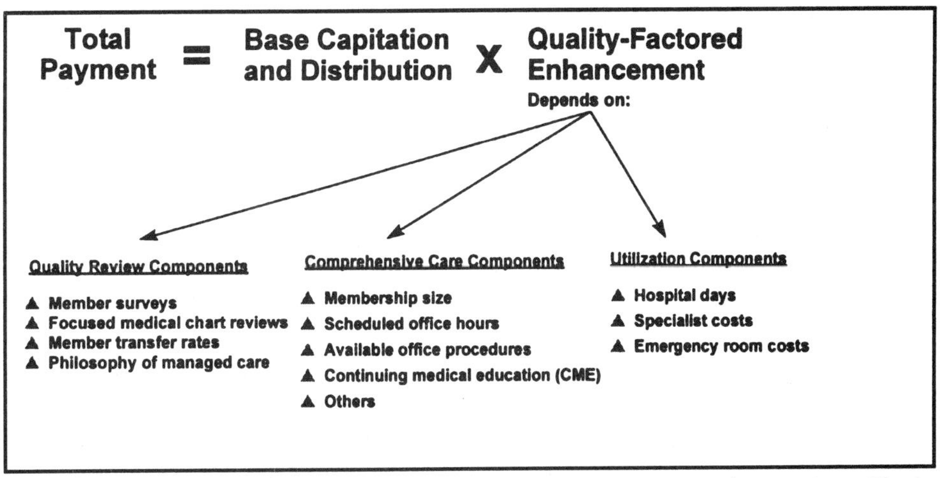

Comprehensive Care components are measures that enhance a PCP office's ability to succeed in a managed care system by evaluating things like office hours, available office procedures, and sufficient internal practice coverage. Utilization components evaluate a PCP office's use of hospitals, as measured in bed days and use of specialist care and emergency rooms.

Each measure within each of the three components is given its own weight. The Quality Review and Comprehensive Care components account for 82 percent of the overall Quality Factor, while the Utilization component accounts for 18 percent. The Quality Factor score can add as much as 29 percent to the capitation amount. The total compensation of the PCP office, therefore, is comprised of several components. The base capitation is dependent on the age and sex distribution of the capitated Aetna U.S. Healthcare members. The enhancement to the capitation is based on the calculated Quality Factor. The base plus enhanced capitation payments are made twice a month to the PCP office.[55,56]

This model does not stand alone as a mechanism to improve quality, nor is it a means to devalue outliers. A comprehensive quality improvement process uses the same data to identify those providers who consistently do not achieve minimal standards. Realigning toward quality-based goals is considered an essential element to ensure the continued value of managed care in our society.[57]

THE FUTURE OF PERFORMANCE MEASUREMENT

Purchasers have increased the scrutiny paid to MCOs through projects such as the HEDIS Quality Report Card. In return, MCOs are holding their providers accountable for the quality and costs of care provided to members. The decision-makers in the care process are the PCPs and specialty care physicians. However, PCPs and specialists are becoming more organized because of the need to manage patient populations. The two basic arrangements are groups of physicians joining together to form single specialty or multispecialty physician organization (PO) or physicians joining the institutions that have been the center of much of their business in the past (e.g., physician hospital organizations). Financing can vary under these arrangements—from independent practices organized in a management and financial relationship to assume risk, to group practices and institutions that are wholly owned by the core entity. These groups can be small (e.g., a group practice without walls) or large (e.g., an integrated delivery system covering a large geographical territory).

Regardless of the management and financial relationship of the units that serve as the building blocks of today's medical delivery system, there is a need to better understand the performance of the group as a unit, along with the individual physicians and other providers that make up the unit. For example, large integrated delivery systems (IDSs) must be able to quantify both the costs and quality of the care they provide to the population of members for which they are responsible. They need to know the who, what, where, why, and how of health care dollars spent. Where do costs seem to be higher than expected and where are they lower? Which physicians appear to practice more cost-effectively, and what can the other physicians learn from these best practices? What are the referral patterns and associated specialty costs of the PCPs, and what are the procedure rates, admission rates, and hospital bed days of the specialists? The IDSs must know this information in the aggregate as well as for each physician. As large IDSs begin to have more accountability for an entire population of patients, they will be responsible not only for the quality of each procedure performed or each patient seen, but also for the entire population of patients and population-based measures, such as cardiac catheterization rates, mammography rates, and immunization rates.[58,59]

It is much more challenging to measure the quality of health care than the costs of health care. The IDSs will become responsible for the same population-based measures of quality for which the MCOs are held accountable (i.e., HEDIS). Given the capitated relationship of members to the IDS or the PCPs of the IDS, population-based measures can be determined. The true winners will be those IDSs that have access to the information systems to capitalize on computerized medical records, real-time decision-support tools, physician and patient reminders, and tools that enable practice patterns to be evaluated and continuously improved.[60] They will practice outcomes management in which the measurement of the outcomes of care can be linked to the processes of care. In health care, cost and quality are inseparable. High-quality care leads to better outcomes but also lower costs; therefore, systems that concentrate only on the costs of care and ignore the quality components of care will not succeed in this new era of accountability.

The future holds enormous opportunities to improve the quality of care for millions of Americans. USQA and the Aetna U.S. Healthcare health delivery system are pursuing these opportunities.

REFERENCES

1. Siu A, McGlynn E, Morgenstern H, Brook R. "A Fair Approach to Comparing Quality of Care." *Health Affairs*, 10 (1990):62-75.
2. Hanchak NA, Murray JF, Hirsch A, McDermott PD, Schlackman N. "USQA Health Profile Database as a Tool for Health Plan Quality Improvement." *Managed Care Quarterly,* 1996; 4:58-69.
3. Ginsburg P, Hammons G. "Competition and the Quality of Care: The Importance of Information." *Inquiry*, 25 (1988):108-115.
4. Hanchak, et al. "USQA Health Profile..."
5. Roos L, Brazauskas R. "Outcomes and Quality Assurance: Facilitating the Use of Administrative Data." *Quality Assurance in Health Care*, 2 (1990):77-88.
6. Hidalgo J. "Development of a Model Longitudinal Data Base to Measure Outcomes and Quality of Care Among Persons with AIDS." *QRB*, 16 (1990):355-364.
7. Weiner JP, et al. "Applying insurance claims data to assess quality of care: A compilation of potential indicators." *QRB*, 16 (1990):424-438.
8. Leatherman S, et al. "Quality Screening and Management Using Claims Data in a Managed Care Setting." *QRB*, 17 (1991):349-359.
9. Goldfield N. "Measurement and Management of Quality in Managed Care Organizations: Alive and Improving." *QRB*, 17 (1991):343-348.

10. Hanchak, NA. "Using Administrative Data to Evaluate the Quality of Care." *Journal of Clinical Outcomes Management* 1996; 3:57-61.
11. Gottlieb L, Margolis C, Schoenbaum S. "Clinical Practice Guidelines at an HMO: Development and Implementation in a Quality Improvement Model." *QRB*, 16 (1990):80-86.
12. Hanchak et al. "USQA Health Profile. . ."
13. Goldfield N. "Measurement and Management. . ."
14. Siu AL et al. "Choosing Quality-of-Care Measures Based on the Expected Impact of Improved Quality of Care for the Major Causes of Mortality and Morbidity." *RAND HMO Quality of Care Consortium*, JR-03 (1992):1-73.
15. Iezzoni LI, Heeren T, Foley SM, Daley J, Hughes J, Coffman GA. "Chronic Conditions and Risk of In-Hospital Death." *HSR: Health Services Research*, 29 (1994):435-46.
16. Von Korff M, Wagner E, Saunders K. "A Chronic Disease Score From Automated Pharmacy Data." *J Clin Epidemiol*, 45 (1992):197-203.
17. Green J, Wintfeld N. "How Accurate are Hospital Discharge Data for Evaluating Effectiveness of Care?" *Medical Care*, 31 (1993):719-731.
18. Nordstrom DL, Remington PL, Layde PM. "The Utility of HMO Data for the Surveillance of Chronic Diseases." *Amer J of Pub Health*, 84 (1994): 995-997
19. Hanchak et al. "USQA Health Profile. . ."
20. The Diabetes Control and Complications Trial Research Group. "The effect of intensive treatment of diabetes on the development and progression of long-term complications in insulin-dependent diabetes mellitus." *New England Journal of Medicine*, 329:977-986, 1993
21. Rubin RJ, Altman WM, Mendelson DN: "Special Article: Health Care Expenditures for People With Diabetes Mellitus." *J Clin Endocrinol Metab*, 199;78 (1992): 809A-809F.
22. Rendell M, Kimmel DB, Bamisedun O, O'Donnell T, Fulmer J. "The Health Care Status of the Diabetic Population as Reflected by Physician Claims to a Major Insurer." *Arch Intern Med*, 153 (1993): 1360-1366.
23. Grana JR, Preston WD, McDermott PD, Hanchak NA. "The Use of Limited Administrative Data to Risk Stratify Asthmatic Patients." Publication Pending.
24. Hanchak NA, Murray JF, Arkans H, McHugh E, McDermott P, Schlackman N. "Improved Outcomes of an Outpatient Pediatric Asthma Patient Management Program in an IPA HMO." *Am J Man Care*, 1996; 2:387-392.
25. Wilson SR, Scamagas P, German DF, Hughes GW, Lulla S, Coss S, Chardon L, Thomas RG, Starr-Schneidkraut N, Stancavage FB, Arsham GM. "A Controlled Trial of Two Forms of Self-Management Education for Adults with Asthma." *American Journal of Med*, 1993;94:564-576.

26. Mayo PH, Richman J, Harris HW. "Results of a Program to Reduce Admission for Adult Asthma." *Annals of Int Med*, 1990;112:864-871.
27. Ash A, Porell F, Grunenberg L, Sawitz E, Beiser A. "Adjusting Medicare Capitation Payments Using Prior Hospitalization Data." *Health Care Financing Review*, 1989;10:17-29.
28. Newhouse JP, Manning WG, Keeler EB, Sloss EM. "Adjusting Capitation Rates Using Objective Health Measures and Prior Utilization." *Health Care Financing Review*, 1989;10:41-54
29. Newhouse JP, Sloss EM, Manning WG, Keeler EB. "Risk Adjustment for a Children's Capitation Rate." *Health Care Financing Review*, 1993;15:39-54.
30. Hanchak et al. "Improved Outcomes. . ."
31. Wilson et al. "A Controlled Trial. . ."
32. Mayo et al. "Results of a Program. . ."
33. Weiss KB, Gergen PJ, Hodgson TA. "An Economic Evaluation of Asthma in the United States." *NEJM*, 1992;362:862-866.
34. Buist AS, Vollmer WM. "Preventing Deaths from Asthma." *NEJM*, 1994;331:1584-1585
35. Grana et al. "The Use of Limited. . ."
36. Weiss et al. "An Economic Evaluation. . ."
37. Donabedian A. "The Quality of Care: How Can it Be Assessed?" *JAMA*, 26 (1988):1743-1747.
38. Brook R. "Quality of Care: Do We Care?" *Ann Intern Med*, 1990;115:486-490.
39. Hanchak, NA. "Managed Care, Accountability, and the Physician." Medical Clinics of North America 1996; 80:245-261.
40. Sennett C, Legorreta AP, Zatz SL. "Performance-based Hospital Contracting for Quality Improvement." *Joint Commission Journal of Quality Improvement*, 1993; 19:374-383.
41. Hanchak. "Managed Care, Accountability. . ."
42. Feinglass J, Handler I, Hughes R. "Using Severity-Adjusted Physician Practice Profiles to Identify Cost-Effective Care." *NLM Publications*, 20 (1987): 99-122
43. Lasker RD, Shapiro DW, Tucker AM "Realizing the Potential of Practice Pattern Profiling." *Inquiry*, 29 (1992): 287-297.
44. McNeil, B, Pederson, S, Gatsonis, C. "Current Issues in Profiling Quality of Care." *Inquiry*, 29 (1992): 298-307.
45. Hanchak. "Managed Care, Accountability. . ."
46. Hanchak et al. "Improved Outcomes . . ."

47. Hanchak NA, Murray JF, Harmon-Weiss S, Schlackman N. "The Effectiveness of an Influenza Immunization Program in an HMO Setting." *The American Journal of Managed Care*, 1996; 2:661-666.
48. Weiner JP, Parente ST, Garnick DW, Fowles J, Lawthers AG, Palmer H. "A Claim-Based Profile of Care Provided to Medicare Patients with Diabetes." *JAMA*, 1995;273:1503-1508.
49. Hanchak NA, Schlackman, N. "The Measurement of Physician Performance." *Quality Management in Health Care*, 1995; 4:1-12.
50. Hanchak. "Managed Care, Accountability. . ."
51. Feinglass et al. "Using Severity-Adjusted. . ."
52. Salem-Schatz S, Moore G, Rucker M, Pearson S. "The Case for Case-Mix Adjustment in Practice Profiling." *JAMA*, 272 (1994): 871-874
53. Morrow, RW, Gooding AD, Clark C. "Improving Physicians' Preventive Health Care Behavior Through Peer Review and Financial Incentives." *Archives of Family Medicine*, 4 (1995): 165-169.
54. Schlackman N. "Evolution of a Quality-based compensation model: the third generation." *Am J Med Quality*, 8 (Summer 1993): 103-110.
55. *Ibid.*
56. Hanchak NA, Schlackman N, Harmon-Weiss S. "U.S. Healthcare's Quality-Based Compensation Model." *Health Care Financing Review*, 1996; 17:143-159.
57. Hanchak. "Managed Care, Accountability. . ."
58. *Ibid.*
59. Hanchak et al. "The Effectiveness of an Influenza. . ."
60. Ellwood P. "Shattuck Lecture(Outcomes Management: A Technology of Patient Experience." *NEJM*, 318 (1988):1549-1556.

Chapter 13

Milliman and Robertson

Demonstrating and Communicating Quality

Frederick W. Spong, MD, MBA

As the turn of the century approaches, all health care providers, particularly managed care organizations, face mounting pressure not only to demonstrate the ability to effectively deliver health care services but also to document and communicate measures of clinical quality and fiscal accountability. Providers, employers, and consumers as well as federal and state regulatory agencies are demanding tangible proof of the claim that the managed care model of delivery and financing is the solution to the problems of spiraling costs and unjustified variation in medical practice patterns.

Discussion and dissemination of quality measures have not been limited to the medical and group health administration literature. Publication of medical outcomes report cards and disease- and procedure-specific morbidity and mortality rates has attracted widespread media attention and sparked controversy. Advocates of the public release of clinical outcomes and other performance measures contend that despite inherent limitations, these studies offer consumers (patients, employers, and payers) the means for comparing providers.

Some skeptics denounce the clinical credibility of scales such as surgical mortality as incomplete indicators of quality. Others speculate that the data are readily manipulated by providers to enhance marketing and contracting opportunities, rendering the reports unreliable guides for health care decisions. Critics cite problems with data collection and risk adjustment of a severity sufficient to compromise the utility and validity of published reports.

The impact of increasingly frequent public release of clinical and cost outcomes and performance measures on consumer and provider decisionmaking, utilization, and the systematic delivery of medical services is not yet fully understood. Anecdotal accounts suggest that some providers labeled as "outliers"—individual physicians and medical groups that fall out of bounds of study parameters—have curtailed selected diagnostic and surgical procedures in response to published reports citing their greater-than-average morbidity and mortality rates.

USING DATA TO MEASURE QUALITY

The use of administrative data to gain insight about patients, physicians, and clinical practice is emerging as a requisite component of MCO quality improvement programs. Managed care plans are leading proponents of the use of administrative data to draw inferences about the quality of clinical care. Administrative data, routinely collected for purposes other than quality assessment, offer MCOs access to a wide range of clinical information to measure and improve the quality of care.

Long-term, the effect of published comparative evaluation of providers on panel establishment, selective contracting, and exclusion from existing plans is uncertain and in many instances may be punitive. Hospitals and medical groups, particularly those in mature managed care markets, may be forced to compete for network inclusion on the basis of standardized performance measures.

Despite legitimate concern about the reliability, validity, and interpretation of data, there is consensus that scrutiny and dissemination of quality data will escalate. To date, consumer interest has focused on individual providers, such as local hospitals and physicians. Employers, choosing between managed care plans involving the same group of participating hospitals and physicians, are requesting plan-specific information to guide contracting decisions. Companies and employer-driven health care coalitions seeking to assemble their own provider networks often rely on physician- and hospital-specific data during the selection process.

With multiple audiences demanding that MCOs perform their own due diligence, the need for multidisciplinary, collaborative processes to generate and analyze key indicators of quality is becoming increasingly urgent. Working together, practitioners and administrators can overcome the shortcomings of available data and can develop their own measures in the absence of universally accepted methods for integrating cost and quality data to yield reliable indices of cost-effectiveness.

The most beneficial use of the data is not for punitive action against providers, but as inspiration and incentive to systematically improve care. When evidence of quality problems is identified, MCOs must be prepared to launch a variety of interventions to address and promptly resolve such problems.

QUANTIFYING HEALTH CARE MANAGEMENT

This chapter describes the collective experience of Milliman & Robertson, Inc. (M&R) in assisting managed care and provider organizations throughout the United States in the identification of key indicators to measure quality and to define benefits. It also elaborates traditional and innovative interventions—implementation-ready strategies—successfully instituted to enhance quality in terms of process and outcomes.

Milliman & Robertson health care management consultants assist provider organizations to intensify the degree to which health care management is applied. M&R considers managed care to be the outcome of judicious application of research—data collection and analysis in concert with proactive management of data, utilization, cases, and quality.

Data management is used to measure and monitor outcomes, to identify the prevalence of best practices, and as the foundation for provider profiling. Utilization management is the process of evaluating the necessity, appropriateness, and efficiency of health care services, preferably prospectively during patient care rather than after care is completed.

Case management is patient-centered intervention aimed at improving health care delivery and outcomes. Quality management enables MCOs to identify deviations from accepted standards of clinical practice, measure outcome standards, support opportunities for improvement, and assist consumers (all purchasers of health care services including prospective patients, payers, employers, and health care coalitions) to understand the relative value of health care purchases. Using these definitions, the degree of health care management is quantifiable and an important measure of the overall effectiveness of the MCO.

The greater the degree of health care management, the greater the amount of fiscally responsible managed care generated. The greater the degree of health care management, the lower the consumption level (utilization and cost of services). This definition resolves confusion about differences in MCO models (e.g., HMO, PPO, EPO, POS) and helps employers and other health care purchasers to interpret the results achieved by various types of MCOs by applying uniform criteria to compare MCOs.

THE CONTINUUM OF MANAGED CARE MODELS

A loosely managed system reimburses providers through traditional fee-for-service coverage sold by a commercial carrier or administered by a third party. By definition, the services provided by this type of delivery system include some medically unnecessary services. Typically, a loosely managed system does not utilize a circumscribed provider network or incorporate comprehensive utilization management techniques.

One benchmark for clinical efficiency is an estimate of medically unnecessary hospital admissions and patient days. Loosely managed delivery systems experience unnecessary admissions in excess of 15 percent and 30 percent unnecessary patient days.

Further along the continuum, and the most prevalent model, is moderately managed care. M&R deems care to be moderately managed when the percentage of unnecessary admissions ranges from 5 to 15 percent and the percentage of unnecessary days is between 15 and 30 percent.

Although few in number, highly evolved MCOs are characterized by minimal or progressively decreasing provision of medically unnecessary services and practice patterns consistent with the best observed performance levels. Well-managed MCOs prospectively can limit medically unnecessary admissions and services to less than 5 percent. Having learned to efficiently manage care without a negative impact on the quality of health care provided, well-managed MCOs use clinical information systems and performance measures to identify and resolve inexplicable variations in clinical practice patterns.

Through education, training, incentivization, and repeated exposure to best practices, they continuously seek to improve adherence to established guidelines. These MCOs can document ever-improving quality as measured in terms of patient satisfaction, health status indicators, and delivery system efficiencies.

ESTABLISHING BASELINE MEASURES USING RETROSPECTIVE REVIEWS

Inpatient chart review is a reliable, primary research method to evaluate the quality of medical care. It is a pivotal first step in a comprehensive assessment of existing practice patterns, critical pathways, and identification of areas where further efficiencies are possible. Inpatient and ambulatory (i.e., outpatient, clinic, and office practice) chart reviews help to quantify the degree of health care management and construct the framework for outcomes analysis.

Milliman & Robertson medical consultants (physician and nurse evaluators) conduct chart reviews to evaluate the extent and type of care provided to patients. Typically, from 100-150 inpatient charts (a random or stratified sample to reflect particular patient mix patterns) are reviewed during a single project.

To determine the extent to which medically unnecessary services were provided to the sample patients, the results of reviews are compared to the best observed practice norms presented in the *M&R Healthcare Management Guidelines*™. These guidelines have gained acceptance as industry standards and are used to define goals and objectives for patients who do well—that is, traverse a predictable clinical course with no unanticipated complications.

In addition to noting the nature and extent of irregularities or deficiencies observed in the quality of care provided, M&R-focused reviews pinpoint the number of perfect stays, medically unnecessary admissions, and medically unnecessary days. Typically, fewer than one-third of stays reviewed are deemed perfect stays. Perfect stays are medically appropriate admissions with lengths of stay that could not be further reduced without having a negative impact on the quality of care.

Experience in numerous clinical assessment projects reveals that medically unnecessary admissions comprise 5 to 25 percent of hospital admissions. These admissions are commonly associated with shorter-than-average lengths of stay. There is significantly greater variation in the percentage of days identified as medically unnecessary. M&R's research projects have revealed as few as 5 percent and as many as 50 percent of medically unnecessary days.

This determination of medical necessity assumes optimal communication between health care providers, especially for patients transferred from one institution to another. It also presumes the availability and use of cost-effective alternatives to acute inpatient care such as rehabilitation or subacute care facilities, rapid treatment units, and professional home health services.

For each stay, the review process entails: a determination of the medical necessity of each admit reviewed; a determination of the medical necessity for each day of each medically necessary stay; a calculation of the number of unnecessary days; a determination of the medical necessity of the services provided during the stay (physician and ancillary health care services that were medically unnecessary); and the estimated cost associated with delivery of medically unnecessary services.

A summation of the temporal sequence and clinical course of care presents appropriate alternatives to continued inpatient care when continuation is considered medically unnecessary. The summary is useful as a teaching tool and may be referenced by other medical reviewers. Combined with other utilization data prepared by M&R actuarial consultants, the results of medical chart reviews can be used to project the extent of medically unnecessary services in the overall population. Actual utilization is compared with geographically consistent information from the health care database, *M&R Health Cost Guidelines*™, to determine the degree of health care management.

Although these reviews are retrospective, the results offer valuable information for prospectively improving an organization's degree of health care management through the institution of more efficient practice patterns. This rigorous approach relies on the clinical facts as presented in the patient charts. It is a dramatic departure from traditional managed care analysis, which, until recently, relied on anecdotal reports and assumptions.

CASE STUDY: INPATIENT CHART REVIEW

The specificity, sensitivity, and results of this type of retrospective research were reconfirmed during an M&R engagement to perform inpatient chart review, targeting selected medical and surgical DRGs, for a prominent New England-area health plan. The impetus for this review was the plan's experience with volume impact and adverse variances between their results and expected lengths of stay.

Overall, inpatient medical care was judged to have been excellent in terms of patient outcomes, although using Milliman & Robertson benchmarks for clinical efficiency, the results were consistent with a moderately managed system. Twenty-nine percent of days and 8 percent of admissions in the reviewed sample were judged to have been medically unnecessary and as such, potentially avoidable. Surgical cases were managed more efficiently than either obstetrics/gynecology or medical diagnoses.

As a result of this review, specific recommendations were made including early discharge planning, vigilant concurrent review, proactive continuity of nursing care, and enhanced case management of patients with chronic illnesses. To facilitate greater flexibility in the use of resources, the managed care plan also was advised to expand utilization management to include physician-designed, prior-authorization protocols for selected admissions.

Alternatives to acute inpatient care, such as rapid treatment units and home health care, were suggested as appropriate for many patients with pneumonia (DRGs 89 and 90). The plan was exhorted to engage physicians, nurses, and other practitioners in a consensus standard to define the most efficiency deliverable. Clinicians and administrators were directed to plot a course of incremental, attainable improvements in efficiency to assist the plan in departing from and improving upon historic practice patterns.

GAINING CONSENSUS FOR QUALITY IMPROVEMENT

Securing organizational and physician commitment to clinical practice guidelines has proved an effective approach to mobilize practitioners to deliver uniform, standard protocols, independent of financial incentives to do so. Further, adherence to guidelines, protocols, and standards can obviate the need for some utilization management activity. Effective, stipulated preadmission communication between physicians, patients, and families creates realistic expectations about the length of stay as well as the need for and nature of postdischarge care.

Congruent expectations about the projected length, course, and location of treatment—inpatient, outpatient, or home care—contribute to higher levels of patient satisfaction. Further, protocols focusing on preadmission and admission assist to identify administrative problems with operations, process, and outcomes (e.g., scheduling delays, telephone response times, protracted days to complete requisite services as opposed to consolidating services into the minimum number of days required).

To jump start the plan's efforts to implement the *M&R Healthcare Management Guidelines*™, M&R provided onsite training to motivate and empower as many plan personnel involved in utilization management as possible. The training emphasized judicious, appropriate use of diagnostic tests, particularly medical imaging services, since imaging procedures constitute a substantial medical expense. It reviewed primary care guidelines for the management of 17 classes of medical and surgical disorders and concluded with a discussion of observation and treatment in rapid treatment units.

Preintervention health outcomes data were compared with postintervention data to measure the effect of adherence with M&R guidelines. Data collection focused on the following aspects of care:

1. **Length of stay (LOS) and cost.** Preprocedure and postprocedure LOS were compared to M&R guidelines. Special emphasis was placed on examination of "units" of high-cost expenditures such as intensive care unit and ventilator patient days.
2. **Patient satisfaction.** Preintervention data primarily consisted of reports of patient satisfaction with care received. For postintervention data collection, an instrument inquiring about perceived problems with care was custom designed.
3. **Health status.** In addition to Medical Outcomes Study Short Form data routinely collected on inpatients as a component of the nursing health history, postprocedure health status data were solicited via questionnaire.
4. **Functional impairment and disease-specific outcomes.** Functional outcomes, such as the Specific Activities Scale (SAS) and New York Heart Association Class data, were complemented by baseline and follow-up collection of diagnosis-specific functional status data.
5. **Diagnosis-specific clinical indicators.** Selected surgical procedures required data collection for key clinical indicators (e.g., type of anesthesia administered, postoperative ventilator use) with the potential to affect outcomes and LOS.

Hospital information systems were used to determine readmission rates for related medical problems at 30, 60, and 180 days postdischarge; the presence of comorbid illnesses; and selected patient sociodemographic information including insurance status and relationship to a primary care provider. Extended care facility days were tracked to accurately attribute true cost savings from reduced LOS as opposed to cost shifts related to increased extended care facility utilization.

Finally, a provider satisfaction measure was developed for administration both before and after the intervention. This pre- and post-test measure assisted M&R in gauging the effect of the intervention on provider perceptions of the impact of optimized lengths of stay.

Consistent with M&R's previous experience with MCOs, large and small, preliminary results of this intervention were decidedly positive. The client MCO gained a clear understanding of the impact of health care management on financial performance, significantly reduced inpatient LOS, secured consensus and enthusiastic support for intensified health care management from providers, and reported favorable patient satisfaction trends.

While many MCOs can and do achieve resoundingly good short-term results from adherence to the *M&R Healthcare Management Guidelines*™, the challenge is to sustain and improve upon these results. If implementation and adherence to guidelines are viewed as a "project" or short-term initiative, then the multiple objectives of effective utilization management will not be fully realized.

Over time, diminishing or absent support for prudent utilization management and ongoing provider participation in implementation (i.e., "ownership" of the process of reviewing, refining, and adapting guidelines in response to changes in local health care delivery, patient mix, or reimbursement) certainly will compromise results. Without the requisite organizationwide commitment to sweeping changes in corporate culture—attitudes and behaviors—clinicians and administrators likely will revert to traditional practice patterns, thwarting the MCO's future ability to succeed in the cost-restrictive medical care marketplace.

Taken together, outcome measurement and adherence to widely accepted protocols and algorithms enable MCOs to effectively satisfy the requirements of the Health Plan Employer Data and Information Set (HEDIS) and respond to requests for data to generate provider-specific profiles and "report cards." Implementing practice guidelines and monitoring variance from these accepted appropriateness criteria not only address external requirements for accountability but also lay the groundwork for improving health care quality.

M&R has been gratified to observe swift and unified physician response to clinical performance issues when in-service education, administrative support, and resources to institute interventions are accessible to support and sustain collaborative quality improvement programs. In-service education has proved effective for speeding acceptance and integration of critical pathways, administrative protocols, and practice guidelines. It may be used to rapidly alter specific clinical practices such as routine utilization of diagnostic tests, prescribing patterns, and referral to home health care and has been applied successfully to reduce inpatient length of stay for selected admitting diagnoses.

The marketing ramifications and short-term consequences of disseminating quality measurement and improvement information provide immediate and tangible positive reinforcement for these efforts. When reports to employer groups and accrediting organizations clearly convey MCO accountability and capacity to effectively address problems, plans and their participating physicians have realized significant increases in market share and penetration.

COMMUNICATING QUALITY TO CREATE OPPORTUNITY

Plans able to demonstrate and communicate quality have experienced overall growth in membership, access to previously "untapped" employer groups and health care coalitions, and enhanced employer support and endorsement. Managed care organizations will continue to demonstrate quality to employers, providers, consumers, and accrediting entities by offering data to substantiate claims of clinical proficiency, patient satisfaction, and cost-efficiency.

Published results of internal quality assessment programs, such as annual member satisfaction surveys as well as the results of consumer surveys and independent quality audits, have been used by MCOs to communicate quality and gain recognition and acceptance among employers and consumers. One example of a corporate expression of support in response to such efforts is the business decision to offer employees financial incentives to enroll in the managed care plan demonstrating superior performance.

Moreover, maintaining and communicating quantifiable improvements in delivery management, health outcomes, and financial performance will be insufficient for MCOs intent on remaining competitive in a marketplace demanding ever-improving results. The most successful MCOs not only will be flexible and responsive, quickly and easily responding to changing clinical treatment protocols, but also accurately will project utilization and the effective use of financial resources to design new programs and services and amend health care benefits.

MANAGING QUALITY TO MINIMIZE RISK

The integration of actuarial, medical, and management sciences also has generated reliable methods for pricing and for the use of quality measures to define and modify medical benefits and health care services. This integrated approach aids MCOs and health care providers in evaluating risk assumption.

For example, a plan or provider group may wish to determine whether a proposed reimbursement arrangement is feasible or want to assess the financial consequences of deviating from risk-neutral reimbursement. Equipped with the results of this research, MCOs and provider networks can confidently decide to undertake or eschew greater levels of risk.

M&R health care consultants, in particular actuarial consultants, have applied risk-assessment techniques to help MCOs and provider groups answer urgent questions such as: Can M&R meet the financial challenges of managed care and remain profitable? Can M&R provide quality health care at a competitive price? Is M&R prepared for capitation and relationships requiring full or partial risk assumption?

Today, there are two interrelated questions about research methods plaguing MCOs. The first concerns a reliable methodology for ascertaining true costs in order to create and institute equitable capitation agreements. The second challenge is how to determine the appropriateness of existing or proposed per diem, case or fixed, monthly per capita rates.

CASE STUDY: FEASIBILITY OF CAPITATED SERVICE AGREEMENTS

A recent engagement with a preeminent teaching hospital illustrates the development of utilization and actuarial cost models to serve as the foundation for capitated service agreements. Radiology, emergency medicine, and oncology services were identified and selected as the first areas to benefit from this systematic evaluation.

The project entailed determination of average charges, projection of utilization, and resulting per member per month claim costs for professional radiology services. Included were projections for loosely managed and well-managed delivery systems for both commercial and Medicare populations, geographically adjusted to mirror the local medical service area. For purposes of comparison, geographic adjustments for several other metropolitan areas relative to the nationwide average also were prepared.

Four actuarial cost models for professional radiology services were created. The models constructed and contrasted unmanaged and optimally managed care for commercial and Medicare populations. The design process relied on actuarial analysis and clinical assessment of information from two major proprietary databases, the *M&R Health Cost Guidelines*™ and *Healthcare Management Guidelines*™. It also utilized other information from data sources developed and maintained within individual M&R consulting practices.

Utilization and charge assumptions were presented by CPT-4 code for professional-only services and combined professional and technical services. Professional-only services are those delivered to inpatients or outpatients and billed separately from the technical component, independent of the setting in which services are provided. Combined services are generated when radiology services are performed in an office, clinic, or other nonhospital, ambulatory setting and reflect billing for both professional and technical components.

Relative value units per service were presented using the McGraw-Hill relative value scale for the commercial population and Resource Based Relative Value Scale (RBRVS) units for the Medicare population. To facilitate comparisons of the impact systematic health care management can and should have on utilization and cost, the CPT codes were grouped and presented with accurate projections of annual utilization per 1,000, average McGraw-Hill units or average RBRVS units, conversion factor, average cost per service, and per capita monthly claim cost.

This project not only provided the hospital with the requisite data to make the informed business decision to capitate services but also with a process for physician involvement in capitation feasibility studies. Together with the client organization M&R established a Capitation Liaison Committee composed of clinical and administrative leaders to ensure comprehensive understanding of the opportunities afforded by capitation and implementation of capitated agreements consistent with the organization's mission, goals, and objectives.

During regularly scheduled meetings of the liaison committee, the essential elements of successful capitation were enumerated and discussed. M&R conferred about key issues including:

1. the responsibilities of financial partners;
2. equitable, fair, and fiscally responsible capitation rates and protocols;
3. the importance of ongoing communication and sharing information about utilization, cost, and premiums;
4. methods for simultaneously managing utilization and enhancing patient satisfaction;
5. education and incentivization of primary care and specialty physicians;
6. obstacles to implementation and known risks; and
7. the role and responsibilities of the liaison committee.

Collaborative Quality Improvement Training

Throughout the feasibility and implementation phases of the capitation development project, M&R designed and gained consensus for algorithms for patient referral and utilization review. M&R also planned continuing education programs to reinforce initial training. Along with tangible deliverables—data-based, equitable, and appropriate capitation rates and pilot protocols for implementation—M&R's intent was to teach the client organization an effective, collaborative process for identifying and addressing clinical and administrative issues and problems.

In a myriad of managed care settings, onsite, intensive training has proved to be a powerful intervention to enhance quality in terms of process and outcomes. The relevant literature and consulting projects with client MCOs demonstrate that training to address problems ranging from formulary use and adherence to practice guidelines to member and provider satisfaction does yield rapid, statistically significant results. While many MCOs have endeavored to introduce quality improvement initiatives such as the use of practice guidelines and critical pathways without organizationwide orientation and training, M&R's experience emphatically confirms the importance of initial, ongoing, collaborative, and continuing medical and administrative in-service education.

The risks associated with launching clinical quality initiatives with incomplete understanding and education are greater than simply unsuccessful or failed quality improvement measures. M&R has observed more than simply physician failure to adhere to practice guidelines and administrators "shelving" notebooks filled with guidelines. The greatest risks are those to relationships—the alliances between MCO administration and participating physicians and the relationships between participating physicians and their patients.

In more than one MCO, the distribution of practice guidelines without adequate training and discussion is assessed by physicians as "relatively unimportant." Physicians in these MCOs perceive protocols and practice guidelines as merely "more paper from the bean counters" and irrelevant to the frontline, professional practice of managed care medicine.

The most disgruntled practitioners are those who do not understand the rationale or impetus for the implementation of this quality improvement intervention. They have scornfully suggested that the guidelines represent "yet another onerous instance of nonphysicians overstepping their bounds to interfere with referral relationships between primary care and specialty physicians and physician-patient relationships."

By far the worst consequence of mandated adherence to guidelines without the prerequisite training is the manner in which some physicians have misrepresented the intent of the guidelines to patients. M&R has heard accounts of physicians using guidelines (and indirectly, the MCO administrators responsible for ensuring compliance with the guidelines and utilization management) as the scapegoats for a variety of patient satisfaction problems ranging from shorter-than-anticipated lengths of stay and delayed access to specialists to the prescription of generic as opposed to brand-name pharmaceuticals.

There is no question that failure to effectively communicate with clinical leaders and participating physicians can sabotage even the most circumspect quality improvement program. Unilateral administrative decisions to alter relationships and referral practices between physicians often are perceived as groundless or punitive by physicians. Such perceptions may act to exacerbate antipathy between clinicians and administrators. Such antagonism erodes the trust and unity of purpose between clinicians and administrators essential for quality management and performance improvement.

M&R's experience with training designed to catalyze attitudinal and practice pattern changes has been extraordinarily successful. The organization has discovered that the majority of physicians are enthused about receiving information about the practices and interventions that optimize outcomes. Enlightened about the necessity and utility as well as the fiscal and clinical propriety of health care management principles, they will embrace and champion the guidelines and protocols that support informed clinical decisionmaking and improved patient care.

An unanticipated benefit of collaborative quality improvement training for several MCO clients has been the cultivation of a physician's ability to establish goals and quantifiable objectives for selected groups (e.g., medical and surgical specialty groups, interdisciplinary utilization management, and quality improvement committees) as opposed to focusing exclusively on individual efforts. Since nearly all performance measurement and quality improvement interventions require cooperation and support from allied health professionals, administrators, and MCO enrollees, the fundamental value of the capacity for teamwork should not be underestimated.

The character, tone, and extent of the training provided vary in response to the goals and objectives of each MCO embarking on or intending to intensify quality measurement and health care management activities. Nonetheless, every individual involved in quality management must be acquainted with cardinal historical information, national trend data, and local market challenges as well as organization-specific utilization and cost data, goals, and measurable objectives.

EMPOWERING PROVIDERS TO EMBRACE QUALITY AS A CORE VALUE

Orientation to the medical marketplace begins with an examination of total national health expenditures, comparison of health care costs (i.e., the relationship between health insurance premiums, medical inflation, workers' earnings, and overall inflation), and physician-controlled health care expenditures. It considers sources of reimbursement for medical care, demographic analysis of health plan enrollment, and trends in HMO enrollment. Also presented are industrywide and plan-specific estimates of wasteful and unnecessary services performed and the prevalence of selected health care management practices including utilization of practice guidelines, outcome analysis, preventative services, and efficient formularies.

Physicians and others participating in the training are introduced to the key factors determining MCO viability and competitive position in the health care marketplace—quality, cost effectiveness, accountability, prevention, and patient satisfaction. The design and rationale for integrated delivery systems, capitation, outcome assessment, and economic credentialing prepare participants for the paradigm shift from the current delivery system directed to "manage sickness" to one intended to "manage health."

The current model is characterized by its emphasis on episodic care; scrutiny and improvement of individual provider performance; clinical efficacy at the time of intervention; and micromanagement of utilization and related health care decisions. The acute care hospital is at the center of this effort to manage sickness.

In contrast, the rapidly maturing managed health paradigm considers the primary care center as the locus of service delivery. It identifies other outpatient settings, including the patient's home, as ideal for an increasing number of preventive, restorative, and rehabilitation services.

Focusing on population health status as opposed to individual health status, participants in this model are given the incentive to optimize system performance, enhance prevention measures, and improve clinical efficacy. Driven by providers, this effort requires self-management based on shared values, unity of purpose, and adherence to administrative and clinical utilization management protocols.

Utilization management is defined as the deployment of treatment guidelines, critical pathways, and protocols to monitor and improve the overall health status of the MCO patient population. The goal of utilization management is to provide timely, appropriate, cost-effective care to each individual without provision of duplicative or unnecessary services.

THE PIVOTAL ROLE OF PHYSICIANS IN QUALITY MANAGEMENT

The new paradigm assigns primary care physicians an increasingly important role in health care management. It anticipates that they will manage between 80 and 85 percent of all presenting medical problems, frequently handling multiple problems concomitantly. Serving as gatekeepers and case managers, they wisely must select and provide medical services consistent with patients' needs and preferences. The success of quality management programs hinges on the capacity of primary care physicians to perform well in this new role.

Primary care physicians are responsible for evaluation, appropriate referral, and authorization of access to specialists, emergency medical services, diagnostic tests, and procedures. They also must engage support of professionals to coordinate services such as case management and the provision of home health care.

Moreover, primary care physicians can and should be empowered to act as ambassadors for the plan and its quality improvement initiatives. They must communicate quality to consumers to generate the congruent expectations, clinical outcomes, and physician-patient relationships that contribute strongly to patient satisfaction.

Until primary care practitioners are trained to perform these new responsibilities, it appears unjust to evaluate their performance in these areas. Early-provider profiling efforts focused on physician specialists, particularly the surgical subspecialists who perform costly procedures. While use and dissemination of crude, unadjusted measures of procedure-related morbidity and mortality were, and continue to be, challenged by physicians and other industry observers, at least these comparisons purported to measure competencies expected of specialty physicians.

Unlike their specialist colleagues, who have not yet been assigned substantial case management responsibilities, gatekeeper physicians must rely heavily on both MCO resources (e.g., systems, personnel, facilities) and capacity to offer timely access to a comprehensive array of treatment options and service delivery settings. For example, in the absence of available alternatives to acute, inpatient hospitalization services primary care physicians can not be expected to excel in case management.

Despite this obvious inequity, there is evidence that increasingly sophisticated provider profiling, which has gained acceptance among payers as a credible measure of physician performance, will include evaluation of the primary care physician's ability to perform gatekeeper and case management functions. This reality underscores the paramount importance of training to support all clinicians, especially primary care physicians, to participate fully and earnestly in the development and implementation of the efficient case management practices and clinical protocols correlated with quality.

PHYSICIAN EDUCATION: A POWERFUL INTERVENTION TO IMPROVE QUALITY

Along with intensive, onsite training, the most progressive MCOs have instituted a variety of innovative communication and in-service education programs to introduce and reinforce practices aimed at addressing and resolving perceived and detected quality concerns. Physician peer counseling, workshops engaging participants in role-play, videotaped physician-patient encounters, and newsletters to familiarize clinicians with aspects of MCO performance measurement and quality improvement activities have met with differing degrees of success.

Prior to assuming the position of senior health care consultant with Milliman & Robertson, this author served as associate medical director of one of the largest HMOs in the Western United States. In this capacity, the opportunity was seized to launch one such novel physician education initiative aimed at improving quality as measured by physician and patient satisfaction.

Case Study: Physician Education

The educational program sought to enhance physician-patient communication and relationships—in view of the direct association between physician-patient communication and MCO member satisfaction, compliance with treatment, and, consequently, clinical outcomes. The specific, quantifiable objectives of the program included:

- Enhancing patient adherence to prescribed treatment regimens to improve clinical outcomes;
- Preventing unnecessary, wasteful utilization by optimizing patient satisfaction with initial encounters;
- Decreasing reported rates of disenrollment attributable to dissatisfaction with the quality of physician-patient communication and relationships; and
- Improving physician satisfaction and preventing physician burnout.

Dubbed "Curbside Consultations"— in deference to the informal consults physicians traditionally trade in hospital corridors, parking lots, and cafeterias—the monthly, interactive direct mail program consisted of a pithy summary of a physician-patient interaction and recommended communication techniques for improving patient and physician satisfaction with the encounter. It was mailed to more than 13,000 primary care and physician specialists representing approximately 200 medical groups and independent practice associations contracted to participate in the MCO.[1]

Each issue depicted a common scenario or response to a frequently asked question, such as a patient frustrated by seemingly endless, administrative delays and problems and a patient demanding duplicative or unnecessary diagnostic testing. Strategies even were devised for handling the patient presenting with a list of problems too long to be read, let alone addressed, in a single office visit.

"Curbside Consultations" copy, punctuated by an amusing, single-panel cartoon, was designed to be readable, informative, and entertaining. Every issue contained a tear-off response card to encourage physician readers to commend, dispute, or offer feasible alternatives to the suggested approach.The piece also invited readers to contribute "patient-pleasing pointers"—their own field-tested approaches for improving physician-patient relationships.

The volume of responses from physician-readers was greater than expected. Direct mail marketers consider any response rate in excess of 0.5 percent to be excellent. The average response rate for "Curbside Consultations" was 1.2 percent. In comparison, the quarterly physician newsletter, distributed in the same manner during the same period, rarely evoked a response. The volume and quality of replies to "Curbside Consultations" provided ample evidence of the program's ability to reach its intended audience.

Readership of "Curbside Consultations," far more difficult to estimate, was believed to be substantially greater than the response rate. Shortly after the program was instituted, authors began to receive unrelated reports of "Curbside Consultations" gracing the walls of medical staff dining rooms along with tales of their use as springboards for discussion of MCO-specific patient satisfaction problems. A handful of responses from physicians outside of the client MCO (physicians who were not on the MCO mailing list) indicated that in at least a few instances, physicians were sharing "Curbside Consultations" with colleagues in other practice settings.

Hundreds of physicians wrote to express support for the intent of "Curbside Consultations." Respondents hailed the case presentations as "plausible" and "true-to-practice." They characterized the recommended approaches as "intelligent," "appropriate," and "workable." Primary care and specialty physicians offered a plethora of suggestions for enhancing patient satisfaction with encounters and requested specific topics for inclusion in future issues.

The overwhelmingly favorable response to this education initiative demonstrated physician receptivity, both to the vehicle—the interactive direct mail format—and its content. Physician readership, receptivity, and enthusiasm consistently increased throughout the life of the program. When it concluded, authors received pleas for its continuation from physicians who believed it had significantly enhanced their abilities to communicate with patients about a range of clinical and MCO-specific issues.

Many respondents credited the utility and relevance of the program to the extensive clinical and administrative practice experience of the author and timely, personal responses to inquiries. The broad appeal and unanticipated success of this format subsequently inspired contemplation of other uses of personal, interactive communication with physicians. It was hypothesized that this vehicle would be equally effective as a communication strategy for introduction and reinforcement of other programs and practices to improve quality.

Recent advances in telecommunications and increasing physician reliance on hospital and office-based computerized management information systems offer new and additional venues for the dissemination and discussion of data and practices related to improving process and outcomes of health care delivery. Today, besides interoffice and postal mail service, physicians regularly receive information through fax transmission and interorganizational voice and electronic mail.

The information superhighway allows physicians access to a variety of medical databases and forums where they can share medical practice experience with colleagues who vary in terms of specialty, location, practice setting, and managed care affiliation. Web sites, university libraries, and discussion groups offer perspectives on public health issues and clinical, continuing medical education in areas ranging from adolescent medicine and infectious diseases to geriatric medicine and long term care.

Despite expanded access to data afforded by advanced electronic information transfer, many physicians continue to suffer and decry the absence of mentors—colleagues, particularly physicians external to their organizations—for immediate council, guidance, and instruction about how to perform health care management responsibilities. As this volume goes to press, plans are under way to offer this kind of advice, education, and support to physicians and MCO administrators on-line, in an interactive format reminiscent of the "Curbside Consultations" direct mail program.

Available at the Milliman & Robertson Web site (www2.milliman.com/milliman), on-line "Curbside Consultations" no longer will be exclusively devoted to the program's previous subject matter—training to enhance physician-patient communication and relationships. The upgraded "Curbside Consultations" will endeavor to provide instruction about the use of health management guidelines, protocols, and clinical pathways as well as performance measurement and quality improvement.

If, as cyberspace pundits predict, the global medical village grows to become a sizable virtual city, then this M&R Web site will be the venue—a "town hall"—for showcasing novel and effective quality improvement programs, airing problems, and engaging in collaborative problem solving. On-line "Curbside Consultations" will facilitate the dialogue between mentor physicians and their less learned colleagues, enabling them to share issues of industrywide importance. They will support changes in MCO corporate culture to improve service quality and reinforce the efforts of individual clinicians and administrators.

Finally, most managed care plans and provider groups seeking to intensify quality measurement and improvement efforts subscribe to the premise that attitudes must change before practices can be amended. M&R's experience confirms the importance of attitude in promoting changes in clinical practice patterns. M&R contends, however, that to improve clinical quality it is preferable to change behaviors—train clinicians and administrators to achieve the desired results of health care management—first.

While understanding and involvement are prerequisites for behavior change, there is mounting evidence that attitudes change in response to favorable experience. Empower providers to achieve measurable improvements in the quality of care first and new philosophies, perspectives, values, and relationships will follow.

Attainment of competence and skills to effectively manage health care organically catalyzes changes in the attitudes of individuals and shifts in corporate culture, resolving many obstacles to productive relationships between clinicians, administrators, and health care consumers. Health care providers proficient in monitoring, identifying, and swiftly intervening to solve problems understand that optimizing quality and cost effectiveness is an unending process.

Change is a constant in the definition and refinement of quality benchmarks. Driven to higher levels of performance, quality-driven organizations will define, establish, communicate, and then promptly exceed industry standards.

REFERENCE

1. Spong FW. "Curbside Consultations: A Novel Vehicle For Physician Education." *HMO Practice*. September 1994; Volume 8, Number 1.

Chapter 14

Ernst & Young LLP

Transforming Quality Measures Into Value

David Plocher, MD, and Linda Davis, RN

Ernst & Young is an international professional services firm with over 10,000 consultants, of which more than 1,000 are devoted to health care. E&Y's customers include providers, integrated delivery systems, payers, suppliers, and manufacturers. This chapter will comment on the models of quality proposed earlier in this book, describe the efforts of E&Y's customers to improve value through quality measurement, and conclude with E&Y's view of the future of quality measurement and value improvement, including its challenges and opportunities.

Ernst & Young serves a variety of industries, including manufacturing, retail, information technology, communications, and health care. A "fused" approach, integrating performance improvement, information technology, culture, and industry knowledge, is required to transform quality measures into value. While measuring quality in health care has lagged behind other industries, managed care has provided the structure, process, and outcome measures not present in a fee-for-service environment to measure quality and improve value. Ernst &Young recently has established a National Managed Care Group, comprised of experts from the disciplines mentioned above and from the managed care industry, to integrate established methodologies from other industries with health care methodologies and improve quality measures and value for its customers.

RESPONSE TO PROPOSED MODELS OF QUALITY

The first section of this book describes formal models for measuring quality in managed care. These models include measures from traditional approaches of quality assurance for hospitals as well as patient-centered outcomes from the Foundation for Accountability (FACCT) and the Medical Outcomes Trust.

Today's market does not reward providers or health plans for quality measures and value improvement. Despite all the rhetoric regarding quality, incentives in place today continue to reward lower costs. E&Y is just beginning to see employers use National Committee for Quality Assurance (NCQA) accreditation as a criterion for selecting health plans. The *Health Care Forum* article, "Managed Care Comes of Age" by Jeff C. Goldsmith, PhD, of Health Futures, Inc. and two Ernst & Young national directors, Michael J. Goran, MD, and John G. Nackel, describes national trends and the evolution of managed care. They state that "as markets mature, managed care plans will increasingly be forced to actually *manage care*." Actually, managing care is described as controlling resource intensity, improving delivery processes, and increasing consumer satisfaction through clinical pathways, outcome monitoring, and TQM/CQI mechanisms, all of which improve value. Their article summarizes how managed care, now in its adolescence, is beginning to mature and will shift from a cost-driven system to one that actually manages care, improves value, and eventually improves health.

Table 1.

Managed Care: Stages of Evolution

	Stage I Event Driven Cost Avoidance	**Stage II** Value Improvement	**Stage III** Health Improvement
Objective Function	Price	Value/customer satisfaction	Health status improvement
Cost Targets	Inpatient days	Resource intensity	Health risks
Locus of Control	External	Peer-driven	"Contract" with family
Focal Point	Inpatient hospital	Physician driven	Home/ neighborhood

The quality models proposed earlier in this book represent evidence that managed care is evolving from Stage I (cost avoidance) to Stage II (value improvement) (see Table 1). Efforts to establish common measures, collect data on agreed-upon indicators, and ultimately improve value are characteristic of Stage

II. The Joint Commission on Accreditation of Healthcare Organizations (JCAHO), the American Medical Association (AMA), and the Health Plan Employer Data and Information Set (HEDIS) reflect Stages I and II by measuring the structure and process of care. Models that measure member- or patient-centered indicators, such as the Medical Outcomes Trust and the Foundation for Accountability, indicate movement into Stage III—health improvement. These diverse models of quality measurement indicate that consensus regarding model of measurement does not exist among the managed care industry, employers, providers, and consumers, but the industry is evolving to Stages II and III. The managed care industry will catch up to other industries when selected indicators are routinely measured and widely known, such as an airline's on-time arrival score or the safety records of automobiles.

While these three stages describe the general shift in focus of managed care at a high level, health care remains locally driven in many aspects. National initiatives related to quality standards, structures, and processes are emerging in health care. However, local forces such as provider supply and purchaser activity continue to determine whether value improvement initiatives make the priority list for local health plans and what form they will take.

The shift to quality and value improvement is not a top priority for many Ernst & Young customers, due to the lack of local market forces. Ernst & Young has developed a Spider Model to describe the complex multidimensional characteristics of local markets. The shift from cost avoidance to value improvement and health improvement varies from market to market, due to a variety of factors. Figure 1 illustrates a hypothetical market's scoring on each axis compared to a mature market.

Figure 1. Spider Model©

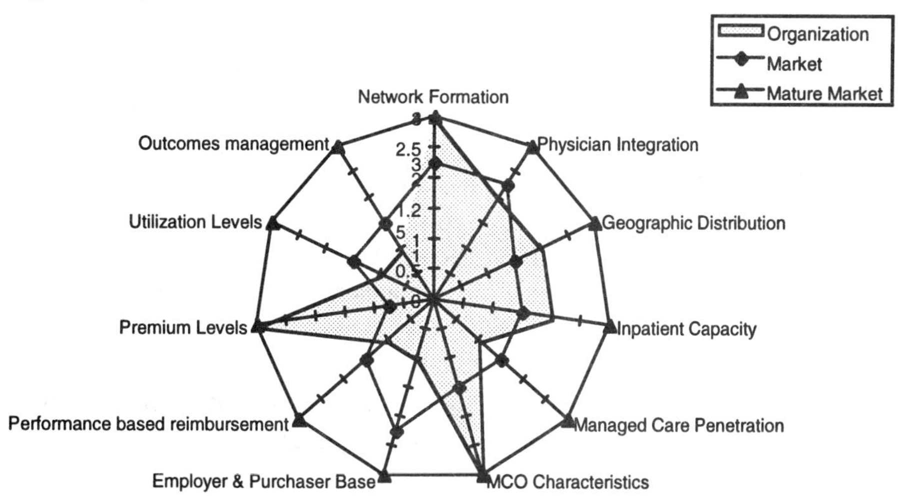

© Used with permission from Ernst & Young.

The "Outcomes Management" axis describes the level of sophistication in managing care and the focus on quality and value. As markets mature, there is increased attention to quality indicators, nonhospital-based utilization, the processes of care (clinical pathways, practice guidelines), and how to measure quality. The more mature markets add disease management to increase continuity across sites of care and demand management to increase patient involvement in their own care. The most mature markets focus on improving the health status of health plan members and the community as a whole. The spider model provides insight to E&Y's clients regarding how readily local purchasers and competitors will support or motivate a major investment in quality measurement and value improvement initiatives.

The models of national organizations described earlier, such as HEDIS, have accelerated each particular market's movement along the outcomes axis where previously no local force existed. Despite HEDIS' shortcomings, including the expense and difficulty in gathering data and the lack of consensus around whether it is measuring the right indicators, it has focused improvement activities on specific processes and measurement of common, consistently defined indicators, as well as provides comparative measures that would not have existed in many markets without a national initiative.

E&Y's responses to these models include the following observations:

- Individuals (principally physicians) and organizations will improve quality when incentives exist and there is consensus on what to measure, e.g., they are paid for it or they lose market share without it.
- Individuals and organizations should be held accountable for those factors over which they have control; in some cases collaboration between organizations is necessary, for example:
  1. Health plans have some, but limited, control over physicians' interpersonal style, which significantly affects member satisfaction. However, they can build incentives to improve service by rewarding physicians with bonuses for improved performance.
  2. Health plans and physicians have some, but limited, control over functional health status. Yet successful outcomes after surgery are directly related to the success of the surgery and may be measured with functional status tools because other conditions, such as chronic illness, socioeconomic status, educational level, marital status, ethnic origin, employment, and other environmental factors have a much greater impact.
- The cost of abstracting relevant medical data from written records is the single largest cost obstacle in quality measurement.
- Multiple stakeholders including health plans, providers, physicians, employers, and consumers must come to consensus around relevant measures.
  1. NCQA only recently formed a focus group of practitioners for input into HEDIS 3.0.

2. Consumers have not been polled routinely regarding what they value and its relative importance to what providers and health plans deem as quality.
3. Employers have departed from the HEDIS measures in their formation of FACCT in order to focus on patient-centered measures.

- Models and information systems must be built for flexibility; what they measure today will change with the increasingly frequent new discoveries in medical science.
- National initiatives such as HEDIS and FACCT will speed the evolution of local markets toward measuring quality.
- Local initiatives related to quality will have limited impact unless market forces are brought to bear and providers and health plans are rewarded for quality either in increased reimbursement or market share.

EXAMPLES OF VALUE IMPROVEMENT

In most cases, Ernst & Young's medical management consultants are called by customers to assist them in managing utilization rather than improving quality simply because health plans still are rewarded for lowering costs—not for improving quality. However, several of E&Y's more recent engagements have been related to improving quality, either because of national or local market pressures or in anticipation of future requirements. The following section will describe examples of engagements related to quality measurement and value improvement, including assessing care management capabilities, improving nonfatal complication rates, preparing for NCQA certification, building information systems capabilities including data warehouses to gather HEDIS and other measures, developing Centers of Excellence, developing risk-assessment tools, and measuring the impact of new programs including nurselines.

Assessing Care Management

The impact of overutilization on quality and value are tightly intertwined. A mathematical interpretation of value can be expressed as the following: (Value= (Benefit/Cost).

Additionally, the relationship is evident when a member suffers a complication while having an invasive procedure that is subsequently revealed to be unnecessary based on explicit evidence-based criteria. Another example is when a member is drawn into a maze of tests and procedures, all prompted by a false-positive screening test—the cascade effect—which also proves to be unnecessary.

Ernst & Young has received numerous requests over several years from health plans and integrated delivery and financing systems (IDFSs) to assess care man-

Figure 2. Interventions in Care Management©

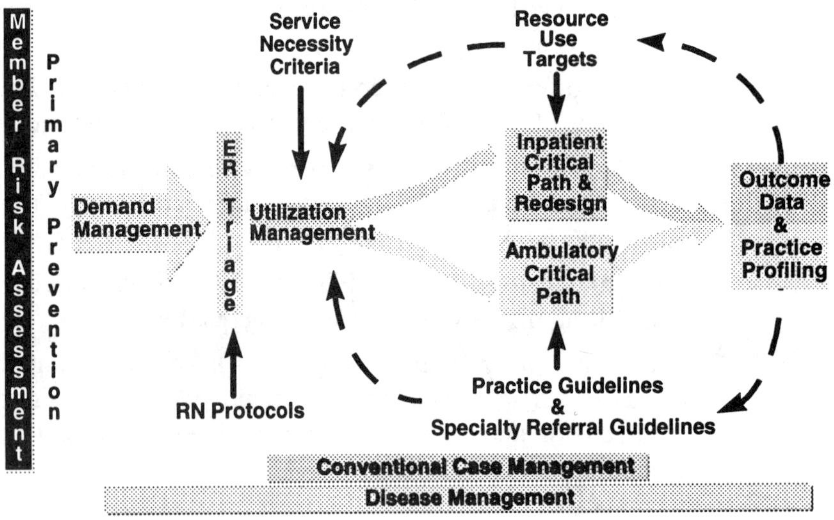

© Used with permission from Ernst & Young.

agement in order to better manage costs and utilization. E&Y has developed a methodology, the Care Management Assessment, to assist health plans in discovering macro and micro causes of excess utilization. More recently, E&Y has added emphasis on studying ambulatory sites, case management, and disease and demand management in addition to institutional utilization. Figure 2 illustrates E&Y's depiction of the relationship of care processes and interventions as well as the scope of review in the Care Management Assessment. Starting on the left side of the diagram with member risk assessment, interventions may range from primary prevention to outcomes analysis.

Figure 3. Interventions in Care Management©

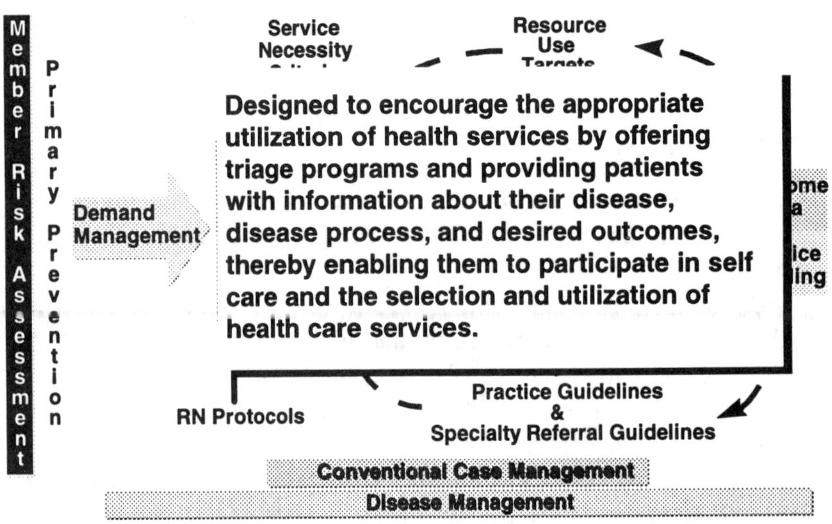

© Used with permission from Ernst & Young.

One of the lessons learned from this assessment is that practitioners, particularly physicians, have preferred learning methods. They do not appreciate lectures, time-consuming books, or laundry lists of terms. Therefore, E&Y created a self-teaching software program where the operator points and clicks on the item needing explanation, which then appears in hypertext with added narrative available if requested, as illustrated in Figure 3.

In this manner, E&Y provides knowledge transfer through tools and techniques in an instantly meaningful array to practitioners. In the words of one clinician in a West Coast HMO after reviewing the illustration: "the lights finally went on!"

E&Y's consulting role usually begins with this kind of knowledge transfer. The company then proceeds with the exploratory assessment process. Figure 4 summarizes the key steps.

Figure 4. E&Y's Care Management Assessment

Engagement Timetable: 8 Weeks

- **Preparation and Kick Off Meeting**
- **Data and Information Request**
- **Site Visit**
- **Information Evaluation and Analysis**
- **Review of Key Findings for Accuracy**
- **Value Propositions**
- **Portfolio Develpment**
- **Written Report**
- **Final Presentation**

The assessment concludes with an organized prioritized portfolio of improvement initiatives and value propositions that identify the benefits and costs of each initiative for the customer. A small excerpt of typical utilization findings compared to industry benchmarks follows in Figures 5-10. The findings come from a 100,000 member IPA-model HMO in the upper Midwest.

Figure 5. Echocardiograms/1,000

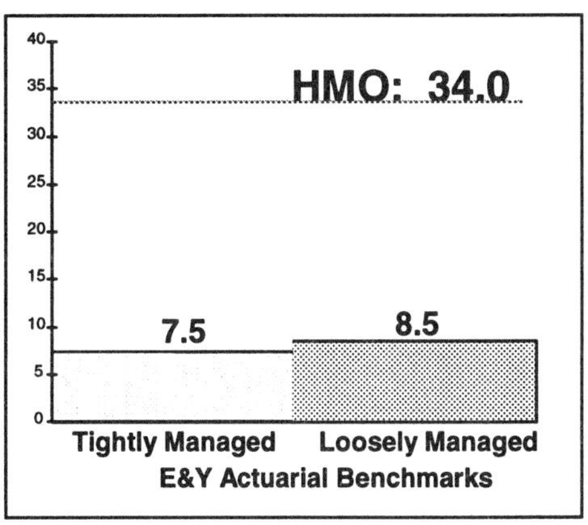

Figure 6. Holter Monitors/1,000

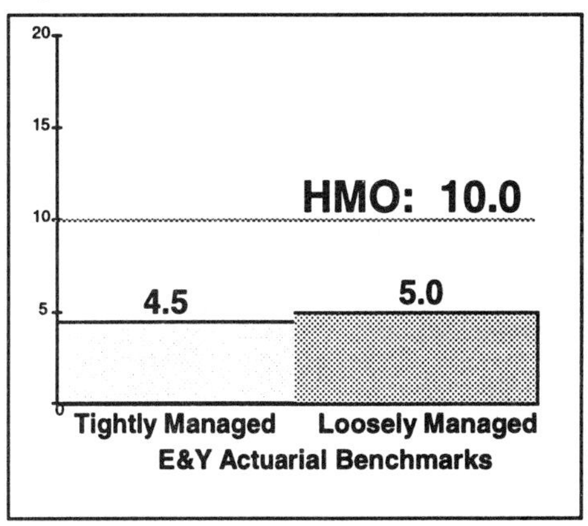

Figure 7. Exercise Tests/1,000

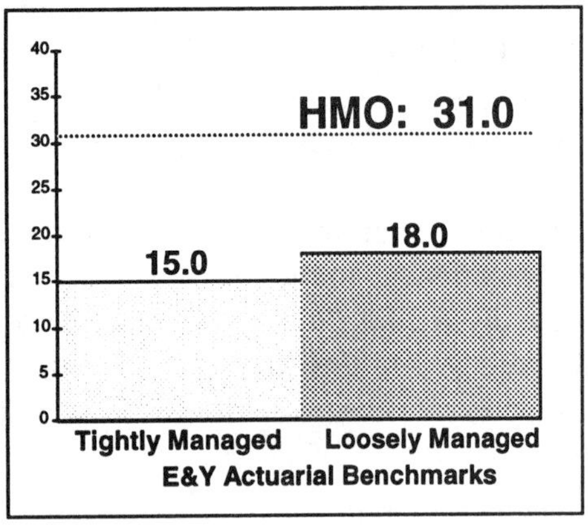

Figure 8. Gastroscopy/1,000

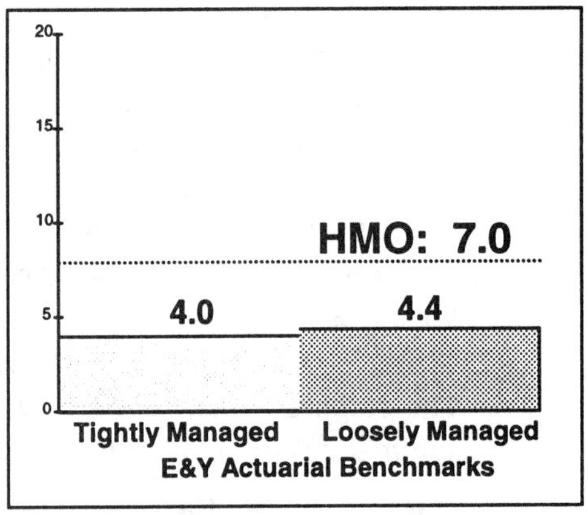

Figure 9. CT Scans/1,000

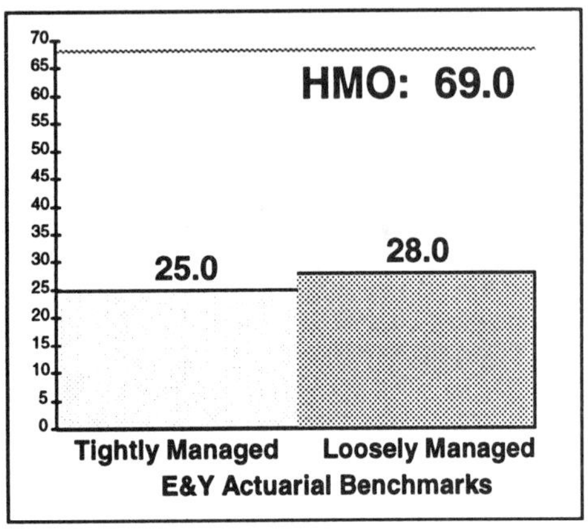

Figure10. MRIs/1,000

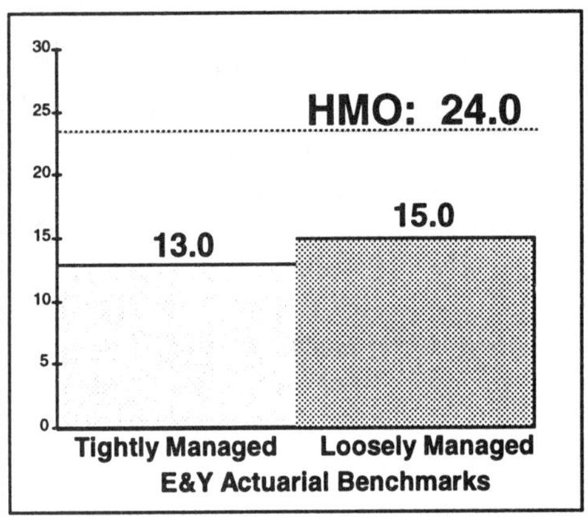

With diagnostic testing rates from 50 percent to almost 400 percent more than even loosely managed markets, the impact of variability and related quality issues is identified and quantified. These data and other information, including provider network configuration, the supply of providers, financial incentives, customer demands, among others help determine which care management tools and techniques will need enhancement. E&Y then projects an expected return on investment for this improvement and delivers an organized and balanced portfolio of projects along with implementation assistance including:

- Process redesign and reengineering;
- Information technology such as vendor selection and installation; and
- Culture change.

The pressure to reduce costs and utilization is not decreasing as markets evolve to value improvement; in fact, it is increasing. At the same time, market demands are adding quality measures such as HEDIS. The Care Management Assessment tool will continue to be important as managed care evolves.

Improving Nonfatal Complication Rates

Several years ago, E&Y advanced from the mainstream of mortality analysis to examination of nonfatal complications. This was based on E&Y's impressions as follows:

- Death may have little to do with the quality of care processes.
- Nonfatal complications are more likely than mortality to reflect on therapeutic misadventure.
- Death occurs too rarely to be useful in comparison studies—huge sample sizes are needed to achieve statistical power.
- Nonfatal complications occur with such frequency that practical sample sizes can be achieved.
- Nonfatal complications cost more than deaths as measured by resource consumption.

E&Y is not suggesting that mortality rates be ignored, but that examination of value and quality will have much greater impact on the overall quality of care if nonfatal complications are studied. However, E&Y is humbled by the difficulties posed by the need to severity-adjust nonfatal complication rate comparisons.

This is the context for one of E&Y's formal outcome studies in 1992. E&Y was asked to assist a prestigious academic medical center in the Midwest to solve the following puzzle for their coronary bypass program:

- High cost;
- Overhead not excessive;
- Low mortality; and
- Market share inroads by lower cost providers with similar mortality rates.

E&Y began performance measurement along several fronts. However, no national, registry-like cardiac database was in use by the customer. Therefore, the study required comparisons of large varieties of outcome data.

The company began with a routine study of charges, cost, length of stay, and mortality for coronary bypass surgery. E&Y used coded disease staging by SysteMetrics for severity adjustment. In a parallel study of Medicare patients only, E&Y corroborated this with adjustment using APR-DRGs.

However, as introductory remarks predicted, this routine analysis of mortality was not particularly illuminating and did not solve the client's problem.

E&Y next summarized the peer-reviewed literature to produce averages (potentially "benchmarks") of procedure-specific, nonfatal, complication rates. Where the better literature specified, E&Y risk-stratified the outcome data. Because E&Y could only compare ICD-9 codes from the customer's administrative dataset, not all of the possible risk-stratification schemes could be used. Unfortunately, validation with extensive medical record review was beyond the scope of the study.

Unfortunately, validation with extensive medical record review was beyond the scope of the study.

Figures 11 and 12 show comparison of nonfatal complications did offer a solution to the problem.

Figure 11. CABG—% Major Nonfatal Complications

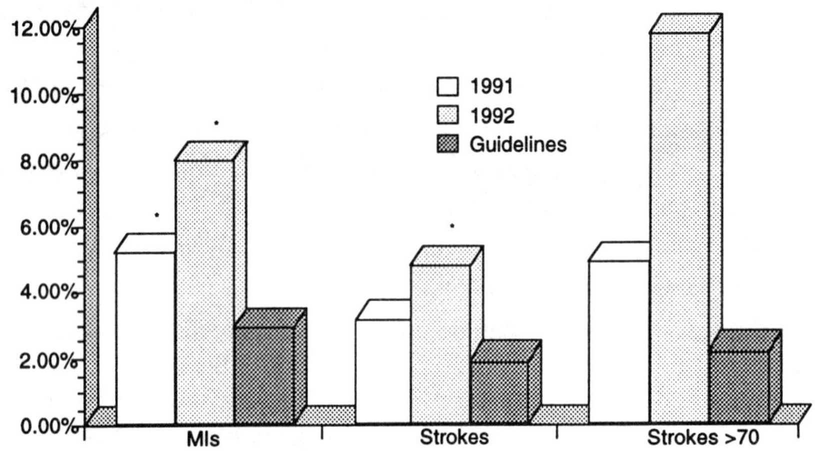

* Rate is significantly different from guideline rate - P < 0.05

Figure 12. CABG—% Minor Nonfatal Complications

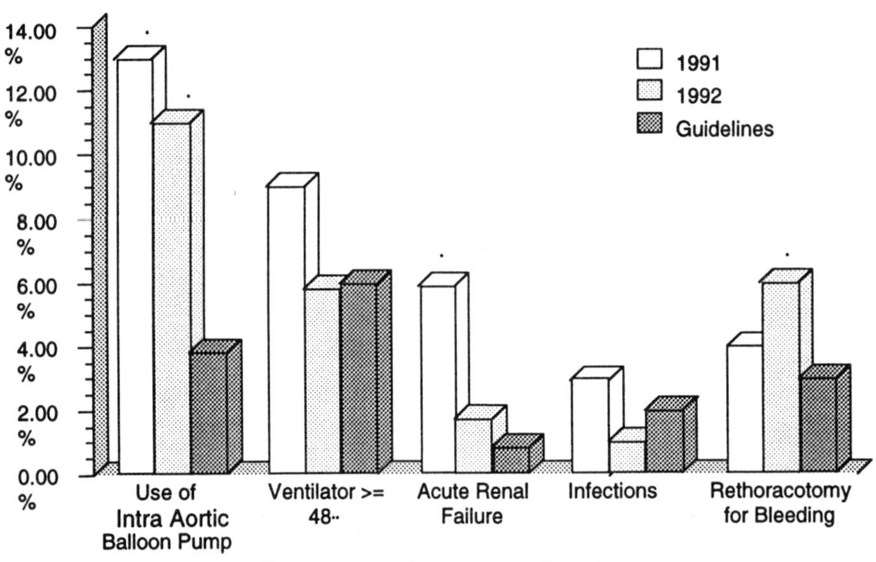

* Rate is significantly different from guideline rate - P<0.05

For years 1991 and 1992, E&Y compared key complication rates with literature-derived norms and included statistically meaningful comparisons. The risk stratification was limited to age (e.g., separating all postoperative strokes from strokes over age 70), excluding patients with prior bypass surgery, emergency bypass surgery, and catastrophic outlier cases.

The customer appreciated the insight into complication rates and cost drivers. For example, excessive returns to the operating room for a repeat thoracotomy due to a bleeder was a huge driver of resource use. The high stroke rate prompted reconsideration of patient selection criteria, as well as prophylactic measures. By this linkage of outcome to process, a complete quality improvement initiative was launched.

Developing Centers of Excellence

Ohio

The preceding discussion on performance measurement and improvement was taken to the next level by an East Coast customer—a large hospital. The setting was, one of the team members quipped, "a one hospital town that happens to have two hospitals." One of the largest payers in the region was not willing to support this excess capacity and began to demonstrate this point with the rationalization and regionalization of coronary bypass surgery in 1993.

E&Y was retained to assist this hospital in responding to a payer's request for proposal (RFP) for a Center of Excellence status. The client had not entered data into formats consistent with any of the national cardiac databases. Therefore, E&Y's role was to collect, organize, analyze, and display performance data for the response to the RFP. E&Y used risk stratification and severity-adjustment techniques similar to the preceding case. For example, in the case of coronary angioplasty, E&Y reduced possible indicators for measurement from the plethora of literature and data to three end-points:

- Acute MI,
- Emergency bypass surgery, and
- Death.

E&Y then risk stratified cases according to:

- Age,
- Gender,
- Emergency versus elective, and
- Number of vessels (with consideration for lesion type).

There was discussion about adding other risk stratifiers, such as diabetes and smoking status, but the argument for simplicity prevailed. The results of the outcome comparisons with the literature suggested that the customer received excellent quality services. Input from the customer suggested the costs were slightly higher than the local competitor.

The final step was to prepare the hospital for the payer site visit. Medical directors from the payer interviewed coauthor David W. Plocher, MD, on topics ranging from performance measurement techniques to data integrity. Several weeks later the customer was awarded the exclusive contract.

Unlike the depiction of Centers of Excellence in the media where cost reduction is the primary driver, E&Y's experience has included situations where careful consideration is given to all known factors affecting quality prior to contracting, including scientific review of risk-adjusted performance data for selected indicators of quality.

Minnesota

In the case of another customer, Blue Cross Blue Shield of Minnesota (BCBSM), quality was the primary driver in selecting providers for its cardiac network in 1993. Criteria included, among others:

- Minimum service volume (both hospital- and provider-specific) requirements for specific procedures (cardiac catheterization, EPS, angioplasty, CABG, valve replacement), which, according to research, are clearly related to the quality of processes and are reliable predictors of superior outcomes for invasive procedures.
- Performance of the physician group linked to a particular institution in order to consider the impact of the "system of care" rather than one part of the system separate from the others.
- Commitment of time, energy, and resources to CQI methods and sharing best practices, including reviewing data and even working with competitors in order to improve performance.

Selected cardiac network providers' performance was adjusted for severity using Medisgroups and was 14.7 deaths per 1,000 procedures compared to 52.6 deaths per 1,000 procedures for nonnetwork providers. Complications included an average of 29.4 heart attacks per 1,000 for network providers after cardiac bypass surgery, a rate far lower that the 105.3 per 1,000 rate among nonnetwork providers.

Global case rates were negotiated to align the incentives of multiple providers by including all costs in one price for a given DRG. In another arrangement, providers agreed to provide care for all complications for CABGs for one year after discharge, which served as an incentive to focus on preventing complications. Financial incentives as well as culture, care processes, and volume were evaluated and considered as drivers of behavior change. Initially, BCBS Minnesota improved value by selecting providers with superior outcomes and reducing costs by almost $15,000 per patient. Currently, efforts are under way to assess performance as the initial contract approaches its third year.

Developing Member Risk-Assessment Methods

Identification of members at risk for specific illness is of increasing interest to health plans, particularly where recent medical breakthroughs and treatments that improve outcomes and reduce costs have been documented in the literature. By more precisely identifying individual members who will benefit from these new treatments or interventions, educating the provider and member, and removing barriers or enabling these new processes of care through technology or other means, health plans significantly can improve value primarily for the member, but also for the purchaser and provider.

The first step is careful identification of the member. Health plans have routinely asked for advice on selecting the best health risk appraisal (HRA) or member risk-assessment tool and vendor (also known as illness risk appraisal, or IRA). E&Y has observed substantial variations in the ability of these tools to predict resource consumption in the near future as well as wide variation in their abilities to predict utilization with various populations and conditions. One instrument may show acceptable predictive validity for seniors, while a different instrument and approach are needed for commercial members. In fact, among commercial members, the high-risk young seem to be the least willing and least likely to cooperate with completing risk assessments. Furthermore, the conventional HRA focus on cardiovascular risk for events that aren't likely to occur for 10-20 years does not warrant the attention of the chief financial officer of an HMO struggling with a high medical loss ratio this year or next year.

As many other plans had learned, their conventional approach to large case management was not sufficiently effective in altering the course of an illness or substantially reducing resource consumption. By using classic case management trigger conditions, they were missing opportunities for value improvement because the catastrophe already had occurred. Arranging for a lower per diem rate or for transfer to home care a day or two sooner than hospital-based case managers had scheduled did not deliver the value demanded by the market or the customer. Managing care sooner and tailoring it to individual needs would deliver increased value to the member, customer, and the client.

It was against this background that E&Y was asked to assist HealthNet, a 1.2 million member HMO in southern California. As E&Y proceeded to design a new program to better identify members who would benefit from case management, E&Y was aware that much more was required than simply selecting an HRA vendor. E&Y needed to design multiple inputs allowing case managers to identify members in their homes or at any site who would soon consume large amounts of health care resources. Furthermore, the intent was to discover those circumstances that had a modifiable course. That is, the 80:20 rule is less useful when a case is already catastrophic and continues its course of resource consumption, unaffected by the case manager.

E&Y began by drawing process flow diagrams of all the possible avenues by which a high-risk member could be identified in the current state, and then brainstormed possible discovery steps in the future state. Nonclinical engineering scientists were key facilitators in this effort.

Another important distinction within the search was that a diagnosis code did not always serve as the most prospective and sensitive "radar." By the time a claim database revealed a worrisome ICD-9, E&Y believed some of the opportunity was lost. E&Y needed the kind of "radar" that searches for high-risk behavior that may not have a narrow, conclusive diagnosis code.

The next step was an analysis of the participating medical groups to determine where the program should be piloted. E&Y prioritized the effort by comparing utilization excesses and aimed for locations with the largest potential for improvement.

In Figures 13 and 14, E&Y outlines example components of this health plan's prospective member identification.

As the pilot is implemented, a tracking methodology will continuously measure the performance of medical groups involved.

Figure 13. Risk Assessment

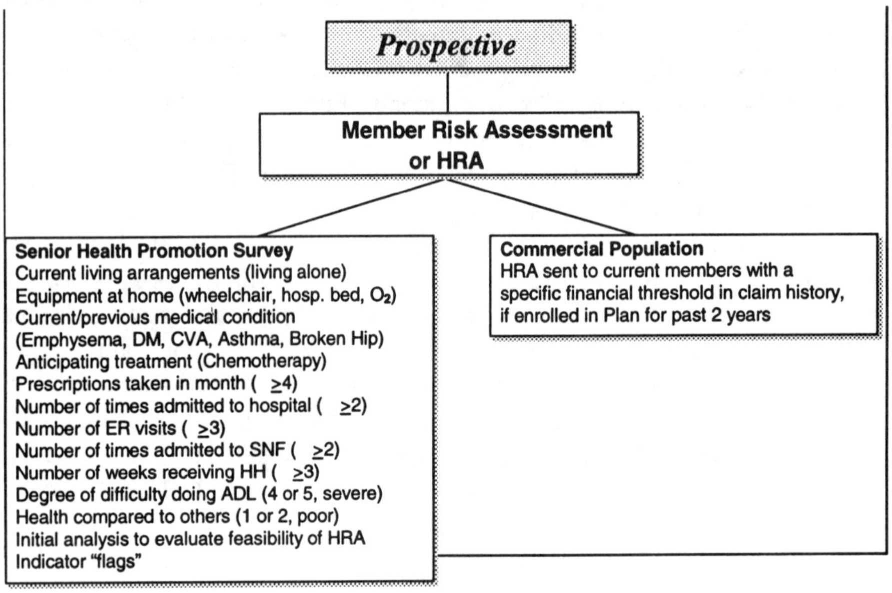

Figure 14. Prospective and Current Sources of Triggers

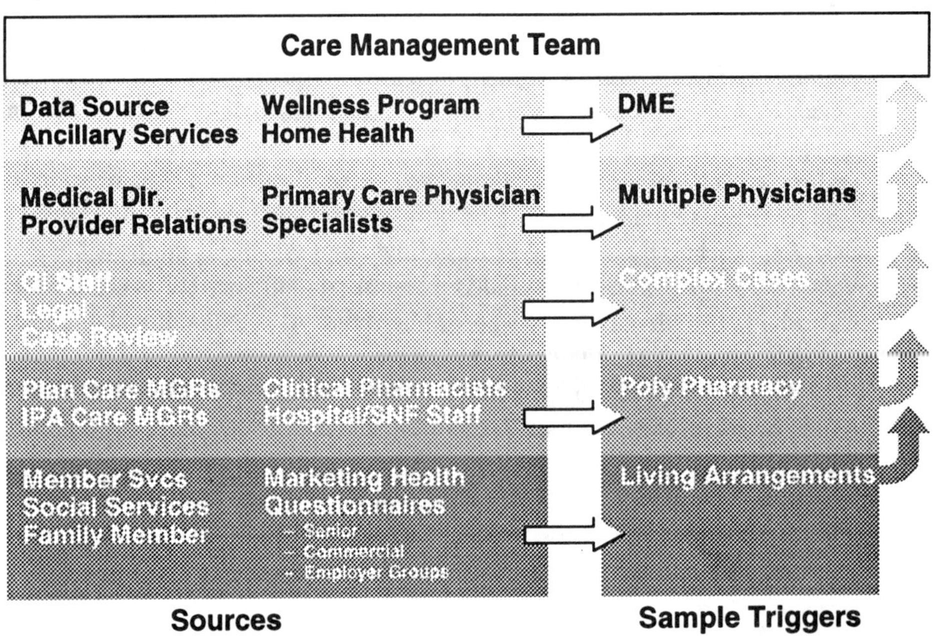

Building Information Technology Capabilities

Ernst & Young has assisted many clients in building information technology systems to improve internal operations, manage data, and produce quality measures. The following section describes how two organizations have approached this challenge.

Missouri

Alliance Blue Cross Blue Shield has made a major investment in information technology to automate care management functions with new utilization management software and to develop a common back-end data warehouse. This warehouse now serves as the primary source of data for measuring diverse types of information including quality indicators aggregated around providers, members, or both.

New utilization review software has taken data that were textual and free form and converted them into over 200 data fields. These fields include predefined quality issues that can be aggregated and analyzed for patterns. Notes now are organized into designated categories and subjects for cross-referencing and aggregate reporting. Criteria and benchmarks are automated, eliminating the need to reference manuals and multiple documents. As a result, performance is expected to be more efficient and consistent.

Extensions have been built to integrate utilization management software and processes with case management, disease management, and pharmacy claims data. Cases now can be referred to disease and case management with no physical handoffs. Triggers have been built to identify members as candidates for disease management programs. Other sources of data include pharmacy claims data and results from health assessments. Lab and x-ray results on HMO members will be available in the near future.

The creation of a data warehouse allows Alliance BCBS to determine, quantify, and prioritize issues. Variations in use and illogical medical use patterns can be identified and prioritized for interventions such as clinical practice guideline implementation, member education, or reminders.

Now that the data warehouse is available to multiple new users, challenges include managing them and providing technical support. "Power users" have been identified and assigned to specific departments to train over 94 users on how to access the warehouse, construct reports, interpret the data, and determine next steps.

Quality improvement efforts are being organized around the needs of newly formed physician groups and their members. The data warehouse enables accurate and prioritized problem identification specific to a given group and compared to other groups. For example, HEDIS scores, the incidence and prevalence of certain diseases, and variation of practices within a group can be identified and communicated to the group. Action plans then can be formulated.

With access to the data warehouse, the health plan is able to identify and prioritize quality issues from an aggregate level. This level of analysis provides scale as well as the ability to identify significance in patterns and minimize bias present when analyzing data from an employer, provider, or other smaller aggregation. The plan then can communicate its findings to parties that are in a position to solve the problems or improve the measures.

Aligned incentives between providers and payers, agreed-upon clinical practice guidelines, and quality measurements support the collaboration necessary to transform quality measures into value.

Ohio

E&Y has had a long-term relationship with the Cleveland-based BCBS plan, assisting it with its two-fold project approach—replacing the staff-model HMO systems with customer server technology and integrating all the processes including administrative and medical data. The latter includes building a large clinical and administrative data warehouse for the entire corporation to integrate all functions and allow data sharing by connecting all facilities through Internet technology. This data warehouse is being populated with data and is scheduled to be complete by mid 1997 for all BCBS's HMOs—approximately half of the hospital providers and selected physicians.

This initiative began approximately 10 years ago. The organization foresaw the competitive marketing advantage of integrating and managing information in order to reduce costs and provide better care and maintained its course with incremental improvements over the interim. Its planning cycle includes five- to eight-year strategic plans with updates every six months.

The resulting system will improve quality measures in two ways—it will provide better, more complete information faster to improve clinical decisionmaking and to improve administrative and care delivery processes that reduce delays and waiting times. Secondly, aggregate and comparative reporting of processes and outcomes will be possible for clinical and administrative data. The result will be an "internal health information network" for BCBS.

For the first time, full functionality is in place for the HMOs, providing the ability to communicate among multiple locations and coordinate scheduling, medical records, ordering, and medical records transcription. Communication with outside providers for referrals is not in place but is slated for 1997.

Preparing for NCQA Certification

NCQA certification has quickly become a requirement for maintaining market share for HMOs. Ernst & Young routinely provides assistance in preparation for an NCQA accreditation. The following case illustrates the importance of culture change and internal champions when pursuing a quality agenda.

In 1994, NCQA accreditation was not a market imperative for a 95,000-member IPA in the Midwest. However, it was anticipated to be a future market imperative, as the IPA began to enroll Medicare risk and Medicaid members and state government employees. The Health Care Financing Administration (HCFA), the

Medicaid regulators, and benefits managers for state employees required either NCQA accreditation or similar standards. In addition, the plan's rural market was beginning to see new market entrants of national players who already have obtained NCQA accreditation.

The health plan had a suboptimal quality program upon initial evaluation. It transformed into an organization with multiple service improvement initiatives and the majority of departments became genuinely excited about their involvement in quality improvement projects.

At the time of E&Y's initial evaluation, the quality improvement focus was on clinical issues and not service. The plan had preventive service initiatives in place and had demonstrated improvements in mammography and Pap smear rates. After initial review of the plan's quality program, Ernst & Young recommended substantial change to the quality improvement program. E&Y found the quality department, operations, service department, and board members resistant to the changes necessary to pass the review. Although there was the beginning of external pressure for NCQA accreditation from employers such as the local state government, because of the resistance of the organization Ernst & Young recommended converting the NCQA visit to a mock assessment.

Subsequently, the internal imperative took the form of a new, 72-year-old, full-time medical director who provided the energy and became the catalyst for change. The new medical director had extensive utilization management experience, was enthusiastic, and was not encumbered by the need to climb the corporate ladder. These factors paved the way for several changes, including:

- Formation of a multidisciplinary improvement committee,
- A board member who had been an obstacle to change agreeing to chair the committee,
- Interdepartmental open houses for staff in order to improve knowledge of each others' processes and communication,
- Identifying and agreeing upon service indicators such as phone answering statistics and turn-around on credentialing, complaints, and grievances,
- Plans to implement a congestive heart failure program,
- Plans to identify for flu vaccine high-risk populations, and
- Plans to implement a diabetes disease management program.

This plan's NCQA site visit now is scheduled for late 1997. By that time it should be much better prepared to meet both the "letter and the spirit" of NCQA's requirements.

Measuring the Effectiveness of Nurseline Services

Health plans and employers have been providing telephonic-based health information to members and employees in one form or another for almost 20 years. Based on the recent explosion in the growth of these services, one can safely assume that delivering health information anytime, to anyone with a phone, is a service that is valued.

Many of E&Y's customers wish to quantify the value in terms of reduced utilization before making the financial outlay and commitment to a vendor that could become a partner in other new care management initiatives. While offering a nurseline is now a market imperative in most places, quantifying the value and finding ways to increase that value remain a challenge.

The primary rationale for nurselines from a health plan perspective is to ensure that the timing and site or intensity of care are appropriate for the member's circumstances; that is, a phone call during the night prompts the nurse to provide "symptom triage," such that a caller with a sore throat may wait until the next morning to be seen for a throat culture and the caller with a specific pattern of abdominal pain will be encouraged to go promptly to the emergency room rather than self-medicate with antacids.

E&Y's health plan customers have asked E&Y to quantify and prove the value of their nurselines in formal and rigorous studies. Although they have heard the anecdotes about reduced emergency room use and seen studies produced to date, the urgent need is for a more complete and replicated study of reduced utilization and cost. Subsequently, E&Y recommends independent studies on satisfaction, access to appropriate services, functional status, and clinical outcome measures.

Key characteristics of the study in progress include:

- Establishing a control group; randomization is not practical in most cases,
- Severity adjusting using ambulatory care groups,
- Comparing experience of two time periods (T1/T2) where a control group cannot be found matching demographics and benefits,
- Adjusting for reduction in utilization already occurring due to other market forces,
- Adding two nested studies:
    1. Emphasizing differences for time-limited, acute symptoms (TLAS)[1] rather than all diagnoses, and
    2. Comparing differences between nurseline eligible users and eligible nonusers, and
- Deliberately excluding any consideration for the difference between the caller's original inclination and the nurse's final disposition (due to subjectivity).

In Figures 15, 16, and 17, E&Y has depicted the study format.

Figure 15. Nurseline Study—Longitudinal Design

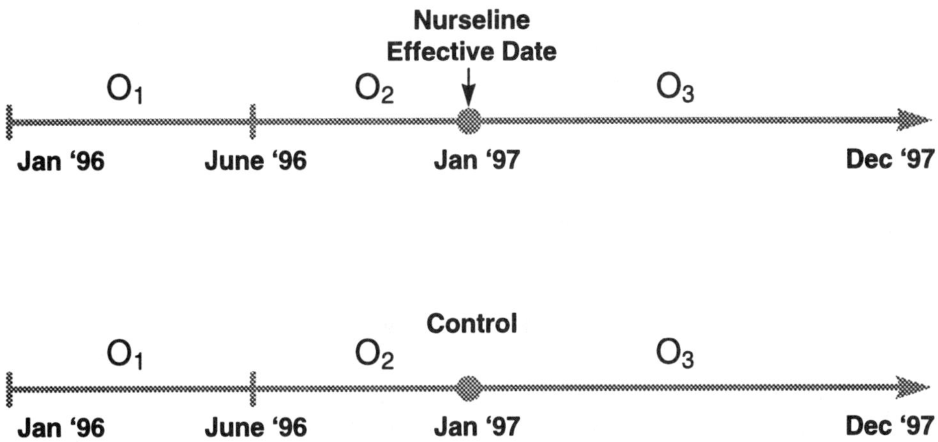

Figure 16. Nested Study #1: Time Limited Acute Symptom Conditions

Identify patients who developed TLAS conditions	Retrospective evaluation of office visits & utilization	Prospective evaluation of office visits & utilization
Nurseline Eligible	*0_1 (Jan - Jun 1996)* *0_2 (Jul - Dec 1996)*	*0_3 (Jan - Dec 1997)*
	Frequency matched (age, sex, condition)	
Control Group (Nurseline Ineligible)	*0_1 (Jan - Jun 1996)* *0_2 (Jul - Dec 1996)*	*0_3 (Jan - Dec 1997)*

Figure 17. Nested Study #2: Nurseline Users Compared to Nonusers

Identify patients who are eligible for Nurseline services	Use of Nurseline services during the study period is documented	Prospective evaluation of office visits & utilization
	Nurseline Users	*0_3 (Jan - Jun 1997)*
	Frequency matched (age, sex, length of membership)	
	Nurseline Nonusers	*0_3 (Jan - Dec 1997)*

E&Y anticipates publishing early results from the nested studies in early 1998. The longitudinal study report will follow. Additional studies related to these types of services are needed to document whether callers experience different outcomes from noncallers and whether those differences are related to health status or other factors.

CONCLUSIONS AND FUTURE NEEDS

The pace and magnitude of change in health care would suggest that prognosticators should proceed with caution. However, the editors have asked E&Y to comment on its view of the future state of health care quality measures and value improvement and how organizations can anticipate and stay ahead of future demands related to quality measures. As E&Y reflects on the examples described in the previous section and the evolution (or revolution) of health care from Stage I (cost avoidance) to Stage II (value improvement) and Stage III (health improvement) the future of quality looks challenging, contentious, yet promising. This section will describe today's current state, barriers, and enablers of change and what will be required of organizations to be winners of the quality contest.

Current State

Several social trends are converging with the changes in health care and in quality improvement. Faith Popcorn, a predictor of marketing trends, includes the "vigilant consumer" as an important new phenomenon. These consumers include aging baby boomers who are accustomed to getting information before making decisions about purchases, routinely have defied authority, have a history of activism, and who feel entitled and deserving of excellent customer service. This prediction is supported by the fact that one of the most popular topics on the Internet is health care, as well as the new importance of satisfaction in HEDIS. These vigilant, aging, demanding consumers will reshape the definition of quality together with physicians, health plans, and employers. The health care providers and plans that meet the expectations of these consumers, especially as they age and use more services, will be the winners.

Several changes in today's health care industry also will weigh in when looking at the future of quality:

- The financial predictions related to Medicare will increase the pressure on managed care to control costs without jeopardizing quality for a population new to many health plans.
- Adopting and implementing new, cost-reducing, yet effective medical interventions quickly, such as ACE inhibitors for CHF, will become the new indicators for quality measurement and value improvement.
- Investment in information technology will require changes in their processes and culture; the organizations that learn how to adapt and use the new information quickly will have the competitive advantage.

- Conversion of nonprofit organizations to publicly traded corporations will increase pressure for quick, positive, financial performance from Wall Street.
- Industry consolidation and strategic alliances with suppliers will create internal focus and distraction from quality measurement and value improvement.
- Growing public concern regarding managed care will increase the importance of accreditation in purchasing decisions.

Barriers and Enablers of Change

There are multiple barriers to transforming quality measures into value:

- There is a lack of consensus on the definition of quality and key indicators among health plans, physicians, employers, and consumers. This lack of consensus is illustrated by the unwillingness of nearly three dozen HMOs to be included in *Newsweek*'s performance score card because of disagreement on the evaluation process and measures. A formalized mechanism for consensus building that includes the public sector would expedite the identification of quality measures that are meaningful to all.
- Self-reported data will require auditing for data integrity and accuracy; independent organizations will be called on to audit and produce indicators such as satisfaction and functional status.
- No organization "has it all" when considering the capabilities required to transform quality measures into value; they are spread among multiple organizations including physician groups, health plans, PBMs, and suppliers of information technology. Therefore, formation of successful strategic alliances will become a core competency.
- Agreement on risk-adjustment methods will become increasingly important as financial arrangements are implemented to reward performance. Valid risk adjustment also will prevent or minimize providers' disincentives to accept sicker or high-risk patients.
- The cost of manually abstracting clinical data from written medical records raises the debate over whether the benefit will outweigh the cost of measurement; the organization that can eliminate this cost barrier, e.g., through links to electronic records, will be the winner. For example, knowing HgbA1c values by member will provide health plans with valuable information in improving targeted, customized, member education programs.
- Wall Street's lack of patience with return on investment in quality, which is expressed today as increased administrative costs, will create barriers for publicly traded companies.

- National organizations such as NCQA and FACCT will accelerate progress in markets with no local driving force.
- Purchasers (Medicare and Medicaid) basing decisions on quality indicators, whether it is NCQA or FACCT, will accelerate the transformation.

Future State Winners

Health care now is straddling two stages: cost avoidance and value improvement. The industry is in need of valid risk adjusters to move into value improvement and away from cost avoidance. Value improvement means simultaneously reducing costs and improving quality. The winner of the value improvement challenge will be the entity that has the following capabilities:

- Owns or has access to the necessary data,
- Understands health care processes (episodes) and can organize the data into useful information and quality measures for process change,
- Understands which care process changes will improve quality measures,
- Understands which quality measures will be defined as value by customers and consumers and focuses on those measures,
- Implements care process (provider and member behavior) change and culture change quickly, and
- Measures and communicates outcomes to consumers, employers, providers, and health plans.

Today's owners and users of data warehouses (most of which include only claims and membership data) are a few health plans and pharmacy benefit managers (PBMs). Acquiring the necessary data from multiple sources is today's challenge. The better-positioned organizations will be those who can identify those individuals who will benefit from targeted interventions, project future costs based on prevalence of conditions in their population, estimate cost savings (or return on investment) from newly implemented care processes, and manage risk for the resulting value improvement.

Future state winners will stay ahead of the evolving demands from NCQA, FAACT, and others for quality measures by:

- Constructing data warehouses that include easily accessible, longitudinal, patient- and provider-focused data;
- Building automated linkages to external data sources such as electronic medical records, satisfaction data, lab results, and others;
- Acquiring staff, skills, and expertise in data analysis and information management;
- Staying informed or involved in national efforts to identify and select new measures and anticipating the new direction these efforts may

take, such as the recent switch by NCQA from prevention measures to measures related to the care of chronic disease and high-cost individuals;

- Keeping in touch with consumer and employer opinion related to value and quality in health care either through consumer focus groups, employer forums, public opinion polls, surveys, or other means of consumer and market research;
- Building alliances with local physician leaders who can provide constructive solutions to information-gathering challenges, offer insights into changing physician behavior, and influence their peers; and
- Collaborating with competing organizations in gathering data from paper-based medical records in order to reduce the cost and improve the quality and efficiency of the data.

In addition to staying ahead of the curve in gathering data for measurement, organizations ultimately will be challenged to improve the measures by changing the behavior of both physicians and members. Staying ahead of this curve will require training staff in, or hiring individuals with, skills in physician and member behavior change. Attention to the three aspects of quality coined by Avedis Donabedian—structure, process, and outcomes—will continue to be necessary. Structure (accreditation and credentialing) and process (clinical practice guidelines) will be as important as outcomes in some cases. Not all incompetent processes are evident from outcomes data; it is often revealed too late, is not related closely to the intervention, or is often confounded by other factors.

If Stage II—value improvement—isn't enough of a challenge, Stage III—health improvement—already is happening in more communities like Minneapolis. Population-specific and community-oriented measures are emerging and collaboration among competing health plans and public health organizations is beginning. Movement into this stage will be accelerated by consolidation of health plans into a few, manageable, large organizations that are positioned to collaborate on key measures, movement of large blocks of publicly funded populations into managed care, and providers understanding what they can and cannot control related to improving health. As with value improvement, the key to accelerating the evolution will include building consensus on key measures, building structures and organizations designed to improve them, managing them, and rewarding organizations' plans for attaining them.

REFERENCE

1. Elsenhans V, Marquardt C, Bledsoe T, et al. "Use of Self-Care Manual Shifts Utilization Pattern," *HMO Practice, The Journal of the HMO Group*, Vol. 9, No. 2, June 1995, pp. 1190-1195.

Chapter 15

The Case of Pennsylvania

Public Release Of Quality Data

Ernest J. Sessa

In fiscal year 1985-1986, overall hospital expenditures in Pennsylvania rose a mere one percent—the lowest increase in six years. Given that figure, one almost wonders what all the fuss has been about. Things weren't always so rosy, which helps to explain why Pennsylvania is in the forefront of a national movement to contain health care costs while improving the quality of care patients receive.

During the 1970s and early 1980s, states such as Pennsylvania became increasingly concerned with rapidly rising health care expenditures. The annual rate of growth in health care spending averaged 15.2 percent a year from 1977 to 1983. Inpatient hospital expenses grew by 14.9 percent a year during this period. The nation spent $75 billion on health care in 1970, $248 billion in 1980, and $458 billion in 1986 (see Figure 1). The percentage of GNP spent on health care continued to increase, topping 10 percent by the mid 1980s and reaching 10.9 percent in 1986.

In an effort to bring these skyrocketing costs under control, the Pennsylvania General Assembly unanimously passed Senate Bill 293 on July 1, 1986. ACT 89, which created a new independent state agency called the Pennsylvania Health Care Cost Containment Council, was signed into law shortly thereafter by then Gov. Richard Thornburgh. ACT 89 took more than three years of effort, driven primarily by a coalition of business and organized labor leaders working together to pass market-oriented health care reforms.

Figure 1. U.S. Health Care Expenses

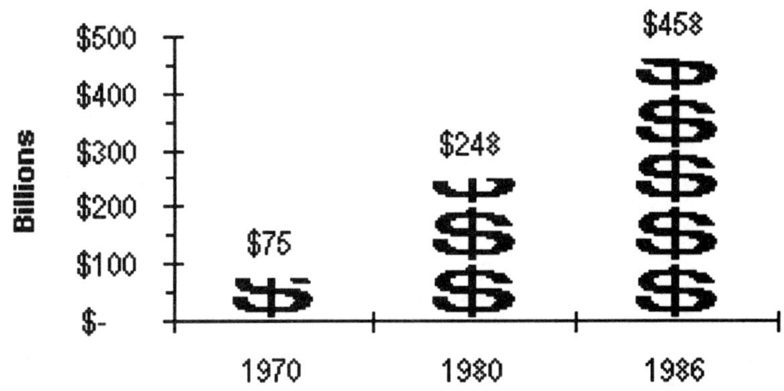

It was the mission of this new agency, under the law, to promote cost containment by stimulating a competitive health care market. This would be achieved by providing group purchasers and individual consumers with consistent, accurate, and credible information about the cost and quality of health care services in Pennsylvania. A unique feature of the law, and the Council's trademark since, was the requirement to report data about the quality of care. This was done so that access to quality care would not be jeopardized in a search for lower costs and in the belief that quality should cost less.

In order to further invest the primary stakeholders in this issue firmly in the process, a 21-member council was created with the intent of functioning as a board of directors. This would include:

- business community representatives (six members),
- organized labor representatives (six members),
- hospital representative (one member),
- physician representative (one member),
- commercial insurance representative (one member),
- PA Blue Cross/Blue Shield plans (one member),
- health maintenance organization representative (one member),
- consumer representative (one member),
- Secretary of the state Health Department,
- Secretary of the state Department of Public Welfare, and
- Commissioner of the state insurance department.

ACT 89 assigned the Council three main responsibilities:

1. Collect from health care providers and other sources data on health care costs and quality and disseminate this information to businesses and other purchasers, consumers, and the general public;

2. Study the issue of health care for the uninsured and develop a plan to address the problems identified during the study; and,
3. Review proposed legislation calling for additional mandated health benefits upon request from the legislative or executive branches of government and make recommendations about their (mandates) cost and medical effectiveness.

Initially this effort was pointed to the development and public release of a document that would allow consumers and group purchasers to make valid comparisons of hospital care based on cost and quality considerations. This publication became known as the Hospital Effectiveness Report.

THE "HOSPITAL EFFECTIVENESS REPORT"

For many years the "Hospital Effectiveness Report" served as the flagship publication of the Council. First published in 1988 as a quarterly regional report, the report evolved to annual reports including a full year's data from 175 of PA's largest hospitals across 55-60 treatment categories (Diagnostic Related Groups), divided into nine regional reports. These reports included severity-adjusted mortality and morbidity rates, patient volumes, average lengths of stay, and average hospital charges for services. The Council utilized Medisgroups™, a severity-adjustment system developed by MediQual Systems, Inc., to risk adjust the data. This system, which every PA hospital was required to install, allowed for the abstraction of numerous key clinical findings from patients' medical records. These records pertained to the patients' condition upon admission to the hospital and then again at about the mid-point of their hospital stay. These findings were assigned certain weights mathematically according to their impact on the patient. Once all the findings were calculated, patients were classified into one of five groups ranging from very sick to not very sick (0-4) for an admission severity score and a morbidity (mid-stay) score.

By December 1990, with the release of the Philadelphia Regional report, reports for all regions in Pennsylvania had been released. These were preliminary reports, designed to acquaint people with the process and to work out the system. The Council cautioned consumers that a quarter's worth of data was not enough upon which to base a decision and that a full year of data was necessary.

In April 1991, the Council released its first full-year report, covering inpatient hospital admissions occurring in 1989. Wide variations in treatment outcomes such as mortality and morbidity rates were shown for more than 125 of Pennsylvania's largest hospitals (see Figure 2). Charges for heart bypass surgery ranged from $40,929 to $86,053 at Philadelphia-area hospitals. Hip replacements ranged from $12,847 to $46,566.

For the first time, consumers, businesses, labor groups, insurers, and the medical community had concrete, comprehensive health care information. These groups now had an essential tool—a tool they could use to ask intelligent questions and, in conjunction with doctors and hospitals, begin to identify the most efficient and effective providers.

Figure 2. DRG 294 Diabetes (Age greater than 35)

Hospital	Number of Patients	Average Admission Severity Score	Age 65 and Over (%)	Deaths		Medically Unstable during first week (major morbidity)			Average Stay (days)	Average Charge ($)
Chestnut Hill Hospital	43	2.0	53.5	2	2.39	1	1.68		7.9	7,078
Episcopal Hospital	68	2.1	29.4	0	1.36	1	1.41		8.1	8,907
Frankford Hospital of Philadelphia	60	1.9	50.0	1	2.36	3	1.22		7.8	9,233
Franklin Square Hospital	66	1.8	27.3	3	0.97	5	0.91	—	7.8	8,200
Germantown Hospital & Medical Center	66	1.5	22.7	1	0.69	0	0.74		5.9	6,452
Graduate Hospital	54	2.2	44.4	2	3.41	3	2.01		5.2	10,549
Hahnemann University Hospital	44	2.0	47.7	0	0.93	0	0.73		7.3	11,028
...										
Philadelphia County	1,336	1.9							7.6	9,088

Source: Pennsylvania Health Care Cost Containment Council, July 1, 1989-June 30, 1990 data

Average Admission Severity Score:
The rating that measures how sick a patient is at the beginning of their hospital stay on a scale of 0 to 4, 0 is not very sick and 4 is very sick.

Statistical Rating:
- + fewer deaths or fewer patients who were medically unstable than hospitals in comparative database
- – more deaths or more patients who were medically unstable than hospitals in comparative database
- ◊ single occurrence of a death or major morbidity in a DRG where death or major morbidity is very rare
- no symbol actual number of deaths or actual number of patients who were medically unstable are not statistically significantly different from hospitals in comparative database

SMALL AREA ANALYSIS

Small area analysis shows hospital admission rates for a large number of medical conditions and surgical procedures for the residents of defined, community-sized areas called "health market areas." Rates also are shown by county and region and include the statewide average. These admission rates can be compared to the rates in neighboring geographic areas and to the state rate. Identifying differences, and changing them where appropriate, can have major implications for health care cost containment and access to care.

The first small area analysis reports, for Region 5 (South Central Pennsylvania) and Region 2 (northwestern Pennsylvania), were released in June 1991. These reports covered hospital admissions during the last three quarters of 1988. The remaining seven regions in the Commonwealth were released by September 1991. Since then, these population data have been incorporated into Council reports on coronary bypass surgery, c-sections, and the treatment of heart-attack patients.

Small area analysis can highlight communities where serious access to care problems, health problems, or overutilization of services may exist. This may be reflected by a higher-than-average admission rate, particularly for certain medical conditions. For example, if residents do not have access to primary care—that which can be obtained from a pediatrician or general practitioner in an office visit and that is more preventive in nature—they must go to the local hospital for treatment.

The Council's data can help communities determine the factors underlying patterns of health care spending and distribution. It provides a valuable information base to hospitals, doctors, businesses, labor groups, insurers, and consumer groups—information that can be used to raise intelligent questions. And the most important question that small area analysis provokes is this: in a community with large variations, are we getting the best value for our health care dollar? If the answer is no, local leaders can access targeted information to use in achieving that goal.

THE "HOSPITAL FINANCIAL REPORT"

In December 1990, the Council released its first "Hospital Financial Report." This report, covering fiscal year 1989, offered to the public, providers, and policymakers of the Commonwealth the first statewide overview of the relative financial performance of hospitals in Pennsylvania. The "Hospital Financial Report" relies primarily on audited financial statements and also uses Medicare and Medicaid cost reports. The report is organized by type of facility: general acute care with 100 or more beds, general acute care under 100 beds, children's hospitals, rehabilitation, psychiatric, and specialty hospitals.

Each facility type is reported by region with two types of tables for the hospitals in each region. The first table reports revenue and expense numbers. They include: gross patient revenue, uncollected charges, net patient revenue, total operating revenue, total expenses, income or loss from operations, nonoperating revenue, and excess or deficiency of revenue over expenses (see Figure 3).

Figure 3. Operating Revenues and Expenses

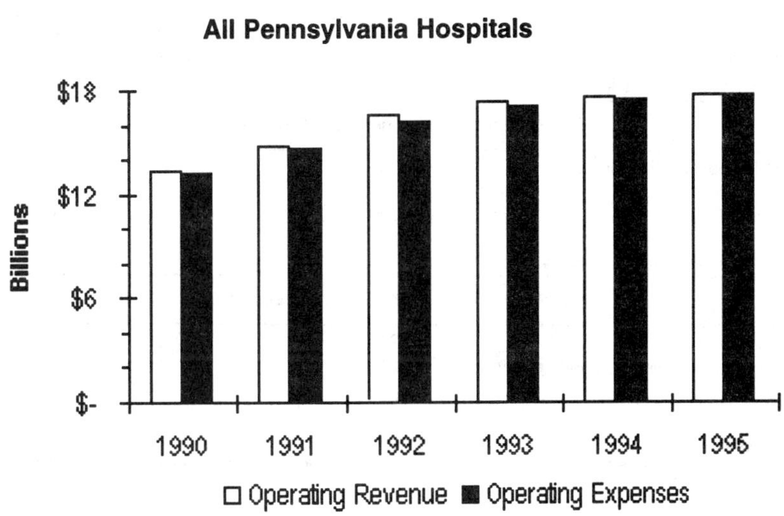

The second table discloses financial and utilization statistics. It includes: operating margin, net margin, gross inpatient/outpatient revenue, percentage of uncollected charges, percentage of occupancy, average length of stay, inpatient days and discharges, debt to equity, and capitalization ratios.

THE CONSUMER GUIDE TO CORONARY ARTERY BYPASS GRAFT SURGERY

On November 19, 1992, the Council released its first physician-specific report: *The Consumer Guide to Coronary Artery Bypass Graft Surgery*. This report—the first of its kind in Pennsylvania and only the second published anywhere in the United States—details patient outcomes (risk-adjusted mortality rates) for 170 PA cardiac surgeons, as well as hospital-specific mortality rates and average costs for 40 certified open heart hospitals (see Figure 4). It was also the first time the Council used additional risk factors to supplement the Medisgroups™ technology. This was done in response to the concerns voiced by providers that the Medisgroups™ system wasn't disease-specific. The Council developed a list of candidate variables based on examination of the medical literature and feedback from its Technical Advisory Group and the medical community.

Figure 4. Hospitals in Which Coronary Artery Bypass Graft Surgery Was Performed

Treatment Effectiveness & Average Charge

Hospital		Patients who Died			Average Charge
Hospitals with fewer number of deaths than expected					
Allegheny General Hospital	954	10	18 - 35	+	$55,879
Altoona Hospital	462	3	4 - 14	+	$37,895
Temple University Hospital	346	5	7 - 18	+	$85,310
Hospitals with similar number of deaths as expected					
Albert Einstein Medical Center	604	22	14 - 30	Δ	$84,746
...					
Graduate Hospital	290	9	5 - 14	Δ	$102,637
...					
Wilkes-Barre General Hospital /WVHCS	403	9	6 - 16	Δ	$32,526
Hospitals with greater number of deaths than expected					
Episcopal Hospital	242	12	3 - 11	—	$55,732
Hospital of the University of Pennsylvania	227	12	2 - 11	—	$86,509
Mercy Hospital of Scranton	416	21	8 - 19	—	$32,461
...					
STATEWIDE TOTAL	17,413	497			$54,569

Source: Pennsylvania Health Care Cost Containment Council, 1993 data

Statistical Rating:
- hospital had significantly fewer deaths than expected
+ hospital had significantly more deaths than expected
Δ the hospital's number of patient deaths was not significantly different than expected

The most surprising finding of the report was that the two hospitals that charged the most for bypass surgery had significantly more deaths than expected, while the hospital charging the least had significantly fewer deaths than expected. These data gained the attention of President Clinton, who noted the statistic in an address to the nation, as well as *The Wall Street Journal*, the *Washington Post*, and the *CBS Evening News with Dan Rather*. Approximately 13,000 copies were disseminated to a variety of consumers and users.

FOCUS ON HEART ATTACK IN PENNSYLVANIA

Heart attack is the single largest killer of Americans and Pennsylvanians. This year as many as 1.5 million Americans will have a heart attack and about one-third of those will die. Over 13.5 million people alive today have a history of heart attack, angina (chest pain), or both. The financial impact is staggering as well. The American Heart Association estimates the annual cost of treatment for heart attack and angina at $66 billion. This includes the cost of physician and nursing services, hospital and nursing home services, medication, and lost productivity resulting from disability. The in-hospital charges alone in the Commonwealth of Pennsylvania amounted to nearly $1 billion in 1993.

For these reasons, the Pennsylvania Health Care Cost Containment Council decided to publish information comparing the quality, cost, and geographic impact of heart attacks in Pennsylvania. *Focus on Heart Attack in Pennsylvania*, a comprehensive examination of 40,000 heart attack hospitalizations, was published in June 1996. The study covers six main areas: consumer education; average treatment charges; risk-adjusted mortality and length of stay data for 189 Pennsylvania hospitals; risk-adjusted mortality data for 191 physician practice groups treating 30 or more cases; hospitalization and mortality rate population-based data for all Pennsylvania counties and significantly different communities; and levels of advanced cardiac services, mortality rates, lengths of stay, and average hospitals charges according to aggregate payer groups (traditional fee-for-service plans, health maintenance organizations/preferred provider organizations, Medicare, and Medicaid). (See Figure 5).

Figure 5. Heart Attack Payer

All Southeastern Hospitals, 1993 data

Payer	# Cases	Mortality Rate		Length of Stay	
		Actual	Expected Range	Actual	Expected Range
Blue Cross	2,265	3.4	3.0 — 4.4	*7.0	6.7 — 6.9
Commercial	1,021	2.7	2.6 — 4.5	6.9	6.6 — 7.0
HMO/PPO	1,355	*5.7	3.7 — 5.5	6.7	6.6 — 7.0
Medicaid	665	4.5	3.6 — 6.2	7.8	7.3 — 7.9
Medicare	7,972	13.3	12.6 — 13.8	*8.7	8.4 — 8.6
Other	218	7.3	3.2 — 7.3	6.3	6.2 — 7.3

* Actual is significantly higher than the expected range

The data in *Focus on Heart Attack* showed that if you have a heart attack, your chances of surviving may depend on the kind of health insurance you have. This was the first Council report to focus on data according to payer type. Patients insured by HMOs and PPOs in southeastern Pennsylvania had significantly higher-than-expected mortality rates. HMO heart-attack patients also received fewer advanced cardiac treatments—cardiac catheterizations, angioplasty, and bypass surgery—than did those in traditional fee-for-service private insurance plans in the same area. In contrast, HMO/PPO members in other parts of the state had significantly lower-than-expected mortality rates. Medicaid patients had the lowest level of advanced services throughout Pennsylvania, with the exception of Medicare patients who were older, sicker, and poorer candidates for advanced services. Providing payer-type information is the Cost Containment Council's primary future objective.

SPECIAL REPORTS

The public reports represent only a small portion of the information that the Council collects and makes available. Special, customer-specific reports are available for a fee based on the number of records and the amount of programming required. Those that have requested Council data or special reports include: businesses, hospitals, insurance companies, HMOs, attorneys, benefits consultants, health service researchers, legislators, and several branches of state government. The Council has filled more than 300 special data requests over the past five years.

DATA COLLECTION AND VERIFICATION

Under state law (ACT 89), hospitals are required to submit select data using the UB-92 billing format. In addition, hospitals were required to install and use the Medisgroups™ severity system and to report admission severity and major morbidity (mid-stay review) scores for all patients to the Council. The severity and morbidity scores formed the basis for developing expected (predicted) morbidity. Beginning with the CABG report, the Council added additional clinical factors to hospital reporting requirements.

The recent *Focus on Heart Attack* project offers the best insight into the collection and verification process.

The AMI data used were submitted to the Council by Pennsylvania hospitals providing treatment for AMI during calendar year 1993. In conjunction with these facilities, the Council conducted extensive verification activities to finalize the dataset. This included ensuring the correct assignment of the attending physician and the physician practice group, as well as the correct payer category assignment.

Hospitals and physicians were given opportunities to examine their patient-level data, submit corrections, and request case exclusions. Specially designed computer software was made available to enable hospitals to make quick and seamless corrections. Final patient-level data were sent to each hospital for review prior to the analysis of the data. Hospitals also were given the opportunity to submit 15 diagnosis and nine procedure codes. (In 1993, only five diagnosis and three procedure codes were required; now nine and six are submitted.) Obtaining these additional codes, along with extensive data accuracy verification, added significantly to the clinical depth of the dataset. In fact, there were only five invalid data entries throughout the entire database. Physicians were given the opportunity to confirm attribution of cases and specialty assignment.

The Council relied on each hospital to carry out data element verification and provided guidelines for them to do so. As an ongoing activity of the public reporting process, the Council identifies data quality concerns related to timeliness, completeness, accuracy, and validity through computerized logical edits, manual data verification checks, and data auditing. These issues are communicated to the hospitals, and specific critical concerns are raised prior to data finalization. After publication of the final report, the Council sends each hospital a data quality report. General data quality issues often are discussed with hospitals upon completion of the report.

WHAT IS QUALITY?

How does the Council define quality? No one in the business of measuring patient outcomes or "quality" can pretend to have a comprehensive definition of quality in health care, let alone a measure to capture it. The Council's interest in doing so far exceeds the tools currently available. Nevertheless, the Council has provided information related to quality issues and concerns that, at minimum, provides a basis for consumers (individual and group) to ask intelligent questions of providers. The data can enhance already-existing quality improvement efforts by medical professionals as well.

When the Council began, there were few systems available that provided a risk-adjusted method of assessing patient outcomes. After an extensive bidding process, the Council decided upon a system called Medisgroups™, a product of MediQual Systems, Inc., of Massachusetts. Medisgroups™ allowed for the abstraction of potentially hundreds of key clinical findings from patients' medical records. Abnormal scores then were assigned weights according to scientifically developed algorithms in conjunction with a national comparative database. Each hospital patient then was assigned two scores—an admission severity score and a major morbidity score based on a second reading taken at about the mid-point of the hospital stay. The classifications ranged from 0-4, with 0 representing a patient who was not very ill to 4 indicating the presence of major organ failure. Because of the depth of the Medisgroups™ system, these severity and morbidity scores were applied to patients grouped in numerous diagnostic related groups (DRGs). Hospitals were required under state regulation to install Medisgroups™ in their medical records departments and to begin reporting these clinical data to the Council. Many Pennsylvania hospitals were, in fact, already using Medisgroups™ prior to the state mandate.

In the "Hospital Effectiveness Reports," the Council defined a quality measure as the comparison of actual mortality and morbidity numbers to expected numbers, given the age and admission severity of the hospitals' patients. The expected numbers were based on Medisgroups™-derived severity scores and a national comparative database. Medisgroups(was based on abstracting abnormal readings among hundreds of key clinical findings and used across 50-60 DRGS.

In the "Small Area Analysis" reports, population-based hospital admission rates for AMI, c-sections, gall bladder removal, and adult pneumonia were used as quality indicators. Significantly high or low hospitalizations, compared to statewide norms and other population areas, pointed to possible over- or under-utilization of health care services and presented quality improvement opportunities to be explored.

In the CABG report, the Council supplemented the Medisgroups™ system with additional risk factors such as age, diabetes, previous AMI, previous CABG, renal failure, cardiogenic shock, and congestive heart failure. Ejection fraction already was captured by Medisgroups™.

In the AMI report, the Council again supplemented Medisgroups™ (now Atlas) with additional risk factors and created separate mortality and length of stay models, as well as separate models for transferred patients and those directly admitted.

The Council's role in this process is to communicate information to the public who must make their own comparisons and judgments. The Council has no clinical investigative role or authority; its job is to point out the result of the process. It is the job of the hospital or quality improvement personnel to determine where, how, and why something went wrong in the process.

MODELING AND STATISTICS

The CABG report presents a good example as to the statistical approach of the Council. The research staff begins with an extensive list of candidate risk variables based on previous or similar reports, review of the scientific literature, and feedback from clinicians and researchers. Logistic regression was the statistical technique used to estimate the probabilities of in-hospital mortality. In logistic regression, each category for each statistically significant clinical or demographic factor is assigned a weight or coefficient. A factor category's weight is higher (lower) if patients with that factor category tend to have a higher (lower) chance of mortality. The weights in this report were determined during the research phase using the 1993 statewide CABG dataset. The weights were used to compute each individual patient's probability of in-hospital death given the risk factors of the patient. To obtain the expected number of deaths for a given hospital or physician, the probabilities of death for each patient for that hospital or physician are summed. If a hospital had significantly more deaths than expected, that is represented in the report by a minus symbol. If the rating is significantly fewer deaths than expected, a plus symbol is used. An average rating (number of deaths is equal or similar to the expected value) is represented by a delta symbol.

IMPACT

What has been the effect of more than 80 public reports and 300 special reports over the past seven years? Is the process of public reporting, and the empowerment of those seeking to restrain costs and improve quality, working? The answer is yes.

The most dramatic example can be observed over the four years (1990-1993 data years) of CABG data published in *The Consumer Guide to Coronary Artery Bypass Graft Surgery*. During those four years, CABG patient mortalities in the study population dropped 26 percent (3.9 percent in 1990 to 2.9 percent in 1993). Total CABG mortalities dropped from 4.9 percent in 1990 to 3.9 percent in 1993. In addition, there were 2,500 more operations performed in 1993 than in 1990. At the same time, there was no corresponding decrease in the number of patients with significant risk factors, debunking the notion that the process is causing surgeons to turn away seriously ill patients. A related quality fact is that five of the seven hospitals that had significantly higher-than-expected mortality rates in 1990 had improved to having rates that were as expected or better. Lehigh Valley Hospital (higher than expected in 1990) improved to lower rates than expected in 1992. York Hospital improved to lower than expected in 1993.

As far as costs are concerned, the average price increase for a heart bypass in a Pennsylvania hospital dropped from 10 percent in 1991 to 4.6 percent in 1993. Overall hospital costs rose only one percent in 1995, the smallest increase in six years.

AUDIENCES

A second way to measure impact is in the use of these data to make decisions. A study released in October 1995 by the federal General Accounting Office found that Pennsylvania consumers who had obtained *The Consumer Guide to Coronary Artery Bypass Graft Surgery* understood it and were using the guide to:

- select the best surgeon or hospital because they or someone in their family anticipated having the procedure described in the report,
- select the best surgeon or hospital for procedures other than those described in the report,
- review the rating of the surgeon who had performed their surgery before they had obtained the report,
- ask more informed questions of their doctors,
- increase their general knowledge,

- provide advice to other, or
- satisfy their curiosity.

GAO further concluded that consumers wanted more of this kind of information about the quality of care. Other examples of users follow.

Purchasers

In late 1991, after receiving a disturbing financial prediction about the long term health of their health benefits trust fund, the Laborers' Council Welfare Fund trustees used Council data to assist them in deciding to move from a traditional indemnity plan with Blue Cross of Western PA to a managed care plan with Aetna. Actuarial estimates predicted a savings of $6 million a year by making the switch. Unfortunately, even with the changes achieved through the Aetna plan, by 1994 the Fund remained unable to keep pace with rising costs. After a bidding process, they selected a point-of-service plan from Blue Cross of Western Pennsylvania as the new plan for their participants.

Hospital

In 1994, the Vantage Health Care Network, an alliance of 13 Northwestern Pennsylvania hospitals (seven owners, six affiliates), joined with New Health Management, a national health care consulting firm, to develop and implement a system of clinical pathways. A clinical pathway can be described as a map that describes the best course of hospitalization or treatment for patients of a similar diagnosis. The seven Vantage owners comprise 1,759 beds, 56,000 admissions, and $407 million in annual expenses. Vantage created a company called The Quality Institute for Medical Care to help the hospitals enhance the quality of patient care. The hospitals' motivations for developing clinical pathways were to decrease lengths of stay and costs and to eliminate the variants of poor quality care.

The Quality Institute decided to develop regional pathways for the top 10 diagnoses and determined that the best source of uniform and consistent financial information was the data that each hospital was required to submit to the Council. Using tapes of these data, a program was developed using the ratio of cost to charges from the Medicare cost reports in order to determine actual costs. This new database, which allowed for departmental cost analysis, consisted of 34,000 total admissions, 128 variables, and a workable dataset. In addition, the Council data contained admission severity scoring.

The Institute's analysis revealed that almost 50 percent of readmissions for congestive heart failure were due to one of two things: noncompliance on the medications or noncompliance on the prescribed diet. In response, Vantage made sure that the home care nurse weighed the patient on a weekly basis and that patients stayed on their medications.

An initial pathway dealt with obstructions. The data revealed variability in the preoperative workups and the timespan from admission to surgical consultation. This analysis was possible only because of the depth of the Council's data. The pathway was written to help the internist decide when to involve the surgeon and to identify problems with scheduling of surgeries. Vantage also has developed guidelines for pneumonia, major joints, major bowel elective procedures, and major bowel obstructions and has estimated $3 million in savings. A pneumonia pathway decreased pharmacy costs by $100 a case, total costs were down $400 a case, and lengths of stay declined by half a day. Vantage has predicted a total potential cost savings of $6 million after additional pathways are completed.

State Government

The Council has filled data requests for Pennsylvania Department of Health projects involving seat belt and motorcycle helmet usage, hospital emergency room data, access to pediatric services in rural areas, hospital transfers, Pennsylvania's progress in meeting the HHS Healthy People 2000 project, subacute care, the incidence of diabetes in Pennsylvania, and an analysis of access and utilization of cardiac services for select geographic areas in the Commonwealth. This makes the Pennsylvania Department of Health one of the most active and innovative users of the Council's data.

Medicaid

For the past several years the Council has been exploring ways to assist the Pennsylvania Department of Public Welfare (DPW) in their analysis of the burgeoning costs of the Medicaid program. In 1994-95 the Council completed the first in a planned series of reports to the Pennsylvania General Assembly and the Governor's Administration about hospital utilization patterns of the Commonwealth's Medicaid population.

A second report is planned to explore trends in hospitalizations over time. A third report is contemplated to examine the utilization of Medicaid recipients who are enrolled in managed care programs compared to fee-for-service plans.

Phase II of this project was continued during 1995-96. Enrollment data from the Department of Public Welfare were loaded and formatted into the Council's database system. Additional work is ongoing with DPW in the development of computer programs needed to match the DPW's enrolled Medicaid population with the Council's inpatient hospitalization data. Future activity and collaborative efforts are being discussed by the Council and DPW.

THE FUTURE IS MANAGED CARE

America's health care delivery system is undergoing radical surgery and reconstruction, most of which is being driven by free-market forces. The business and medical news is filled with almost daily reports of consolidations of various kinds. Hospitals are merging with other hospitals. Physicians are organizing and marketing themselves as new health plans. Health plans are gobbling up physician practices in record numbers. Providers are angling to become insurers and insurers are angling to become providers. Much of this changing environment can be chalked up to the increasing management of care and the pressure on providers and insurers alike to be more competitive. One result of these dynamics is that the respective roles of the hospital you go to, the physician who treats you, and the insurance company who pays the bill are becoming increasingly difficult to distinguish.

Another factor is the tremendous growth in the number of Americans enrolled in managed care plans. In 1995, membership in HMOs was expected to reach 56 million—up almost 20 million since 1990. Today, 20 percent of all privately insured Americans belong to more than 570 HMOs. Millions more belong to preferred provider organizations, another form of managed care. Some experts predict that the number of HMO enrollees could easily double by the year 2000.

Yet even those most closely associated with these changes cannot claim to fully understand their implications and consequences. Consumers, purchasers, and policymakers will need all the information they can get to understand how the changing nature of health care delivery will affect them.

Clearly the Council has had an impact through the process of public reporting about the results of physicians and hospitals. However, the health care system is in a state of upheaval, and it is clear that the delivery of health care is no longer simply about doctors and hospitals anymore. There are new players, new arrangements, new rules, and new expectations. The Council needed to change as well to adapt to the restructuring of the health delivery system.

Late last year, then-Council chair and business community representative William Lehr of Hershey Foods Inc., convened a strategic task force to chart the Council's future direction. After a series of meetings, the Council decided to shift the mission of the agency to developing ways to provide information about Pennsylvania's changing health care delivery system, with particular attention to the impact and influence of managed health care plans.

HMOs and other kinds of managed care programs, which are currently offered by 79 percent of American employers, first rose to prominence because of their ability to control costs through an emphasis on preventive care and closer management of doctors and patients.

And costs are coming down. According to the Pennsylvania Economy League, costs are low for Pennsylvania employers—ninth lowest among 13 states surveyed. Increases in health benefits paid by employers dropped nationwide from 12.1 percent in 1991 to 2.1 percent in 1995.

Is there an adverse effect on the quality of care HMO members receive? No, according to a 12-year study by RAND—an independent research organization in Santa Monica CA—which found that patients who belonged to HMOs experienced up to 40 percent fewer hospitalizations and saved up to 28 percent on health care costs compared to those enrolled in fee-for-service plans.

On the other hand, a recent study found that elderly and poor HMO members received worse care than other HMO patients. Another recent study of 90,000 patients by University of Pittsburgh researchers found that managed care plans offer no savings over traditional fee-for-service plans when it comes to treating those in intensive care.

Recent media stories about physician gag rules and financial incentives to deny care do nothing to reassure the public. And there are questions. As managed care continues to grow, will the emphasis of some companies shift more strongly from quality care to cutting costs? Will quality decline and costs escalate as HMOs include older and sicker patients, as they are already doing through programs like Medicare, Medicaid, and employer-paid retiree health benefit plans? In Pennsylvania, Medicare and Medicaid account for about 70 percent of all hospital days.

Certainly there is a role for credible objective information. Managed care has been portrayed both negatively and positively. *Focus on Heart Attack* shows that it's not managed care, generically speaking, that's good or bad, but that it's important to pay attention to picking the right plan. Credible data are necessary to help people do that.

The Council's new goal is to provide the public with information about the changing health care delivery system, especially as it pertains to the impact of managed care. At the time of this writing, the Council was going through a process to agree on the specifics of its "managed care strategy" and lay out its short-term priorities.

AUDIENCES

Who are the audiences for and potential users of information about managed care?

- **Payers.** While payer's own data can be helpful in making decisions, the Council can provide comparative data.
- **Purchasers.** Most purchasers choose from among options including complete indemnity plans, point-of-service plans, provider networks, and group- or staff-model HMOs. If purchasers have additional and comparative information about the cost and quality of care provided through these options, their health benefit strategy may be enhanced.
- **Policymakers.** Government has an interest in structuring incentives and disincentives in the managed care market for those receiving medical assistance, those receiving Medicare benefits, those enrolled in public employee benefit plans, as well as the general public.
- **Health care providers.** There is increasing interest on the part of the public in knowing the effect of the widespread hospital mergers and alliances seen in recent years on the cost and quality of care. The Council may be able to provide systemwide data about these new institutions. Additionally, providers are interested in the impact of managed care on cost and quality.

- **Consumers and the general public.** There are questions about managed care programs. How do they compare to traditional fee-for-service plans? To other managed care programs?

In considering the needs of these audiences, a number of goals can be identified:

- To assist payers in identifying opportunities for cost containment and quality improvement within their own networks of providers and their enrolled populations;
- To continue to stimulate market-driven competition based on cost and quality indicators;
- To assist employers in choosing health plan options and in monitoring plan performance over time;
- To assist employers and individual consumers in choosing high-quality, cost-efficient health plans; and
- To raise general public awareness about issues related to health plan performance as well as about the changing nature of health care delivery.

OUTCOME MEASURES

The Council has traditionally focused on the outcome of patient care, rather than the process of care, in its reporting of quality issues. That primarily is due to the availability of data, not a judgment regarding the merits of process versus outcome measures. On the other hand, coordination with other Pennsylvania state agencies or private entities such as the National Committee for Quality Assurance might provide other data.

INTERACTION WITH OTHER DATA ORGANIZATIONS

At the time of the Council's creation in 1986, the efforts to measure quality in any way were few and far between. Now, the relevant question is not if it will be done, but how. It seems every time one turns around a new organization springs up with the intent of measuring quality in health care. Most are concerned with providing information about the quality of health plans.

Many of these organizations collect data unavailable to the Council. On the other hand, the Council also collects unique data and has a unique public mission. So, in the interest of providing as comprehensive a picture as possible, how best can the Council's data be used in a coordinated and complementary fashion with these other datasets? There are several possibilities.

First, the information can be used in a data repository. For example, a health plan could access data about its enrollees from a centralized data repository. This will be especially important when measures such as HEDIS 3.0 must account for the history of the patient prior to enrollment in the plan.

Second, the Council's data can provide a vehicle for measuring provider performance within and across health plans. Instruments such as HEDIS emphasize the performance of a health plan in managing the care of an enrolled population; they focus less on measuring the performance of providers for the entire population or a specific population. The Council can measure provider performance for the entire population or for a specific population. Ultimately, it's not enough to know simply whether a plan is performing better or worse than expected; you must know *why*. Once risk and health status are controlled for, the quality of care in a plan may be driven by administrative decisions or by clinical performance. It's important to drill down to the cause.

The third possibility involves benchmarking. To the extent that plans do measure the performance of providers, they typically are doing so with their own enrollees. The Council data can be used to compare the performance of those providers to that of a larger population.

DIFFERING ROLES

As a state agency, the Health Care Cost Containment Council has broader public objectives than most accrediting agencies. The accrediting agencies can certainly serve to complement the functions of state-licensing bodies that have specific responsibility for certain delivery mechanisms, such as hospitals and health maintenance organizations. The Council, however, has a broader mandate to report on the "quality" of health care services and is not limited to a specific delivery system, provider, or data source.

It is, however, limited by the data available to it under statute. As a government agency, it can only expand its database by developing new regulations or by seeking amendments to its enabling legislation—a process that inhibits its ability to innovate or to respond quickly to new developments. By coordinating with other organizations to obtain their data, the Council can serve the public in a more efficient, timely, and comprehensive manner. The Council clearly will seek to do this in the future.

What To Measure?

Initially, the topics and measures should affect relatively young patients (those under 65) since most managed care plans are likely to have had higher numbers of younger enrollees in 1995 (the first data year likely to be used by the Council). As managed care penetration increases in the Medicare and Medicaid populations, issues related to these groups will become more important. Initially, outpatient data would not be used but would be incorporated when it becomes available.

In-hospital mortality has been used as the primary outcome measure in most Council reports. For initiatives on managed care, however, this measure may not be the most appropriate. The following are a list of other possible measures to be included in a managed care report.

Bed Days. Are managed care companies reducing hospital utilization? This may be measured by correlating increased managed care penetration to the number of bed days.

Casemix. If utilization is declining as a result of the influence of managed care, how is this occurring? Is it due to a decrease in or the prevention of unnecessary hospitalizations, or is it a result of restricted access to specialized services? Casemix is a method of adjusting for different admission patterns at different facilities. Hospitals that admit more patients to resource-intensive illness categories will have a higher casemix.

Lengths of stay. Are lengths of stay decreasing for managed care patients as compared to fee-for-service patients?

Ambulatory sensitive conditions. These are causes of admissions that should be preventable if there is adequate access to primary care. The hypothesis would be that the percentage of admissions for these conditions would be lower among managed care plans.

Referral sensitive conditions. Are higher numbers of certain procedures performed when an insurer is willing to pay for them? A lower percentage of these cases could indicate success in reducing unnecessary admissions; however, it also might indicate underutilization of services.

Patient risk. Patients with a low-risk level for some medical conditions may be an indicator of inappropriate admissions. A lower percentage of these cases among managed care plans compared to indemnity plans could indicate a reduction in unnecessary admissions.

Charges. While charges may not be the most useful tool for cost comparisons among hospitals (although they are almost universally used for such purposes), a charge comparison (adjusted for casemix and regional differences) of different types of health plans could presumably provide some insight as to whether managed care is doing a better job of controlling in-hospital resource use. The assumption that the facility mix would be the same for both payer groups should negate some of the problems with charge comparisons.

CONCLUSION

The Council will undoubtedly move to reports comparing specific health care plans. In the interim, the Council has published *Buying a Health Plan*, a guide for employers, labor union officials, and health benefits administrators in how to go about choosing the right plan for their company, members, and participants.

Consumers and purchasers can be empowered with the ability to ask intelligent questions and make more informed decisions about health plans just as they have—in Pennsylvania at least—about hospitals and doctors. Severity-adjusted outcome data are contributing to improving the cost and quality of health care. Yet we are only at the beginning of what is possible—more effective delivery systems are yet to be explored; more widely accessible sources of consumer information through the Internet and other cyber opportunities will become available; and data about outpatient, psychiatric, and rehabilitation treatments, just to mention a few other important areas, will be developed.

We are entering a brave new world indeed. As the health care delivery system changes dramatically, it will be increasingly important for those who consume, purchases, and provide health care to understand the implications and consequences of the changing nature of health care, including the dual responsibilities that now permeate the system. *Focus on Heart Attack in Pennsylvania* is an important step in helping the public understand what is going on, what's working, and what's not, and will raise important issues related to the restructuring of our health care system.

Chapter 16

The National Press

Communicating Managed Care Quality

George Anders

Call it the Charles Dickens syndrome. As managed care sweeps across the United States, depictions of this health care revolution diverge so much that they call to mind the opening sentences of *A Tale of Two Cities*. Some articles and broadcast programs tell of great progress in measuring and improving medical quality. In these accounts, it is "the best of times." At the same time, reports of medical disasters are proliferating, linking managed care's cost controls to tragic stories of patients who couldn't see the right specialist, could not get to the emergency room on time, or were denied insurance coverage for costly but potentially life-saving therapies. In those media reports, it is "the worst of times."

For some long-time pioneers in medical quality research, this mixed message is profoundly frustrating. At a September 1996 conference in Washington DC, David Eddy, MD, the renowned epidemiologist at Duke University, described with some bitterness his attempts to interest a panel of journalists in his work. "All they wanted to talk about was horror stories," Eddy recalled. "They didn't want to hear anything we were saying."[1]

Yet other leaders in the managed care community find instructive lessons in this schism. Alan Hoops, chief executive officer of PacifiCare Health Systems Inc., meets regularly with reporters from major news organizations—partly to brief them on progress at his health maintenance organization, but also to learn about potential "hot button" issues that may be catching reporters' attention. Top executives at HMOs can become too insular, Hoops observes, spending most of their time with people who share their views. Journalists, by definition, talk with a wide range of interested parties. Meetings with reporters become "an early warning system," helping PacifiCare identify concerns that doctors, patients' rights groups, regulators, or other parties might be sharing with the media.[2]

As we shall see, the national press's coverage of managed care quality issues has evolved greatly in the past few years and is continuing to evolve. At first, managed care quality was an esoteric topic, covered mostly by reporters whose main sources were epidemiologists, executives in the managed care industry, and a few pioneering managers of corporate benefits programs. Early articles by these reporters conveyed the almost utopian optimism of these experts: a belief that better data would soon build a much better health care system.

With the very rapid growth of HMOs in the early and mid 1990s, skeptical parties also began seeking the media's attention. Doctors phoned reporters with stories of managed care bureaucracy that was hampering their work. Patients in distress (and their family members) contacted news organizations, asking for investigations of what they regarded as HMO blunders. Trial lawyers also invited media coverage of medical calamities with a managed care component. The result has been significant press attention to what one benefits manager calls "the dark side of managed care"—to wit, cases where managed care protocol may lead to bad outcomes.

More recently, a middle path has emerged as increasingly sophisticated journalists try to blend input from all these sources to provide a fuller picture of managed care quality. Such accounts make room both for current-day HMOs' successes and for their shortcomings. Among the most notable versions are detailed guides to choosing an HMO, which appeared in publications as diverse as *Consumer Reports*, *Newsweek*, and *The Wall Street Journal*. These articles draw on a wide range of sources—including some important new commentators—so that medical quality can be viewed more comprehensively. The resulting stories are less judgmental, more realistic, and more inclined to view the quality debate from a wide variety of perspectives. As *Newsweek* writer Ellyn Spragins put it, different consumers will want to differentiate between "an HMO that's great at answering the phone, and one that's doing a great job of detecting breast cancer."[3]

This multistage model of media coverage isn't unique to the managed care debate. In recent years, leading journalism quarterlies have documented similar progressions—and change in emphasis—for press coverage of long-running, complex subjects as diverse as the Vietnam war or the corporate takeover craze of the 1980s. In fact, a pioneering article in the Fall 1996 issue of *Media Critic* begins to build a framework for analyzing press coverage of managed care over the past 15 years. That article, "HMOs: From Cure-All to Curse," demonstrates how much the pendulum has swung in press coverage over an extended timespan.[4] Some key points of that article contribute to the model presented in Figure 1.

Figure 1.

Stage 1: 1970s-1994	Stage 2: 1993- 1997	Stage 3: 1996-
Getting Started With Report Cards	Bad Outcomes; Big Stories	Getting It Right
• Few Reporters Cover the Story • They Rely Mostly on Academic Sources • Stories Focus on Aggregates • Coverage Tends to Be Upbeat	• Print and TV Coverage Escalates • Sources Include Irate Patients, M.D.s • Case-Study Approach Predominates • Coverage Tends to Be Critical	• Newspapers and Magazines Lead the Way • Sourcing Is Very Diverse • Stories Blend Examples, Statistics • Coverage Cites Pluses and Minuses

As any news-reporting cycle plays out, some people see the press as an actor in its own right, while others regard the press more as a clearinghouse for people who champion specific views. From this author's experience as a staff writer at *The Wall Street Journal* since 1981, it seems that there is some validity to both views, but that the "clearinghouse" metaphor generally is more apt. It should be noted that efforts to gain media coverage often are made by people eager to expose what they perceive as bad policy or outright wrongdoing. Such personal appeals for coverage have been particularly pronounced in the debate over managed care quality issues. In some cases, journalists' own experiences as patients in a managed care plan have added to the immediacy of news coverage—as has the quality of care provided to friends and relatives. Health care, after all, is a unique area for the media, touching people's lives in intimate and ubiquitous ways even as it poses multibillion-dollar policy questions.

These issues are discussed in detail in *Health Against Wealth: HMOs and the Breakdown of Medical Trust.*[5] The book's early and middle chapters deal with the promises and pitfalls of managed care, paralleling the first two stages of press coverage described above. The book's concluding chapters look at ways to make managed care work better, in keeping with the goals of the more sophisticated "third stage" coverage.

Many of the examples that follow in this chapter are drawn from that book.

STAGE I: GETTING STARTED WITH REPORT CARDS

The American press's interest in health care quality can be traced back at least as far as 1910, when Abraham Flexner issued his landmark report on the status of American medical schools. With the passage of the federal HMO Act of 1973, managed care quality attracted intermittent attention from journalists in the 1970s and 1980s. Most press coverage of health issues, however, was focused at the time on two different themes: the frightening escalation of medical costs and the exciting breakthroughs of new medical technology. The managed care industry simply didn't command much attention from the media.

Things began to change around 1990. Prominent academic researchers, policymakers, employers, and health insurance executives began talking with one another about the chance to gather meaningful data about health plan quality—and to use that information both to improve the U.S. medical system and make it more affordable. Many of the leaders in this movement, such as Paul Ellwood of the Jackson Hole Group, William Roper of Prudential Corporation, Robert Brook of the Rand Corporation, and David Eddy of Duke University, freely shared their ideas with a select group of business and health journalists who grew interested in the same subjects. Concurrently, employers and several large HMOs began the brainstorming sessions that led to the first HEDIS measures of health plan performance and to the establishment of the National Committee for Quality Assurance (NCQA) as a serious HMO accrediting group. Pioneers in that movement, such as benefits managers Helen Darling at Xerox and Kathleen Angel at Digital Equipment, also opened a dialogue with reporters from *The New York Times*, *The Wall Street Journal*, *Fortune* magazine, and other opinion leaders.

A flurry of press coverage ensued, most of it blending factual accounts of these early initiatives with some ebullient—even giddy—descriptions of the great opportunities that lay ahead once better medical data were available to consumers. In *Fortune* magazine in mid 1993, for example, veteran health writer Edmund Faltermayer sketched out a health care paradise that could arrive as soon as the year 2005, based on a belief that within a half generation, medical outcomes data would be timely, accurate, abundant, and freely shared. "Far from feeling hopelessly passive, as in the dark ages of 1993," Faltermayer wrote, "medical consumers revel in an explosion of information—much of it electronic—that helps them to dispute doctors' proposals for treatment and to decide whether to switch from one health organization to another at the yearly sign-up time."[6]

Other publications picked up those cheery themes, encouraged by no less authorities than the top health care strategists of the Clinton Administration. In late 1993, for the first time, several leading HMOs published data showing their record in administering immunizations, cholesterol checks, and other broad-based aspects of primary care as specified in the HEDIS system. Those early report cards—issued by Kaiser Permanente, U.S. Healthcare, and United HealthCare—were widely praised as a sign that trustworthy data were starting to emerge from the HMO industry and that it would soon lead to better care.

When *The Wall Street Journal* in November 1993 put three of the early HEDIS report cards side by side, a major part of its article consisted of encouraging remarks by Walter Zelman, then a senior health care policy adviser in the White House. Zelman was among the many Administration officials hoping to sell the country on President Clinton's version of health care reform, and he saw the HEDIS report cards as a useful step in that direction. "Report cards should help all around in improving the quality of care," Zelman told the *Journal*. "Consumers will know more about how their health plans are doing, and they will be better able to choose between different sets of providers."[7]

Similarly favorable commentary surrounded early coverage of health plan accreditation by NCQA. In a brief report about NCQA in the early 1990s, *Money* magazine's Lani Luciano wrote: "Until recently, consumers trying to choose among health maintenance organizations had to settle for word-of-mouth investigations of their own. But now help is on the way." Journalists generally accepted NCQA's assessment that plans with full, three-year accreditation were better for consumers than plans with provisional or one-year accreditations, let alone those that were denied accreditation.

An important cautionary note was sounded in 1994, however, by *Wall Street Journal* reporter Ron Winslow. Champions of better medical data might be excited about their progress to date, he observed, but so far consumers weren't nearly as impressed. In a May 19, 1994 article headlined: "Health Care Report Cards Are Getting Low Grades From Some Focus Groups," Winslow reported on a series of consumer feedback sessions run by the Joint Commission on Accreditation of Healthcare Organizations. At those sessions, Joint Commission officials asked ordinary consumers to critique the report cards developed to date. To the surprise and disappointment of JCAHO officials, consumers said that the report cards weren't highly useful to them. The data were either too complex or too far removed from their own immediate health concerns.

As Winslow put it, the consumers' chilly response "amounts to a reality check for the burgeoning movement to provide consumers with report cards on the quality of care delivered by doctors, hospitals and health plans. A gap exists between the kind of information employers and policy makers consider important and what consumers want." Winslow went on to add that other health care organizations were encountering similar consumer resistance or apathy to HMO report cards—at least in the 1994-vintage versions. He noted that a survey by Harvard Community Health Plan found that HEDIS measures ranked last in usefulness among five types of information made available to consumers. Respondents said they would much rather have information on which doctors belonged to the health plan. They also said they would prefer knowing what care is covered and how satisfied other members were with their care.

Such listless responses from consumers made it inevitable that if journalists continued to write about managed care quality, their range of sources would broaden beyond the epidemiologists and health plan officials who were the early experts. New voices would be sought out. As it happened, journalists didn't need to look far to find people with strong opinions about managed care quality.

STAGE 2: BAD OUTCOMES, BIG STORIES

During the winter of 1994-95, *New York Post* investigative reporter William Sherman stayed fit by playing indoor tennis matches on the weekends with a few physician acquaintances.[8] Always a diligent journalist, Sherman periodically asked his tennis partners what was new in their field. The answer surprised him. Managed care was coming to the New York metropolitan market in a big way, and the doctors didn't like it. Not only did it threaten their incomes and their autonomy, they told Sherman, but it might impede patient care. As these conversations continued, Sherman decided he had found his next big investigative project. For the next few months, he interviewed dozens of doctors and patients in New York, looking for stories of managed care gone awry. He combed through subscriber-complaint offices in the state capital, Albany, to see how HMOs looked in regulators' eyes. Finally, in September 1995 he had enough material to launch a five-part series in the *Post*, capturing a banner page one headline each day.

"HMO's Cruel Rules Leave Her Dying for the Doc She Needs,"[9] one front-page headline proclaimed. "What They Didn't Know About Their HMO May Have Killed This Baby,"[10] another headline said. Inside, the *Post* presented more than 20 stories that week on cases where patients or their families alleged that managed care bureaucracy had blocked appropriate care. Examples ranged from growth hormone for a very short child to nonsurgical treatment for an older man's prostate cancer.

The *New York Post*'s series signaled the beginning of a barrage of hard-hitting press and broadcast reports about managed care problem cases. Over the next few months, publications as diverse as *Time* magazine, the *Los Angeles Times*, and *Glamour* magazine presented detailed accounts of medical tragedies involving HMO members. In the summer of 1996, one of *The New York Times*'s columnists, Bob Herbert, declared: "The managed care horror stories are piling up. No one should be surprised. To a frightening extent, the practice of medicine has already been hijacked by inflexible, cold-hearted corporate types whose interests are in profits, not patients."[11]

Suddenly, managed care executives were on the defensive. After years of being positioned as some of the nation's brightest hopes in improving medical quality, HMO leaders now had to explain to television crews and state legislators that they weren't killing babies in the name of saving money. Puzzled and upset, managed care executives began spinning theories about why, in their view, the press had suddenly turned on them. "There are people who have a vested interest in undermining us," said Susan Pisano, a spokeswoman for the American Association of Health Plans, the main HMO trade group, in early 1996.[12] Many high-paid medical subspecialists saw managed care as a threat to their incomes and their way of life, she explained. Rather than bend with the times, she concluded, these doctors were in the midst of an "aggressive attempt" to discredit the HMO industry and were seeking out reporters who could help air their concerns.

Pisano's analysis captured one element of the evolving media portrayal of managed care, but it glided past two other equally important factors. Early efforts to write about managed care quality had been so heavily tilted toward preventive and early-stage diagnostic care that they essentially overlooked health plans' treatment of serious illness. That void needed to be filled. If the HMO industry and academic researchers weren't stepping forward to discuss care of the sick, someone else would. The likeliest candidates were doctors and patients who felt they had an alarming story to tell.

Second, managed care's record in treating serious illness did have its gaps. Researchers at the Harvard School of Public Health and the Kaiser Family Foundation published studies in 1995 showing that sick, poor, or elderly patients were more likely to be dissatisfied with their medical coverage if they were enrolled in a managed care plan, as opposed to traditional fee-for-service care. Mathematica Inc., in a major 1993 study for the Health Care Financing Administration, had raised questions about HMOs' ability to handle recuperative care for elderly stroke patients. And studies presented at the American Heart Association conference in Anaheim CA in November 1995 suggested that HMOs sent their pediatric heart surgery cases to medical centers with worse-than-average mortality rates. Those studies attracted coverage in their own right—and compelled some reporters to probe further.

In some cases, journalists' personal experiences soured them on HMOs, leading them to take a critical view of managed care. In Florida, cartoonist Don Wright grew outraged when a managed care plan tried to discharge his ailing mother-in-law from a hospital hours before a hurricane was due to hit. "She wasn't capable of sustaining herself," a family member angrily recalled. "We really had to fight them to keep her in." After that debacle, Wright began a series of devastating portrayals of managed care mischief.[13] His best-known sketch for *The Palm Beach Post* showed a phone clerk at "KuddlyCare HMO" telling a distraught caller that her husband didn't qualify for emergency coverage. "Gasping, writhing, eyes rolled back in his head?" she said. "Doesn't sound all that serious to me. . . . He's dead? Then he certainly doesn't need treatment, does he?" The dialogue was invented, Wright readily admitted. But it drew from his family's own anger at being shunted about in an insensitive managed care system. "I really wanted to create someone who was terribly efficient and terribly cruel at the same time," Wright later explained. "It sums up what happens to people."

More broadly, press critiques of managed care tended to pinpoint one of three potential problems: restricted coverage of emergency services, sick patients' difficulties in getting to the right specialist, and seemingly excessive cuts in hospital stays.

In airing those concerns, journalists usually gave brief acknowledgment to managed care's successes in handling routine cases more efficiently and more cost-effectively than the older, fee-for-service system. But routine care no longer was the centerpiece of the "managed care story." Reporters focused more on the exceptional case—on the belief that it provided a noteworthy stress test of managed care's capabilities. *Time* magazine, for example, attracted wide attention in January 1996 with a cover story examining several women's inability to get their HMO to pay for high-dose chemotherapy and a bone-marrow transplant as a last-ditch treatment for metastatic breast cancer.[14] Such therapy has erratic results and high costs; the price tag for BMT treatment was more than $100,000 at the time the women were seeking care. (Costs subsequently have declined to about $60,000 per patient.) Yet this therapy often is seen by desperately sick young women as their best hope of overcoming an otherwise fatal disease. As a result, health insurers' handling of BMT cases has been a simmering controversy all through the 1990s. *Time*'s cover story was widely seen as sympathetic to the breast-cancer patients and critical of their health plan's decisions. It attracted more than 200 letters from readers—including many physicians—with sentiment overwhelmingly tilted toward indignation about managed care's limits.

When asked why they turned the spotlight on managed care problem cases, several journalists explained that they wanted to address what they believed was a lack of public awareness about these new health plans' performance in a crisis. "People are happy with HMOs if they are healthy," remarked Joanna Breen, a New York-based producer for the ABC television network.[15] "But the people we focus on are very sick. They were treated as if they were healthy, all the way through, until past the point of no return." Breen's showcase example was the death of a 28-year-old Milwaukee woman, Karin Smith, from cervical cancer that had gone undiagnosed for years, even though Smith reported abnormal bleeding to her HMO doctors and underwent several Pap smears. As ABC reported, the lab reading Smith's slides failed to detect early signs of cancer; its quality assurance programs later came under fire. From that example and others, ABC's Breen said, she concluded that the managed care system "is rife with opportunities for failure."

Typically, these stories portrayed HMOs as the ultimate decisionmakers, deciding who got care and who didn't. In fact, if journalists had probed further, they might have found that corporate benefits managers—by demanding cheaper premiums for employee health insurance—were setting the stage for a controversial ratcheting-down of traditional medical benefits. Even so, few media reports traced medical austerity to its ultimate source: increasingly frugal corporate buyers of health insurance.

The reasons for this omission are complex. In some cases, journalists who focused on the human drama of a medical calamity simply weren't interested in the broader economic milieu. Other times, reporters found it difficult to write about health care purchasers with any degree of vividness. HMO executives made better copy. But even if reporters suspected that tight-fisted payers had an important background role in these dramas, few managed care plans cared to confirm this. Privately, HMO managers might grumble about the tough choices they were forced to make as premiums came under pressure. In public interviews, however, HMO executives were loathe to criticize the corporate managers who steered millions of dollars of business their way. HMO executives also didn't want to suggest that their decisions about "medical necessity" could be swayed by the richness, or stinginess, of their budgets. Instead, the managed care industry preferred to publicly position itself as making the appropriate medical choices in all cases, regardless of the underlying financial dynamics. Faced with an HMO industry that took full credit—or blame—for its coverage decisions, most reporters decided that their accounts needn't include much detail about the purchasers' role in the managed care boom.

The flurry of media coverage about managed care problem cases gained new urgency as state governments began singling out apparent areas of abuse.

Traditionally, states had regulated HMOs mostly for financial solvency. But as an ever-larger percentage of the population entered the world of managed care, state officials from 1994 onward felt more of an obligation to patrol the quality of care delivered by health plans. When state investigations uncovered serious problems—even if they involved only a few patients—reporters covered those cases prominently.

A notable example arose in California in late 1994 when the state's main HMO regulator, the Department of Corporations, announced a $500,000 fine against TakeCare, a Northern California HMO that was subsequently acquired by FHP International. TakeCare and its contracting medical group were faulted for refusing to pay for a pediatric-cancer specialist to operate on nine-year-old Carley Christie, a girl with Wilms' tumor, a rare form of kidney cancer.[16] The girl's parents paid for the top surgeon themselves and then filed a protest with state authorities. California regulators ordered the plan to pay the family's bills as well as the fine. The story got national attention, and most reporters quoted from a statement by California's top HMO regulator at the time, Gary Mendoza, who accused TakeCare of "failure to provide appropriate access to quality medical care, putting in jeopardy the life of a young patient."

Similarly, regulators in Rhode Island in June 1995 cracked down on a mental health managed care company, accusing it of denying necessary care to patients. To resolve the state's complaint, the plan agreed to pay more than $100,000 in various penalties and to oust its top two officials. The main newspaper in the state, the *Providence Journal-Bulletin*, closely followed the state's investigation and periodically suggested that the target company's problems might be indicative of wider quality problems in the industry.

In a Dec. 11, 1995 editorial, the *Journal-Bulletin* wrote: "The weakness of managed care is that the company that decides who gets treatment is also the company that benefits from denying care. That makes managed care in large part a squeaky-wheel system: Complain loud and long enough about your right to care, and you probably will get it. Placing the burden on the mentally ill—on someone paralyzed by depression, for instance—is simply wrong. And unless we change the system of financing health care, it will be up to subscribers and government overseers to make this plain."

Another noteworthy controversy involved health plans' efforts to reduce coverage for maternity stays to 24 hours after a normal vaginal delivery, rather than the customary 48 hours. Experts were divided about whether the shorter stays would have any deleterious effects on newborns or their mothers. HMO officials cited studies suggesting that shorter stays weren't associated with greater deaths or readmissions. The main obstetrical and pediatric societies disagreed, saying that they saw potentially greater risks of jaundice and undetected heart problems in infants, as well as potentially missed complications in mothers. Pediatricians, in particular, bandied about a report by Judith Frank,[17] associate professor in the Department of Pediatrics at Dartmouth Medical School, which looked at 15,000 newborn discharges in New Hampshire and found a 50 percent higher readmission rate among babies discharged after less than 48 hours.

With academic researchers locked in a classic "battle of the studies," journalists looked for other ways to cover the maternity-stay debate. Most often, reporters took their cues from legislative hearings, at which the star witnesses were parents with tragic accounts of newborns sent home under the 24-hour-stay rule, only to sink into dire health within days and sometimes to die. The pathos of those stories dominated the debate—and eventually led to state and national legislation mandating 48-hour coverage of maternity stays for healthy mothers.

One of the most forceful writers on this subject was First Lady Hillary Rodham Clinton,[18] who in 1995 began her own syndicated newspaper column. In one of her columns, she told of a New Jersey baby's death after a 24-hour discharge, arguing that legislation was needed to avoid more such tragedies. In her words: "No insurance company accountant should make the final judgment about what is medically best for newborns and their mothers." Her sentiments were echoed by columnists and editorial writers around the country, many of whom suggested that managed care's cost controls were going too far.

STAGE 3: GETTING IT RIGHT

When *BusinessWeek* writer Keith Hammonds began a major survey of clinical quality issues in early 1996, he found plenty to be concerned about.[19] "Many patients aren't satisfied with managed care," he wrote. "The jihad on health care costs went too far."

But the bulk of Hammonds' article departed from the then-customary practice of ticking off dramatic examples of managed care failures. Instead, Hammonds pinpointed steps that major corporate employers, hospitals, and health plans were taking to improve medical quality while lowering costs. He praised companies such as USAir, Xerox, and PepsiCo, which had begun demanding that HMOs produce outcomes data showing how patients with serious illnesses fared. He cited initiatives by Oxford Health Plans Inc. to spend more on early-stage care of diabetes and asthma. Those actions, he observed, were improving patients' health while reducing giant bills for emergency-room visits and treatment of unwelcome complications. Overall, Hammonds wrote: "Hospitals, doctors and insurers, attended by a growing coterie of consultants and information systems suppliers, are rediscovering quality."

That *BusinessWeek* article was part of a sober-minded reassessment of managed care quality issues, taking place at many of the largest and most influential U.S. news organizations. Reporters no longer portrayed simple primary care report cards as the gold standard of medical quality. Yet writers also moved beyond the other extreme of judging managed care plans solely by their most gruesome failures in handling the very sick. Instead, journalists assembled a more sophisticated synthesis—that made room both for managed care's successes and its shortcomings. These articles blended statistics and anecdotes in ways that conveyed the breadth of the managed care experience, without losing sight of the human dimension.

Some of the most substantial reappraisals of managed care came in the form of consumer guides to choosing a health plan. Publications ranging from *Consumer Reports* to *Boston* magazine to *The Wall Street Journal* put teams of reporters at work, asking them to help consumers find their way in the medical care maze. The result: major packages of stories, often totaling more than 10,000 words, with charts and tables that tried to identify the best health plans, while warning readers of potential hazards.

In its August 1996 issue, *Consumer Reports* adapted its classic ratings format to 37 of the country's largest HMOs. It assessed plans by the HMO industry's classic yardstick—delivery of preventive services—but also asked subscribers about issues that might matter more to the seriously ill patient, such as how often members weren't able to get needed care or how satisfied they were with their choice of doctors. Ultimately, *Consumer Reports* ranked plans by an overall satisfaction index. Blue Cross Blue Shield of the Rochester (NY) area was at the top of the list; PruCare of California was at the bottom.

In the accompanying text, the magazine's editors took a very wide-ranging view of health plan quality. As they put it, a plan "should be able to handle a sudden, acute illness, and try to keep you as healthy as possible by offering excellent preventive services and an outstanding disease-management program that can help you cope with a chronic condition." *Consumer Reports* acknowledged that no plan fully met those tests, and its series included disturbing examples of HMOs that fell far short of those goals. Its conclusion: "HMOs have the potential to deliver good care and control costs at the same time. But in the current environment of unmanaged competition, that hasn't always happened."

In a June 1996 cover story, *Newsweek* magazine took a similarly comprehensive approach.[20] It rated 43 of the largest HMOs in the United States, once again using criteria that ranged from preventive screenings to member satisfaction surveys and the frequency of complaints. "While evaluating HMOs is still an inexact exercise," *Newsweek* declared, "these ratings provide a good start." To design its measuring system, *Newsweek* turned to an outside expert: David Lansky, president of the Foundation for Accountability, an Oregon-based group advising major corporations on managed care quality issues.

Lansky's participation in *Newsweek*'s project was significant for two reasons. It helped the magazine delve into complex, technical areas where journalists alone might lack the expertise to evaluate data intelligently. And it signaled the emergence of an important new type of source for journalists covering the managed care story: the dispassionate expert who could help journalists balance different perspectives on managed care quality.

Most of these new experts were regulators, HMO accreditation specialists, and big corporate purchasers of health care—people whose own jobs required them to make judgment calls about what managed care did well and poorly. Some of these sources actively sought out journalists, inviting them to press conferences and offering background briefings. Others let the press find them. Either way, these sources were willing to share insights, on the belief that skeptical but fair-minded coverage of managed care issues was in everyone's interests.

In July 1996, *The New York Times* ran a front-page article declaring: "The Grading Becomes Stricter on HMOs."[21] In that piece, staff reporter Milt Freudenheim surveyed different attempts to gather data about HMO quality, pointing out that employers themselves weren't satisfied anymore with process measures and wanted more information on patients' outcomes. A major source for that piece was FACCT's Lansky, who was quoted as saying, "We are trying to move an enormous trillion-dollar health care system in a more consumer- and patient-oriented direction."

Similarly, participants in the development of the HEDIS 3.0 measures invited reporters' calls in the summer of 1996. They talked about their hopes that the new yardsticks would provide a fuller gauge of HMOs' ability to care for the sick. *The Wall Street Journal* in July 1996 reported that the HEDIS 3.0 measures would "call for HMOs to disclose more information about their care of patients with illnesses ranging from breast cancer to heart attacks." The *Journal*'s article quoted Louise Novotny, a health-benefits specialist with the Communications Workers of America, as saying that the new standards "move us into some areas more immediately relevant to consumers."[22]

Some of the most persuasive new experts were corporate benefits managers. They acknowledged that their earlier emphasis on primary care report cards was incomplete—and vowed to look at a wider set of quality measures in assessing health plan performance. As Fran Bastien, head of health benefits at Digital Equipment, put it: "We have a responsibility to our employees, now that we have them in managed care, to show them how the plans are performing."

Reporters took a keen interest in the new quality-assessment techniques championed by these benefits managers. American Express, for example, attracted notice with a program to run spot checks on health plans, including simulated phone calls on behalf of a member with AIDS seeking additional care.[23] Those spot checks became "a good way to find out if health plans were referring cases properly or just trying to minimize utilization," explained LuAnn Cash, head of employee benefits at American Express. American Express had moved 70 percent of its workforce into HMOs from 1992 to 1995, Cash observed. The switch saved the company money and had the potential to provide high-quality care. But Cash and her colleagues were determined to police these health plans to make sure they were delivering the full range of necessary care. "It's nice to keep everyone healthy and to focus on prevention," Cash remarked. "But when you ask employees what matters most, they don't care about cholesterol or mammograms. Their fear is that when they get sick, HMOs won't take care of them."

Valuable as each of these experts were, none of them could claim to be truly impartial. As the 1990s were drawing near a close, HMO quality measurement was becoming an intensely controversial subject in academia and in the business community. Different groups vied for attention, each championing a somewhat different set of quality yardsticks. Journalists who relied too heavily on any one set of experts ran the risk of choosing sides and forfeiting some of their profession's traditional neutrality.

Most reporters found their way around that potential hazard, however. When leading quality-measurement groups—such as NCQA, FACCT, and the Joint Commission—differed on which approaches to emphasize most, their variances were widely publicized. Journalists seeking experts from any one of these organizations generally leavened their input with comments from a competing organization or with an indirect acknowledgment of varying methods.

By widening their horizons to look at different approaches to quality measurement, reporters inevitably made their stories more complex. It wouldn't be easy anymore to single out any individual HMO—let alone the entire managed care system—for unalloyed praise or chastisement. But many reporters appeared comfortable with this more nuanced approach to covering managed care quality.

The *San Francisco Chronicle*, for example, in the summer of 1996 called on its veteran medical writer, Carl Hall, to survey all the HMO quality data available to consumers.[24] In the opening section of his article, Hall wrote: "Experts caution against relying too much on any single indicator for what is by nature a deeply personal choice." Hall went on to quote Keith Bishop, the newly appointed head of the Department of Corporations and Gary Mendoza's successor as the state's chief HMO regulator. "It's probably a mistake to assume that one day there will be one survey everyone can rely on," Bishop told the *Chronicle*. "People are measuring different things for different purposes. So everybody needs to look at it in terms of their own particular needs." Even so, Hall concluded that the information he was about to present to readers—ranging from NCQA accreditation to consumer satisfaction scores—could be a useful start.

STAGE 4: WHERE DO WE GO FROM HERE?

Any major trend has its exceptions and anomalies. In offering an overview of media coverage of managed care issues, this author realizes that any diligent researcher can find counterexamples. Scan through a week's worth of print or broadcast coverage and even today there are bound to be reports that still conform much more closely to the early stages described above than to the more comprehensive approach of Stage 3. There are periodic cases where newspapers, magazines, or TV stations will let go of the Stage 3 approach in favor of a simpler story that dwells mostly on utopian promise or worst cases. It is important to realize that the press isn't monolithic; even a single publication or broadcast station is full of correspondents with widely different views of what is "news." Furthermore, intellectual frameworks for covering a story can be swept aside by fresh, unexpected developments. As regulators and employers root out problem areas in current-day managed care, there may be times when HMO missteps call for the stark coverage described in Stage 2.

Broadly, however, this author is confident that the more sophisticated approach described in Stage 3 will emerge as the most common way to cover managed care quality issues. It takes a realistic view of managed care's pluses and minuses in a way that squares with journalists' own sense of everyday experience. It makes the broadest and most intelligent use of a wide range of experts and interested sources. Most importantly, this approach is particularly useful to readers and viewers. Each week about 160,000 people sign up for an HMO, either because they want to or because their employer or government insurer (Medicare or Medicaid) is strongly encouraging them to do so. Those consumers are eager for practical, realistic information about the managed care bargain and how it will affect their lives.

The articles that result will acknowledge that HMO quality isn't a simple subject and that it will mean different things to different people. Reporters will find themselves working with a wide range of sources, including some people who welcome managed care and others who fear it. Yet that complexity needn't stand in the way of clear, well-researched reporting about managed care and medical quality.

At this juncture, it is still too early to say whether one set of HMO quality measures will become the industry's "gold standard," and if so, which parties will develop them. The managed care industry itself is in a great deal of flux, and the science of measuring health plan performance is evolving at least as rapidly. But if one package of measures does prevail, it will do so because those benchmarks prove to be widely trusted by payers, providers—and by patients.

In this battle for acceptance, the media will have a deservedly important role. Doctors and hospital administrators will constantly alert reporters to strengths—and flaws—of various measuring systems. So will payers. Most importantly, consumers will look to magazines and newspapers for clear, reliable gauges of HMO performance. Some inward-looking developers of quality measures might prefer to work in private until everything has been perfected and then launch flawless measures to universal applause. Other developers, however, are likely to see media scrutiny as ultimately helpful to their efforts. Shortcomings can be spotted and fixed more quickly. Strengths can win public praise—and thus speed the acceptance of the measures that work best.

For those reasons, it seems hopeful that the journalistic community and the people who care most about managed care quality can find effective ways to work together. As the final chapter of *Health Against Wealth* observes: "Expertise about the most worthwhile parts of managed care is developing among doctors, employers and patients' rights groups, rather than remaining the secret preserve of HMOs." As these experts' perspectives enter the public debate on managed care quality, the nation at some point should "be able to figure out how to run a cost-effective medical system without abandoning compassion."[25]

REFERENCES

1. David Eddy's remarks: as described by Eddy at a Kaiser Permanente conference September 16, 1996 in Washington DC.

2. Alan Hoops's meetings: cited by Hoops in an interview February 27, 1995.
3. "An HMO that's great . . .": *Newsweek*, June 24, 1996.
4. Framework for analyzing coverage: "HMOs: From Cure-All to Curse," Nancy Meis and Brant S. Mittler, *Media Critic*, Fall 1996.
5. Anders, George. *Health Against Wealth: HMOs and the Breakdown of Medical Trust*, Houghton Mifflin, 1996.
6. "Health care paradise," *Fortune*, June 14, 1993.
7. HEDIS report cards: *The Wall Street Journal*, November 16, 1993.
8. William Sherman's tennis games: phone interview with Sherman, April 1996.
9. "HMO's Cruel Rules . . ." *New York Post*, September 17, 1995.
10. "What They Didn't Know . . ." *New York Post*, September 14, 1995.
11. "The managed care horror stories . . ." *The New York Times*, July 15, 1996.
12. "There are people . . ." as cited in George Anders, *Health Against Wealth*, Houghton Mifflin, 1996, p. 241.
13. Don Wright's outrage: as cited in *Health Against Wealth*, p. 241-2.
14. Breast-cancer cover story: *Time*, January 22, 1996
15. "People are happy . . ." as cited in *Health Against Wealth*, p. 240.
16. Carley Christie case: as cited in *Health Against Wealth*, p. 228-9.
17. Judith Frank's study: as cited in *The Wall Street Journal*, September 20, 1996.
18. Hillary Rodham Clinton's column: as cited in *The Wall Street Journal*, September 20, 1996.
19. Keith Hammonds' survey: *BusinessWeek*, April 8, 1996.
20 *Newsweek*'s rankings: *Newsweek*, June 24, 1996.
21. "The Grading Becomes Stricter . . ." *The New York Times*, July 16, 1996.
22. Louise Novotny's views: *The Wall Street Journal*, July 16, 1996.
23. Spot checks by American Express: as cited in *Health Against Wealth*, p. 234-5.
24. Carl Hall's survey: *San Francisco Chronicle*, September 23, 1996.
25. "Expertise about . . ." *Health Against Wealth*, p. 260.